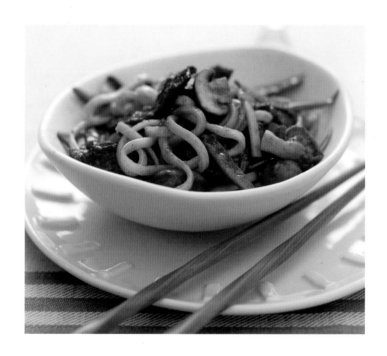

the **diabetes**
cooking book

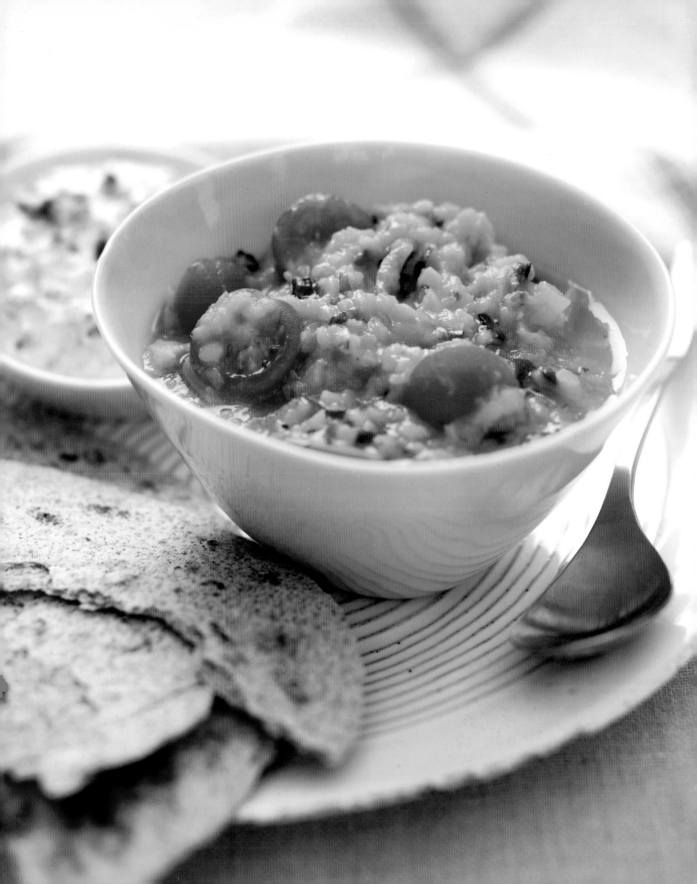

the **diabetes** cooking book

LONDON, NEW YORK, MELBOURNE, MUNICH, AND DELHI

Photography William Shaw

Project editor Robert Sharman
Designer Katherine Raj
Senior Creative Art Editor Caroline de Souza
Managing editor Dawn Henderson
Managing art editors Christine Keilty, Marianne Markham
Category publisher Mary-Clare Jerram
Art director Peter Luff
Production editor Ben Marcus
Production controller Poppy Newdick
Creative technical support Sonia Charbonnier

DK INDIA
Designer Devika Dwarkadas
Senior editor Saloni Talwar
Production manager Pankaj Sharma
Design manager Romi Chakraborty

Important Every effort has been made to ensure that the information contained in this book is complete and accurate. However, neither the publisher nor the authors are engaged in rendering professional advice or services to the individual reader. Professional medical advice should be obtained on personal health matters. Neither the publisher nor the authors accept any legal responsibility for any personal injury or other damage or loss arising from the use or misuse of the information and advice in this book.

First published in Great Britain in 2010
by Dorling Kindersley Limited
80 Strand, London WC2R 0RL
Penguin Group (UK)

A CIP catalogue record for this book is available
from the British Library

ISBN 978-1-4053-4178-3

Colour reproduction by MDP Ltd
Printed and bound in Singapore by TWP

Discover more at **www.dk.com**

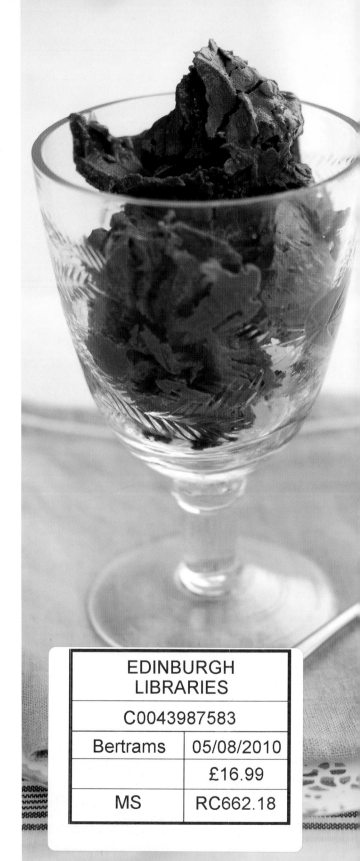

CONTENTS

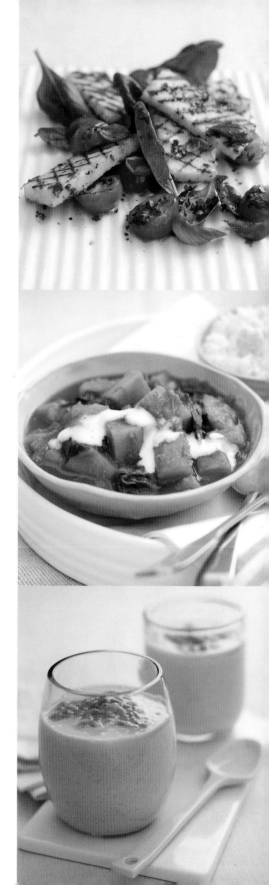

EATING WELL WITH TYPE 2 DIABETES

Food plays a crucial role in determining our health, vitality, and well-being. Various foods we eat are broken down into glucose, which passes into the bloodstream. Our blood glucose level should not become too high or too low, so to regulate it, the pancreas produces insulin. If you have Type 2 diabetes, you'll know that your pancreas isn't producing enough insulin, or the insulin isn't doing its job properly. (If you have Type 1 diabetes, your body isn't making any insulin at all.)

It is important for everyone to eat healthily, but when you have Type 2 diabetes, diet is even more relevant. Choosing the right foods will help you to manage your condition and reduce the risk of other health problems associated with diabetes. In one study, people with Type 2 diabetes were able to reduce their blood glucose levels by an average of 25 per cent just by following a simple diet plan similar to

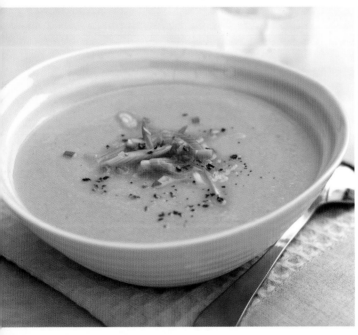

Carrot and Ginger Soup (page 74)

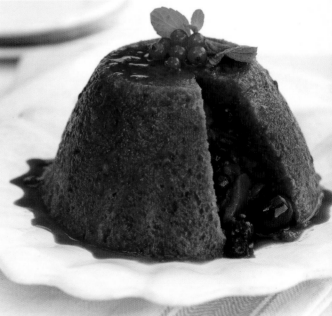

Summer Pudding (page 314)

the one we recommend. Although people often talk about healthy and unhealthy foods, there is no such thing as a good or a bad food: it is the balance of foods that you eat throughout the day that is important.

HOW THIS BOOK CAN HELP

The recipes in this book are designed to help you achieve a healthy, balanced diet that includes wholegrains, low-GI carbohydrates, lean protein, dietary fibre, low-fat dairy products, and plenty of vegetables and fruit. They are also lower in salt, fat and sugar. All this equals a great diet, whether you have Type 2 diabetes or not.

Where the book goes further is in providing "Guidelines per serving" for each recipe (see right), which show you whether the dish is relatively high (3 dots), medium (2 dots) or low (1 dot) in GI, calories, saturated fat, and sugar – the four key dietary areas to watch when you have Type 2 diabetes. For information on how to use these charts to balance your diet and ensure that you are eating appropriately, see page 53.

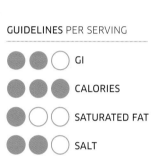

GUIDELINES PER SERVING

● ● ○ GI
● ● ● CALORIES
● ○ ○ SATURATED FAT
● ● ○ SALT

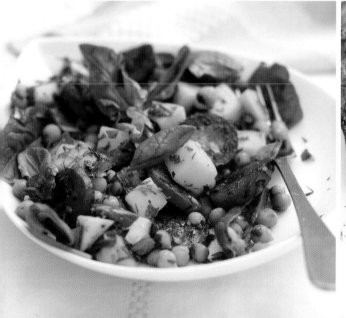

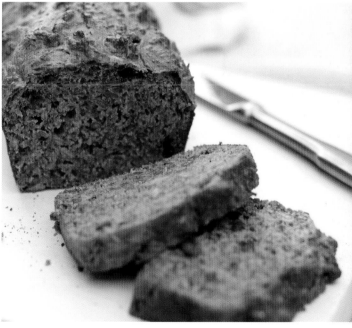

Chorizo, Chickpea, and Mango Salad (page 146)

Fruit and Seed Soda Bread (page 340)

YOUR FOUR HEALTH GOALS

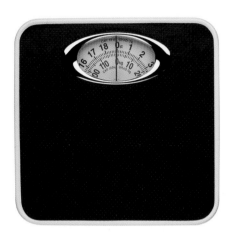

MANAGE YOUR WEIGHT

1 To give yourself the best chance of controlling Type 2 diabetes, and avoiding some of the many health risks it can expose you to, it is important that you are a healthy weight. People who are overweight can improve their diabetes control, lower their blood pressure, and reduce levels of fats in the blood, including cholesterol, by losing weight. The two key factors in controlling your weight are a healthy diet and regular exercise. This book will help you adapt to a healthier diet, and also allows you to monitor your calorie intake, so you can see how much energy you need to be using up through exercise. For more information on healthy weight loss, see pages 34–37.

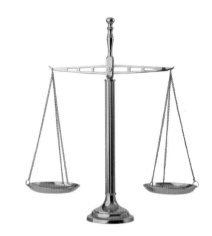

BALANCE YOUR BLOOD GLUCOSE LEVELS

2 Keeping blood glucose levels within a healthy range is a vital part of managing diabetes. If you have too much glucose in the blood for long periods of time, it can damage the vessels that supply blood to vital organs such as the heart, kidneys, eyes, and nerves. The type and amount of carbohydrate you eat are the main dietary factors that determine blood glucose levels. Slow-release carbohydrates keep blood glucose on an even keel; carbohydrates that are digested rapidly cause unwelcome surges in blood glucose levels. See pages 16–17 for more about carbohydrates, and pages 18–19 for information on the glycaemic index.

If you've been diagnosed with diabetes, make these four health goals your priority. They will help you to manage your condition and live life to the full.

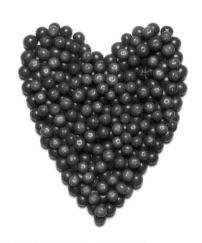

LOOK AFTER YOUR HEART

3 People with diabetes are five times more likely to suffer from heart disease or a stroke, so it is vital to eat the right foods to keep your heart healthy. One of the most important steps you can take is to reduce your intake of saturated fat. Saturated fat causes the body to produce cholesterol, and in the same way that hard water can clog water pipes and appliances with limescale, cholesterol clogs the blood vessels and causes them to narrow, restricting the flow of blood to the heart and brain. See pages 20–21 for more information on fats. Other important routes to heart health are to give up smoking, take regular exercise, and prevent high blood pressure.

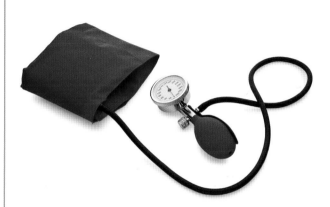

CONTROL YOUR BLOOD PRESSURE

4 High blood pressure increases the risk of heart disease, stroke, and kidney problems. A diet high in salt is a major factor in the development of high blood pressure (see pages 22–23 for ways to reduce your salt intake) – but salt isn't the whole story. The DASH study (Dietary Approaches to Stop Hypertension) carried out in America found that people who had a moderate sodium intake, but who increased their intake of potassium, calcium, and magnesium by eating plenty of fruit, vegetables, and low-fat dairy products, showed more significant reductions in blood pressure that those who simply restricted sodium. Ask your doctor to check your blood pressure regularly.

FIVE-POINT EATING PLAN

Choosing the right diet is a vital part of managing diabetes. A healthy diet will help you to control your blood glucose levels, cholesterol, blood pressure, and weight. It will also help to improve your energy levels, digestion, and immunity. The good news is that eating well when you have diabetes doesn't have to be boring or hard work, and you don't have to miss out on the foods you enjoy. There are five areas of your diet where you can boost your health and well-being by making a few changes. Learn more about these by turning to the relevant pages.

EAT MORE FRUIT AND VEGETABLES

1 Fruit and vegetables are the cornerstone of a healthy diabetes eating plan. They provide vitamins, minerals, and phytochemicals which, among other benefits, will help to keep your heart and eyes healthy; potassium, which helps to lower blood pressure; and dietary fibre, which encourages the digestive system to function smoothly (see pages 12–13).

CHOOSE THE RIGHT CARBOHYDRATES

2 Carbohydrates are converted into glucose, which causes the level of blood glucose to rise. The level to which it rises and the length of time it remains high depend on the type and amount of carbohydrates that you eat. Certain carbohydrates are digested more slowly than others, keeping blood glucose levels even and sustaining energy levels. Understanding the effect of carbohydrates on blood glucose levels is the key to living with diabetes (see pages 16–17).

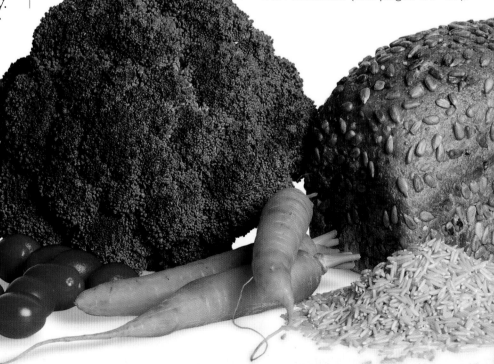

SWAP BAD FATS FOR GOOD

3 Reduce your intake of "bad fats" – saturated fats and trans fats – which increase the risk of heart disease and stroke. Eat more "good fats", such as unsaturated oils, which have a protective effect (see pages 20–21).

REPLACE SALT WITH GOOD FLAVOURINGS

4 A diet high in salt is believed to be a major factor in the development of high blood pressure – something that people with diabetes are at greater risk of having. Experts have calculated that by reducing our intake of salt to no more 6g a day, it can reduce the risk of stroke or heart attack by a quarter. Instead of relying on salt to make food tasty, experiment with other ways to add flavour (see pages 22–23).

LOWER YOUR SUGAR INTAKE

5 Sugar provides what nutritionists call "empty calories" – calories that provide nothing in the way of protein, fibre, vitamins, or minerals and so offer no health benefit. Eating large amounts of sugar will cause your blood glucose levels to rise and in the longer term can lead to weight gain. You do not need to avoid sugar completely, but cut back on it as much as possible and try other ways to sweeten food (see pages 24–25).

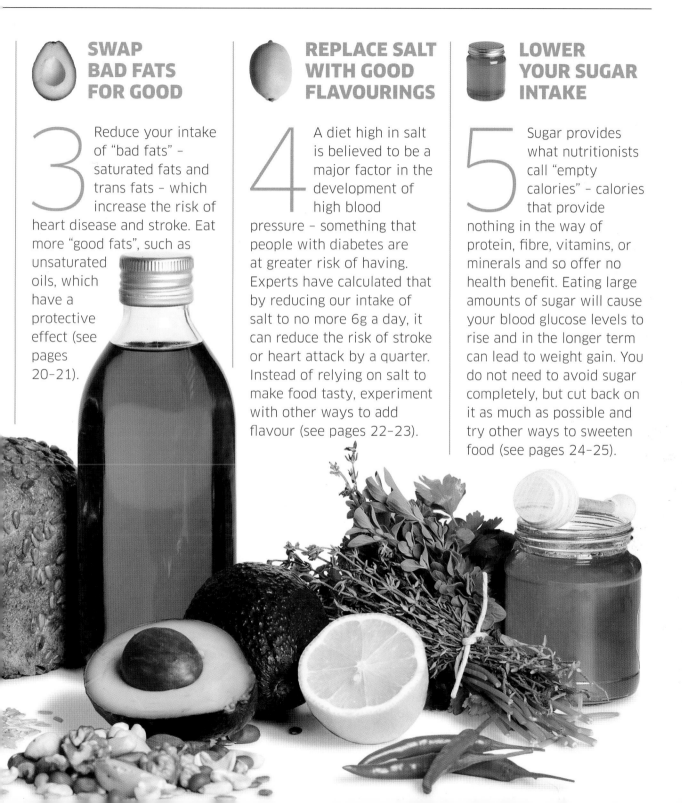

1

EAT MORE FRUIT AND VEGETABLES

A HEALTHY REGIME

One of the easiest ways to improve your diet is to eat more vegetables. Ideally, at mealtimes, around half of your plate should be filled with vegetables. However, don't just think of them as an accompaniment: regard them as an ingredient that you can incorporate into your favourite recipes.

As well as being low in calories and a good source of fibre, vegetables are an excellent source of antioxidant vitamins, minerals, and photochemicals, and can help reduce the risk of many of the health problems associated with diabetes.

Fruit is also a great source of vitamins and minerals, and may lower the risk of heart disease, certain cancers, and digestive problems. However, fruit also contains natural sugars that can affect your blood glucose level, so take care not to eat too much all at once. Dried fruit in particular is a very concentrated source of these sugars, while fruit juice releases its sugar into the bloodstream very quickly, so it is preferable to eat whole fresh fruit.

THE FIVE-A-DAY TARGET

Healthy eating guidelines recommend that we should all eat at least five portions of vegetables and fruit a day. A portion is approximately 85g (3oz). For a quick visual guide, clench your fist – that's about the size of a portion. Five is the minimum number of portions you should be eating each day; the more you can cram into your diet, the healthier you'll be. Aim to eat a variety of vegetables and fruit.

10 EASY WAYS TO EAT MORE FRUIT AND VEGETABLES

1 **Add a handful of vegetables.** Mix chopped vegetables such as carrots or peppers into spaghetti bolognese, shepherd's pie, or lasagne.

2 **Give salad a fruit boost.** Add apple, pineapple, or pear to a green salad; a few raisins, pomegranate seeds, or dried apricots to rice, pasta, or couscous.

3 **Serve roast pumpkin instead of roast potatoes.** Roast chunks of pumpkin, drizzled with a little oil, at 200°C (400°F/Gas 6) for 30–40 minutes.

4 **Breakfast wisely.** Spread mashed banana on toast instead of marmalade. Add a few chopped apricots or a handful of fresh berries to cereal.

5 **Serve meat or fish with a spicy salsa.** Mix finely chopped red onion, chilli, and tomato with avocado; or try onion, chilli, mango, and cucumber.

6 **Give pizzas an extra topping.** Pile pizzas high with vegetables such as spinach, peppers, artichokes, and mushrooms.

7 **Serve healthy snacks at parties.** Instead of crisps, offer pieces of raw carrot, pepper, celery, or cauliflower with a yogurt dip or salsa.

8 **Keep a bowl of fruit on your desk at work.** It means you've always got a healthy snack close at hand, and will help you to resist sweets and biscuits.

9 **Swap your lunchtime sandwich for a bowl of vegetable soup.** Increase your nutrient intake further by adding some beans and pulses to it.

10 **Choose healthy snacks.** Keep a plastic container or ziplock bag filled with washed and prepared vegetables in the refrigerator.

EAT A RAINBOW

Fruit and vegetables of different colours contain different vitamins, minerals, and phytochemicals. These all help to keep you healthy in various ways, so try to eat at least one serving of fruit or vegetables from each of the colour bands every day.

RED	ORANGE	YELLOW	GREEN	BLUE/INDIGO/VIOLET
Strawberries, raspberries, apples, watermelon, red peppers, tomatoes	Carrots, pumpkins, oranges, mangoes, papaya, apricots	Bananas, melons, pineapples, grapefruit	Broccoli, spinach, peas, kiwi fruit, kale, spring cabbage, celery, green beans, cauliflower	Aubergines, blueberries, blackberries, prunes, red cabbage, plums, red onions, beetroot

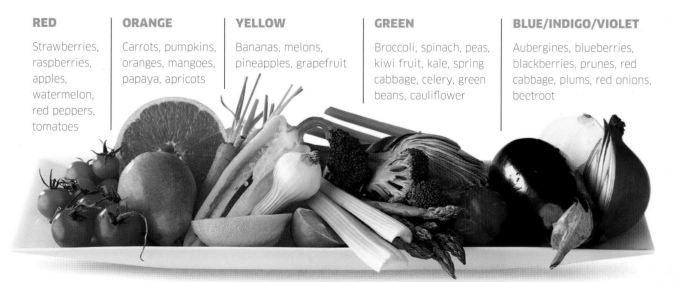

Satisfying hunger

USE LOW-CALORIE FOODS TO FEEL FULL FOR LONGER

When you are trying to lose weight by cutting down the amount of food you consume, it can be a problem making sure that you don't feel hungry. The feeling of fullness, or being sated, that you get after eating depends on what you've eaten. At a technical level, there is a system for ranking foods based on their ability to satisfy hunger – this is called the satiety index (see Useful Websites on page 352). On a simpler level, one of the most important factors is just the volume of food you consume. Think about it – if you snack on cheese, you will need to limit yourself to a tiny portion because of the amount of calories it contains. You are likely to find this less satisfying than if you choose fruit and vegetables, as their lower calorie count means you can crunch your way through a much larger amount.

The examples here compare quantities of different foods that contain the same number of calories. As you will see, if you choose the healthy fruit and vegetable options on the right, you will be able to enjoy a far greater volume of food, keeping you satisfied until your next meal.

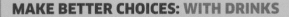

MAKE BETTER CHOICES: WITH DRINKS

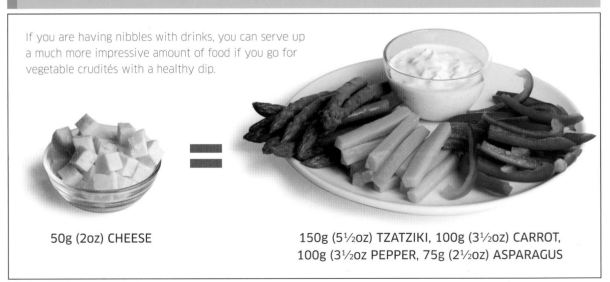

If you are having nibbles with drinks, you can serve up a much more impressive amount of food if you go for vegetable crudités with a healthy dip.

50g (2oz) CHEESE

150g (5½oz) TZATZIKI, 100g (3½oz) CARROT, 100g (3½oz PEPPER, 75g (2½oz) ASPARAGUS

MAKE BETTER CHOICES: SALAD

When you are making a salad, you might consider adding a few chopped peanuts. If you would prefer a greater quantity though, you would be well advised to leave these out and opt for cherry tomatoes instead.

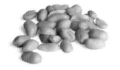

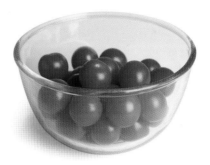

15g (½oz) PEANUTS

450g (1lb) CHERRY TOMATOES

MAKE BETTER CHOICES: BREAKFAST

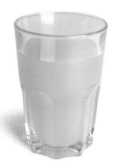

At breakfast, you might find a glass of apple juice refreshing, but will it fill you up as much as two whole apples?

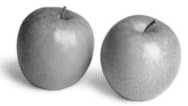

250ml (9fl oz) APPLE JUICE

2 APPLES (100g/3½oz EACH)

MAKE BETTER CHOICES: SNACKS

A small amount of dried fruit makes a good snack, but opt for fresh and you can enjoy a lot more food for the same number of calories.

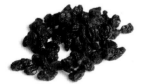

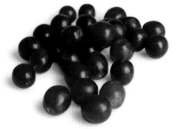

30g (1oz) RAISINS

140g (5oz) GRAPES

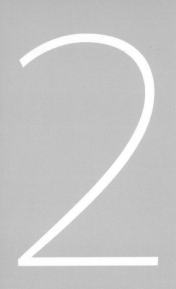

CHOOSE THE RIGHT CARBOHYDRATES

WHAT ARE CARBOHYDRATES?

Carbohydrates are an essential source of energy in our diet. This group of foods can be divided into two main types: starchy carbohydrates and sugars. Starchy carbohydrates include bread, potatoes, pasta, rice, noodles, and cereals. Sugars include sucrose (table sugar), lactose (the sugar found in dairy foods), and fructose (the sugar found in fruit).

Starchy carbohydrates can be divided into two groups – refined carbohydrates such as white bread, white rice, and products made with white flour; and unrefined, wholegrain carbohydrates, such as wholemeal bread and brown rice.

CARBOHYDRATES AT WORK

Refined carbohydrates release their energy quickly and can cause a surge in blood glucose levels. Unrefined, wholegrain carbohydrates release their energy slowly, and this keeps blood glucose levels even. People with diabetes should eat a diet that is high in slow-release carbohydrates which are good sources of energy and nutrients. Some carbohydrates are also better than others at making you feel full for longer after eating.

The glycaemic index (GI) is a way of measuring the effect of a food on blood glucose levels. Low-GI carbohydrates are converted into glucose slowly and so release glucose into the bloodstream gradually. They produce less of a spike in blood glucose levels, which is better for your health. See pages 18–19 for more about the glycaemic index.

Q&A

ARE CARBOHYDRATES FATTENING ?

Although carbohydrates such as bread and potatoes have a reputation for being fattening, they are low in fat and relatively low in calories. It's only when they are eaten with lots of fat – pasta with a rich, creamy sauce, fried potatoes, chips, or bread spread thickly with butter – that they become highly calorific.

Carbohydrates are an important part of a well-balanced diet. Aim for a third of the food you eat every day to consist of carbohydrates, and eat at least one food from this group at every meal.

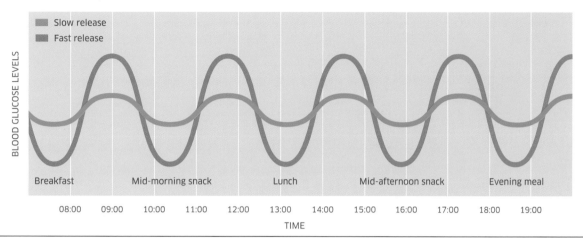

The illustration below shows how your blood glucose level might fluctuate over the course of a day depending on your choice of slow or quick release carbohydrates. The steadier effect of the slow release carbohydrates is better for your health and energy levels.

Slow release
Fast release

BLOOD GLUCOSE LEVELS

Breakfast   Mid-morning snack   Lunch   Mid-afternoon snack   Evening meal

08:00   09:00   10:00   11:00   12:00   13:00   14:00   15:00   16:00   17:00   18:00   19:00

TIME

WHY WHOLEGRAINS ARE THE SMART CHOICE

Most of the carbohydrates we eat should be starchy carbohydrates, fruit and vegetables, and some dairy products. For people targeting a healthy diet, wholegrain products are by far the best starchy carbohydrates. When grains are refined, they lose fibre, vitamins, and minerals. If you eat refined carbohydrates, you are missing the opportunity to consume more of these important nutrients.

Wholegrains can be milled into flour to make foods such as bread and pasta. The fibre in wholegrain foods slows the conversion of starch into glucose, and this helps to balance blood glucose levels. Fibre keeps the digestive system healthy, and a further benefit of choosing wholegrains is that they may also lower the risk of heart disease and cancer.

GI and GL

WHAT IS THE GLYCAEMIC INDEX?

The glycaemic index (GI) is a system that ranks carbohydrates according to how quickly they are converted to glucose in the body, and the extent to which they raise your blood glucose level after you've eaten them. Foods with a high GI (70 or above) are broken down very quickly, resulting in a rapid rise in blood glucose – which people with diabetes need to avoid. Low-GI foods (55 and below) are absorbed more slowly into the bloodstream, causing a steadier, more controlled, rise in your blood glucose level.

CALCULATING GLYCAEMIC LOAD

Glycaemic load (GL) is based on similar information to GI but also takes into account the overall quantity of carbohydrate in a food. Multiply the GI by the amount of carbohydrate in a portion, and you get the GL. Although GI is more commonly used, in certain cases GL can be a better predictor of how a food will affect blood glucose levels. For example, carrots and chocolate both have a GI of 49 – but you don't need to be a nutrition expert to know that carrots are better for you. In this case, the foods' respective GLs confirm that carrots are the healthier choice.

WHAT ARE THE HEALTH BENEFITS OF A LOW-GI DIET?

Low-GI diets were originally developed to help people with diabetes achieve better control of their blood glucose levels, but they have also been shown to help to reduce the risk of heart disease and because they can help control appetite and delay hunger, they can help with weight management.

↟ **Cherries** have a low GI and are rich in vitamin C and fibre.

Q&A

HOW DOES PROCESSING FOOD AFFECT ITS GI?

All types of processing affect the GI of a food, because they make it easier for the digestive system to break down carbohydrates. Processed food therefore has a higher GI than unprocessed food. For example, canned tomatoes have a higher GI than raw tomatoes, and mashed potato has a higher GI than whole new potatoes eaten with their skin.

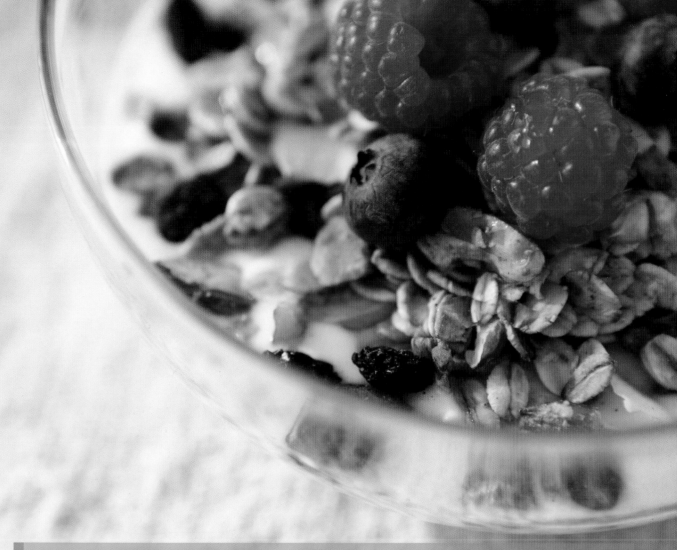

SIX EASY WAYS TO REDUCE THE GI AND GL OF YOUR DIET

1 DON'T OVERCOOK PASTA Eat pasta *al dente* – it has a lower GI than soft pasta, because it takes digestive enzymes longer to break down the carbs.

2 REDUCE THE IMPACT OF HIGH-GI FOOD If you eat a high-GI food such as a jacket potato, combine it with a low-GI food such as beans.

3 CHOOSE RICE CAREFULLY Basmati rice has a GI of 57, compared with long-grain white rice (GI of 72), and jasmine rice (GI of 89).

4 USE VINAIGRETTE INSTEAD OF CREAMY SALAD DRESSING It's lower in fat, and the vinegar's acidity slows digestion and lowers the GI of the meal.

5 WATCH YOUR PORTION SIZES The larger the portion of a carbohydrate, the more it will increase your blood glucose, regardless of its GI.

6 OPT FOR MINIMALLY PROCESSED FOOD The less a food is processed, the lower its GI. Think about the food that you buy, and the way that you cook it.

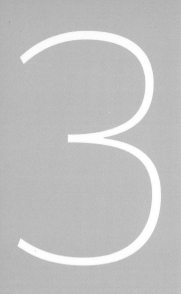

SWAP BAD FATS FOR GOOD FATS

KNOW YOUR FATS

Nutritionists distinguish between two main types of fats: saturated fats and unsaturated fats. Unsaturated fats can be monounsaturated or polyunsaturated; polyunsaturated fats can be subdivided further into omega-3 and omega-6 fats. There is also a further group: trans fats.

The types of fat you eat can affect your health, so fats are often referred to as "bad fats" and "good fats". A diet high in saturated and trans fats – bad fats – will encourage the body to produce cholesterol, which can clog blood vessels and arteries and increase the risk of heart disease and stroke. Polyunsaturated and monounsaturated fats are considered to be good fats. Monounsaturated fats help to reduce cholesterol. Omega-3 fats protect the heart by making the blood less likely to clot, by lowering blood pressure, and by encouraging the muscles lining the artery walls to relax, improving blood flow to the heart. It's important to have a balance of omega-3 and omega-6 fats in the diet. Most of us eat too much omega-6 fat and not enough omega-3 fat.

You should remember that, despite the health benefits of unsaturated fats, all types of fat contain twice as many calories as protein or carbohydrate, so eat fats – even good fats – in moderation.

GOOD FATS

MONOUNSATURATED FATS These are found mainly in olive oil, rapeseed oil, nuts, and avocados.

Q&A

DOES MARGARINE CONTAIN LESS FAT THAT BUTTER?

Both margarine and butter contain the same amount of fat, and the same number of calories – around 37 calories per teaspoon. They differ, however, in the type of fat they contain. Butter is classified as a saturated fat; margarine is available in monounsaturated or polyunsaturated versions.

Low-fat and reduced-fat spreads contain less fat and fewer calories than margarine.

POLYUNSATURATED FATS Omega-6 fats are found in vegetable oils and margarines such as sunflower, safflower, corn, and soya bean oil. Omega-3 fats are found mainly in oil-rich fish such as salmon, fresh tuna, sardines, and mackerel. Plant sources include linseed (flaxseed) and its oil, rapeseed oil, soya bean oil, and walnuts.

BAD FATS

SATURATED FATS Found in full-fat dairy products (cheese, yogurt, milk, cream), lard, ghee, fatty cuts of meat and meat products such as sausages and burgers, pastry, cakes, biscuits, coconut oil, and palm oil.

TRANS FATS These occur naturally in small amounts in meat and dairy products, but they are also produced during hydrogenation, a process that food manufactures use to convert vegetable oils into semi-solid fats. Although, chemically, trans fats are unsaturated, in the body they behave like saturated fat. In fact, some research suggests they are more unhealthy than saturated fat.

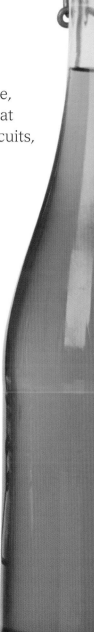

« Make the most of good fats by including them in a tasty salad dressing. Choose from a variety of oils such as olive, avocado, or pumpkin seed.

« Walnut oil is a light oil and a good source of omega-3 fat.

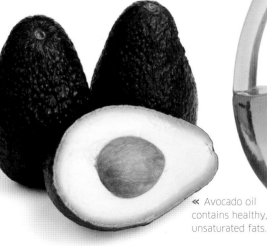

« Avocado oil contains healthy, unsaturated fats.

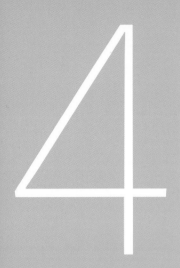

REPLACE SALT WITH GOOD FLAVOURINGS

WHY CUT DOWN ON SALT?

If you have diabetes, you are already more likely than most people to suffer from heart disease or a stroke. To reduce this risk it is important that you control your blood pressure, and one of the key ways to do this is to minimize the amount of salt you eat. Salt is composed of sodium and chloride; sodium is the component that damages health. Most of the sodium in our diet comes from salt, but some comes from additives such as flavour enhancers and preservatives.

Small amounts of sodium occur naturally in many foods, including meat, fish, vegetables, and even fruit. Although cutting back on the salt we add during cooking and at the table will reduce our intake, around 75 per cent of the salt we consume comes from processed foods. Check whether products are high in salt by reading the labels before you buy, but remember that they often list sodium content rather than the total salt content. To convert the figure given for sodium, multiply it by 2.5 to give the amount of salt.

LESS SALT DOESN'T MEAN LESS FLAVOUR

Many people eat more salt than the recommended 6g per day. The more salt you eat, the less sensitive to it your taste buds become. However, you can retrain yourself to enjoy foods with less salt. If you gradually reduce the amount you add to meals, your taste buds will adapt, the salt receptors on the tongue becoming more sensitive again. This usually takes 2–3 weeks. Experiment with other flavourings instead of salt, using the ideas opposite as a starting point.

Q&A

IS NATURAL SEA SALT BETTER THAN ROCK SALT?

Although sea salt contains traces of minerals such as magnesium, calcium, and potassium – which you don't find in ordinary (rock) salt – it doesn't contain enough of these to make a significant contribution to your diet.

Many chefs prefer to use sea salt because they believe it has a better flavour than rock salt, but in terms of dietary salt content and health, there really isn't any difference.

EASY WAYS TO BOOST FLAVOUR

CINNAMON

Try cinnamon in meat dishes such as stir-fries, stews, and casseroles. It may also help to regulate blood glucose.

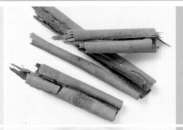

CITRUS FRUIT

Citrus flavours enhance chicken and fish. Add lemon zest to rice or vegetables, orange peel to a stew or casserole.

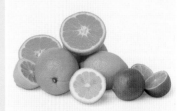

MUSTARD

Add grainy mustard to mashed potatoes, or use a pinch of mustard powder to pep up cheese sauce.

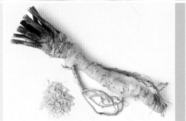

CARDAMOM

Add crushed cardamom pods to rice dishes such as pilaf or rice pudding; flavour stewed apple with ground cardamom.

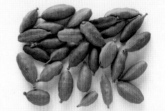

HORSERADISH

Grated horseradish gives mashed potatoes a kick. Mix it with mayonnaise to use as a spread in sandwiches.

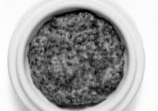

NUTMEG

Has a sweet, spicy flavour. Add a little freshly ground nutmeg to cheese sauce, stewed fruit, or rice pudding.

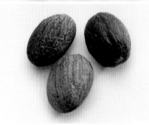

GINGER

Use in stir-fries, salad dressings, or salsas. It works well teamed with meat, fish, or shellfish flavours.

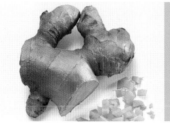

CHILLIES

Chillies range from mild to fiery. Try adding a little finely chopped fresh chilli to tomato sauce or tomato salsa.

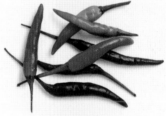

PEPPERCORNS

There are several varieties: experiment with pink, green, and Sichuan peppercorns as well as black ones.

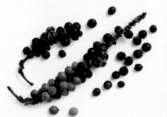

CARAWAY SEEDS

Add a pinch to potato salad or coleslaw; works well with cheese, vegetables, or in bread.

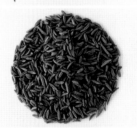

STAR ANISE

Its warm, aniseed-like flavour enlivens a fruit salad; or add a pinch of ground star anise to roasted vegetables.

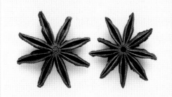

LEMONGRASS

Crush or "bruise" this Asian herb and use it to flavour stews, curries, rice dishes, soups, and marinades.

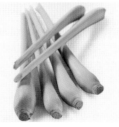

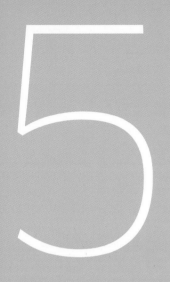

LOWER YOUR SUGAR INTAKE

LOW SUGAR – NOT NO SUGAR

There are two common myths: eating too much sugar causes diabetes, and people with diabetes need to avoid all forms of sugar. In reality, it is the amount and the form in which you eat sugar, plus the other foods you eat it with, that determine the effect it has on your blood glucose level.

People with diabetes should avoid consuming large amounts of foods that are a concentrated source of natural sugar, such as fruit juice and dried fruit. Small amounts of sugar are fine, particularly when combined with foods that are high in fibre (this helps to slow down the rate at which it is absorbed into the bloodstream).

Desserts, biscuits, cakes, and confectionery are not forbidden but because they are usually high in calories, fat, and sugar, and most people with diabetes need to control their weight, eat them in moderation. When there are sugar-free and low-sugar options, it makes sense for you to choose them.

SWEET CHOICES

Sometimes there is no getting away from the fact that a dish requires table sugar or another high-calorie sweetener such as honey or fructose. This tends to be in recipes where the sweetener needs to provide bulk and texture as well as flavour. If on the other hand you just need to sweeten a food without adding bulk, a low-calorie or calorie-free sweetener may be the best option. See the table opposite for information on the various options.

Q&A

WHAT IS THE DIFFERENCE BETWEEN NATURAL AND ADDED SUGAR?

Sugars can be divided into two groups – natural sugar, such as the sugar found in fruit, and the sugar we add to foods. The body treats both types of sugar in the same way.

Concentrate on reducing added sugar in your diet. You could start by giving up stirring sugar into drinks and sprinkling it on cereal.

Enjoy foods containing natural sugar, such as fresh fruit, because you get the benefit of other nutrients, such as vitamins and minerals, at the same time. Dried fruit is also fine in small quantities.

TYPES OF SWEETENER

TABLE SUGAR (E.G. CASTER, BROWN, DEMERARA)	1 tablespoon of sugar contains 59 calories, so it is important to control how much you eat. Sugar has properties other than sweetness that can affect a recipe's success though, so be aware that simply substituting another sweetener may not always work.
HONEY	In health terms, there is little benefit to using honey rather than table sugar. Honey, being denser, contains slightly more calories per spoonful, but it is also slightly sweeter, meaning you usually use less of it.
AGAVE SYRUP	Produced from South American cactus, this is about 30 per cent sweeter than sugar or honey, so you should use a third less. If using this in recipes, reduce the quantity of liquid by about twenty-five per cent and the cooking temperature by 10°C (50°F).
FRUCTOSE	This can be used in the same way as table sugar, although it browns quicker so you may need to reduce cooking temperatures by 25°C (75°F). Its benefits are a lower GI than table sugar and the fact that you need less of it to achieve the same sweetness.
SACCHARIN (E.G. HERMESTA)	This calorie-free sweetener is heat stable so can be used in dishes cooked at high temperatures. However, it does not have the same properties as sugar, and is used in much smaller quantities (it is 300 times sweeter), so cannot be substituted in baking.
SUCRALOSE (E.G. SPLENDA)	Made from sugar, but not recognized by the body as sugar, this calorie-free sweetener has no effect on blood glucose levels. 600 times sweeter than sugar, it is extremely resistant to heat and cold, so useful for flavouring frozen desserts as well as cooking.
ASPARTAME (E.G. NUTRASWEET)	200 times sweeter than sugar, this is used in such small amounts it contributes negligible calories. At very high temperatures it is broken down and loses its sweetness, so it is not ideal for dishes that require high-temperature cooking.

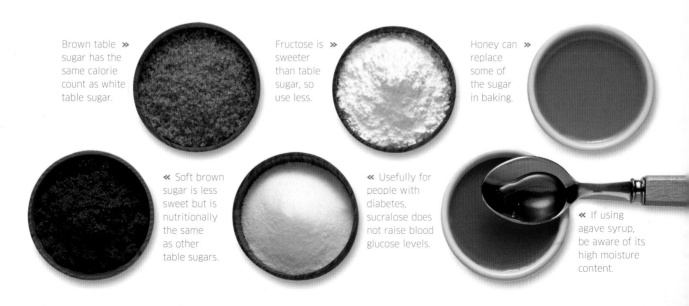

Brown table » sugar has the same calorie count as white table sugar.

Fructose is » sweeter than table sugar, so use less.

Honey can » replace some of the sugar in baking.

« Soft brown sugar is less sweet but is nutritionally the same as other table sugars.

« Usefully for people with diabetes, sucralose does not raise blood glucose levels.

« If using agave syrup, be aware of its high moisture content.

A HEALTHY SHOPPING BASKET

It's very easy to opt for convenience rather than nutritional quality, so take some time to review the contents of your shopping trolley. Making small changes – such as switching from full-fat to semi-skimmed milk, and from white to wholemeal bread – can make a real difference to your health, and help you to manage diabetes.

BE A SAVVY SHOPPER

1 Walk around the perimeter of the store first: the fresh foods are usually there. Approach central aisles with caution: highly processed foods lurk here.

2 Compare brands of processed food to find which has least fat, salt, and sugar, and the most fibre. Look at the figures per 100g rather than per serving.

3 Choose fresh and minimally processed foods, such as 100 per cent fruit juice or all-wholegrain items.

4 Try to avoid foods with added salt or sugar; if necessary, you can add it sparingly yourself.

5 Look at ingredients – the longer the list of additives, the less healthy a food usually is.

6 Don't forget frozen vegetables – they save you time because they are already prepared, and they often contain more vitamins than fresh vegetables.

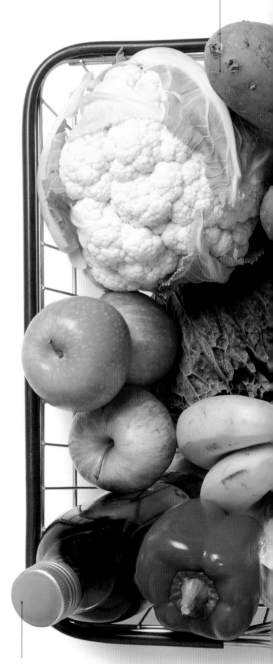

FRUIT AND VEGETABLES
Eat from a wide range of fruit and vegetables for different vitamins, minerals, and phytochemicals. Fresh, frozen, canned, and dried varieties all count towards your five a day.

OIL
Use unsaturated oils such as olive, rapeseed, walnut, avocado, linseed (flaxseed), and soya bean for omega-6 and omega-3 fats.

EGGS

If you don't eat oil-rich fish, choose eggs that advertise themselves as especially rich in omega-3 fats. Eggs are also a good source of iron.

BREAKFAST CEREALS

Choose wholegrain breakfast cereals without added sugar, with at least 3g fibre per serving. Alternatively, make muesli from oats, seeds, nuts, and dried fruit.

DAIRY PRODUCTS

You can obtain a good supply of protein and calcium from dairy products; go for low-fat versions if possible.

RICE

Choose basmati or brown rice, which has a lower GI than long-grain white rice and is a good source of B-vitamins.

OIL-RICH FISH

Oil-rich fish such as mackerel, salmon, and fresh tuna provide omega-3 fats, which help heart health. Eat at least one portion a week; choose a different type of fish for another meal during the week.

POULTRY AND LEAN MEAT

Choose chicken and lean meat rather than fatty cuts of meat. Keep portions modest – 100–140g (3½–5oz) is more than enough for one person.

CANNED BEANS

Beans are high in fibre and have a low GI. Look for the ones canned without salt or sugar; if canned in brine, rinse thoroughly before using.

BREAD

Buy wholegrain bread. It is more nutritious than white and has a lower GI.

EATING FOOD ON THE RUN

Sometimes you can't avoid buying lunch or a snack while you are away from home. Look at the nutrition information on the food labels before you buy, to make sure that you pick products that are as healthy as possible.

HOW TO READ FOOD LABELS

Guideline Daily Amounts (GDAs) tell you how much fat, salt, sugar, and fibre a food contains; also how many calories it provides, and how that contributes to the total amount you can or should eat in a day - lunch should provide around 30 per cent of your GDA, while snacks should total about 10 per cent. You can use this information to make sure that your diet is balanced; if, for instance, you eat a food that is high in fat or salt at one meal, you can choose foods that are low in fat or salt during the rest of the day.

GDA FOR ADULTS	WOMEN	MEN
Energy	2,000kcal	2,500kcal
Total fat	70g	95g
Saturated fat	20g	30g
Sugar	90g	120g
Salt	6g	6g
Fibre	24g	24g

For foods that don't carry GDA labelling, refer to the nutrition panel on the packaging. Look at the figure for a particular nutrient per 100g and then check the table below to find out if it is high or low in that component.

	HIGH	LOW
Fat	20g or more	3g or less
Saturated fat	5g or more	1.5g or less
Sugar	15g or more	5g or less
Salt	1.5g or more	0.1g or less
Fibre	more than 3g	0.5g or less

LUNCH

OPTION 1

WHOLEMEAL SANDWICH »

If opting for a sandwich, choose one made with wholemeal, granary, or rye bread with a lean protein filling such as chicken, fish, shellfish, or hummus; add salad or vegetables.

OPTION 2

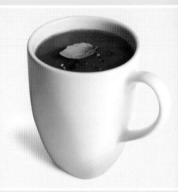

OPTION 3

BROWN RICE SALAD »

If you want a change from sandwiches, try a salad made with brown rice, pasta, barley, or quinoa.

OPTION 4

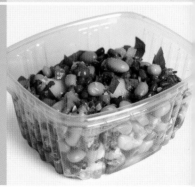

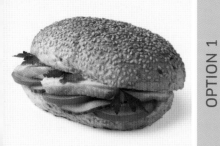

THREE DRIED APRICOTS »

A small, healthy snack in the middle of the morning and afternoon helps to keep your blood glucose level stable and hunger pangs at bay. Dried fruit can be high in sugar, however, so keep portions small.

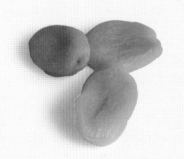

OPTION 1

« SOUP

Soup is a healthy and filling option, but it can be high in salt, so check the label. Choose soups made with beans or pulses and avoid those containing cream or coconut milk – these are high in calories and fat.

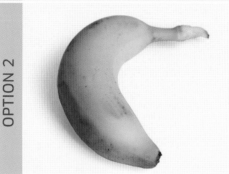

OPTION 2

« BANANA

Make sure that snacks do more than satisfy hunger. They should also provide nutrients such as vitamins and minerals, and fibre. Bananas are a great source of potassium, which helps to control blood glucose.

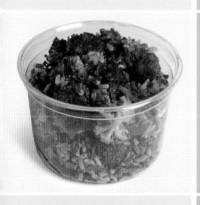

LOW-FAT YOGURT »

A small pot of low-fat yogurt provides protein and calcium, making it a great, hunger-busting snack. It will also help to keep your bones healthy.

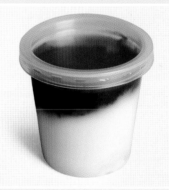

OPTION 3

« BEAN SALAD

Aim to have at least one serving of fruit and one serving of vegetables at lunch. A mixed bean or lentil salad will count towards your five-a-day target and is a good low-GI option.

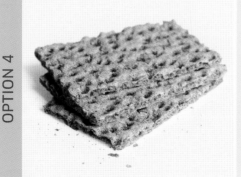

OPTION 4

« CRISPBREAD

For a fibre-rich snack, reach for a couple of crispbread or oatcakes; team with reduced-fat hummus, salsa, or low-fat soft cheese.

10 TIPS FOR DINING OUT

	TIP	WHY?
1	**AVOID BUFFET-STYLE SELF-SERVICE RESTAURANTS**	Studies show that the greater the choice of food on offer, the more calories we're likely to eat. If you are faced with a buffet, don't try a little of everything – limit yourself to three or four dishes.
2	**BEFORE YOU ORDER, LOOK AROUND TO SEE WHAT OTHER PEOPLE'S MEALS LOOK LIKE**	If you're in a restaurant that serves up huge portions of food, it might be best to limit temptation by taking steps to make sure that you aren't faced with a mountainous plate. For example, you could think about ordering two starters or side dishes to constitute the main course.
3	**ASK FOR WATER AS SOON AS YOU SIT DOWN**	Ask the waiter to bring a jug of water. Drink a large glassful before you start eating, and it will take the edge off your appetite. Drinking water will also help you avoid drinking large quantities of alcohol.
4	**ASK QUESTIONS ABOUT THE MENU BEFORE ORDERING**	It's not always easy to tell how healthy or fattening a dish will be, so ask the waiter how it is prepared if you have any doubts. Don't be afraid to request vegetables served without butter, or fish or meat without a rich sauce – make sure you specify when giving your order.
5	**BE THE FIRST TO ORDER**	We may enter a restaurant full of good intentions to select the healthy options on the menu, but we're often swayed by other people's less than healthy choices. To help you stick to your resolution to eat healthily, order your meal first.

Dining out needn't be an ordeal when you are sticking to a healthy eating strategy. Follow these tips to stay on the straight and narrow while enjoying your food.

	TIP	WHY?
6	START YOUR MEAL WITH SOUP OR A SALAD	Soup helps to fill your stomach so you won't eat as much for the main course. One study found that when people had soup as a first course, they ate 20 per cent fewer calories for the overall meal. In summer, begin with a salad (with fat-free dressing), which works in the same way.
7	GET AN EXTRA SIDE ORDER OF VEGETABLES	Most restaurant food is short on vegetables. To make sure that your meal includes a healthy dose of vitamins and minerals, order a portion of vegetables on the side, or add a salad.
8	DON'T LOAD UP ON BREAD BEFORE YOUR MEAL ARRIVES	If bread arrives and you know you won't be able to resist, ask the waiter to take it away. If you want to nibble on something while you're waiting for your order, ask for olives.
9	DON'T ALLOW THE WAITER TO TOP UP YOUR WINE GLASS BEFORE IT IS EMPTY	Alcohol is high in calories so you should keep track of how much you are drinking. If your glass is constantly being refilled, it becomes difficult to do this.
10	YOU DON'T HAVE TO MISS OUT ON DESSERT	Desserts don't have to be a no-go area: just choose wisely. Stick to fruit-based puddings, or ice cream, or share a dessert with your dining partner. Don't add extra fat and calories by drenching the dessert in cream.

MAKE-OVER RECIPES

	TIP	WHY?
1	**ADD A CAN OF BEANS OR LENTILS**	Beans and lentils are full of fibre and have a low GI. Add them to salads, soups, stews, and casseroles. For recipes that specify minced meat, halve the normal quantity of mince and add an equal amount of canned lentils.
2	**SNEAK IN EXTRA VEGETABLES WHENEVER POSSIBLE**	Bulk out meat dishes such as chilli con carne or spaghetti bolognese by adding vegetables such as sweetcorn, diced carrots, or frozen peas. This allows you to use less meat; it also increases your veg intake. Add chopped spring onions, steamed spinach, cabbage, or puréed carrot to mashed potato.
3	**WHEN BAKING, REPLACE SOME OF THE FAT WITH PRUNE PURÉE**	Use prune purée to replace up to 50 per cent of the butter or oil in baked goods such as biscuits, muffins, and cakes. To make the purée, put 225g (8oz) of ready-to-eat pitted prunes and 6 tablespoons of hot water in a food processor or blender and process to make a smooth purée.
4	**USE WHOLEMEAL FLOUR FOR BAKING INSTEAD OF ORDINARY FLOUR**	If haven't used wholemeal flour before, start by substituting it for half the white flour in a recipe. As you get used to cooking with wholemeal flour, you can gradually increase the proportion. Wholemeal flour is a little drier than white flour, so you will need to add more liquid than usual.
5	**USE A SPRAY OIL FOR DISHES THAT REQUIRE LIGHT FRYING**	Oil expands once it gets hot, so when you are softening onions or vegetables, you don't need to add as much as you might think. A spray coats the pan with a film of oil, giving you a saving on fat and calorie content.

Don't abandon your favourite recipes: with a few additions and straightforward changes, it's easy to adapt them to your new goals.

	TIP	WHY?
6	**USE SWEET POTATOES IN PLACE OF WHITE POTATOES**	Sweet potatoes have a lower GI than white potatoes and are an excellent source of betacarotene. You can use them in exactly the same way that you would use white potatoes. Try them baked in their jackets or peel, boil, and mash with a little butter and a touch of cinnamon.
7	**USE FILO PASTRY RATHER THAN SHORTCRUST PASTRY**	Filo pastry has just 3.6g fat per 100g compared with 28g fat for shortcrust pastry, and 36g for flaky pastry. If you're making your own filo pastry, use vegetable oil rather than melted butter to brush the sheets of pastry.
8	**ADD A SQUEEZE OF LEMON JUICE**	Lemon helps to reduce the need for salt. It also helps to slow the breaking down of starch into sugar, and so will lower the GI of a meal. Vinegar and other acidic foods have the same effect.
9	**USE RAPESEED OIL FOR COOKING**	Olive oil is a good source of monounsaturated fats, but it can be expensive. Rapeseed oil offers many of the same benefits at a fraction of the price. It has a mild flavour and can used for sautéing, baking, or salad dressings.
10	**MAKE CREAM LIGHTER**	Reduce the fat content in recipes that call for double cream by using half the stated quantity of cream mixed with an equal amount of Greek yogurt. Choose a reduced-fat version to lower the calorie content still further.

WEIGHT MANAGEMENT

Being overweight makes it more difficult to manage diabetes, and puts you at greater risk of developing some of the complications associated with diabetes, such as heart disease. So if you are overweight you should make weight loss your number one priority. To ascertain whether you are overweight, the body mass index (BMI) chart below provides a quick reference. If you have a lot of weight to lose, the prospect of trying to get down to your ideal weight can seem rather daunting; however, even losing 5–10 per cent of your weight will bring significant health benefits.

BODY MASS INDEX (BMI)

ARE YOU A HEALTHY WEIGHT?

The body mass index (BMI) is a ratio of weight to height. Locate yourself on the graph below, where your height and weight cross, to find out whether or not you are a healthy weight. Alternatively, calculate your BMI by dividing your weight in kilograms by the square of your height in metres.

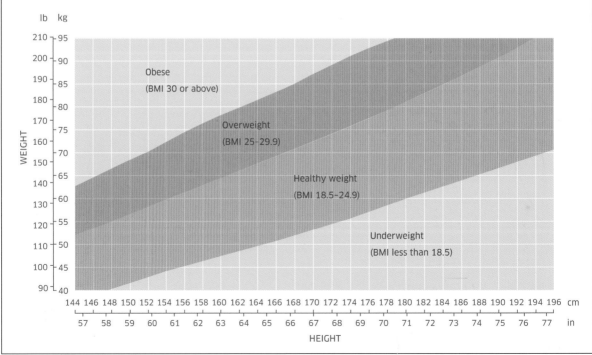

YOUR WAIST MEASUREMENT

Your BMI is only part of the story when it comes to assessing and managing your weight. Fat stored around the middle increases the risk of developing heart disease, high blood pressure, and diabetes. You can check the distribution of fat on your body by measuring your waist. Find the bottom of your ribs and the top of your hips. Measure your circumference midway between these two points (for many people, this will be the tummy button). Make sure that the tape is parallel to the floor and taut, but not pressing into the skin. Breathe out normally and take the measurement at the end of this breath.

The guidelines of the World Health Organization advise that men should not have a waist measurement exceeding 94cm (37in). Above this, the risk of heart disease, high blood pressure, and diabetes is increased. A measurement of over 102cm (40in) puts a man at high risk of these conditions. For women, the thresholds are lower: a waist measurement of 80cm (32in) or above warns of increased risk, and a measurement of 88cm (35in) or above sounds the alarm for high risk.

There is slight variance between ethnic groups, the most significant being that Asian men are advised to taget a slightly smaller waist, as a measurement of 90cm (36in) or above can bring increased health risks.

THE ENERGY BALANCE EQUATION

Your weight is determined by a simple equation. To maintain weight, you need to use up the same amount of energy (calories) you take in from food and drink. If you consume more calories than your body uses, the surplus is stored as fat. Eating even a small amount in excess of our needs will result in a slow but steady weight gain – if we eat just 100 calories a day more than we need (the equivalent of 1½ digestive biscuits), it will result in a weight gain of 4.7kg (10½lb) in a year.

To lose weight, you need to tip the balance the other way, so that you use more calories than you consume; in this situation, the body will draw on fat reserves to provide the energy it needs. You can lose weight by restricting the number of calories you eat, or by increasing the number of calories you use – being more active. Without doubt, the best way is a combination of diet and exercise.

10 STEPS TO WEIGHT LOSS

	TIP	WHY?
1	**SET REALISTIC GOALS**	If you set unrealistic goals for losing weight, you're more likely to become disheartened and quit. Aim for a slow, but steady weight loss of 0.5–1kg (1–2lb) a week and you're more likely to keep the weight off.
2	**PLAN AHEAD AND BE ORGANIZED**	If you plan a week's menu in advance, it means that you don't have to make decisions about what to eat at the end of the day, when you're tired and vulnerable to making poor choices. You'll also save money, because ingredients are carefully planned and nothing will be wasted.
3	**SPRING-CLEAN YOUR REFRIGERATOR AND CUPBOARDS**	Get rid of anything that will tempt you into unhealthy food choices. Make sure that you've got plenty of healthy snacks such as oatcakes, low-fat yogurts, fruit, and vegetables.
4	**LOOK AT FOOD LABELS**	Processed food often contains hidden fat and sugar, so check the calorie count on the packaging. It's also worth comparing brands, because they can vary considerably. Remember that foods labelled as low-fat, reduced fat, or reduced sugar are not necessarily low in calories.
5	**START THE DAY WITH A HEALTHY BREAKFAST**	Skipping breakfast in an attempt to cut calories is a false economy: by kick-starting the metabolism, breakfast ensures your body uses up more calories during the morning than it would otherwise. If you skip breakfast you are also far more likely to be reaching for the snacks by mid-morning.

Making small changes to the way you shop, cook, eat, and think about food can be the key to losing weight and, more importantly, keeping that weight off.

	TIP	WHY?
6	**TAKE A PACKED LUNCH TO WORK**	If you usually buy lunch from a sandwich shop or other take-away, make it at home instead and take it to work. You can control what you put into your lunchbox, and won't be tempted by unhealthy choices in a shop. You can use the time regained from shopping by going for a brisk walk.
7	**SIT DOWN TO EAT**	If you have a tendency to pick at food, make a rule that you can only eat when sitting down at the dining room or kitchen table. This will help you to restrict the bulk of your eating to mealtimes and cut out unconscious nibbling.
8	**SLOW DOWN AND FOCUS**	If you eat too quickly, you miss the signals that the stomach sends to the brain to say that it's full. Chew food thoroughly and put down your knife and fork between mouthfuls. Distractions such as the television can also cause you to miss these signals, so switch it off at mealtimes.
9	**GET THAT MINTY-FRESH TASTE**	As soon as you have finished eating, brush your teeth, rinse your mouth with mouthwash, or chew some sugar-free gum. The minty taste in your mouth will signal that the meal is at an end and stop you picking at leftovers.
10	**HARNESS THE POWER OF POSITIVE THINKING**	A recent study found that people who believed they could lose weight and keep it off were more likely to succeed. Try to visualize a new, slimmer and healthier version of yourself and keep that image in your mind.

KEEPING A FOOD DIARY

We eat for all sorts of reasons, and often it has nothing to do with being hungry. We use food to celebrate, to relieve boredom, or to make us feel better when we're unhappy or lonely. Certain people, places, moods, and situations can also prompt us to eat. Keeping a food diary will help you to identify the external triggers that cause you to eat when you're not really hungry. This will help you to manage your weight, and to substitute healthier choices when snacking.

HOW TO DO IT

Buy a notebook and divide the pages into columns, as shown on the opposite page (or you could take photocopies if you prefer). Start noting down each snack you eat and what time it was when you ate it. Record where you were, how hungry you were, who you were with, and how you felt after eating. At the end of a week, review your diary and make a list of all the triggers that prompted you to eat when you were not really hungry. Once you've identified these, you can start to work out strategies that will help you to avoid or change the way you behave when faced with these triggers.

If, for instance, you find that when you get home after work you're so hungry that you end up eating a family-sized pack of cheesy snacks whilst preparing the evening meal, have a healthy snack such as banana or a yogurt before you leave the office, so you won't be so hungry when you get home. If your food diary reveals that you use food as a way of making yourself feel better when you're unhappy or depressed, make a list of activities – unrelated to food – that will help lift your spirits when you're feeling low. Rather than reaching for a chocolate bar, watch an engrossing film, have a manicure, or take a long, leisurely bath. Old habits are hard to break, and changing ingrained behaviour patterns is not something you can achieve overnight, so allow yourself plenty of time to adjust to a new regime.

TIME	WHERE I WAS	HOW HUNGRY	WHO I WAS WITH	WHAT I ATE	HOW I FELT AFTERWARDS

SAMPLE DAILY FOOD DIARY **DAY:**

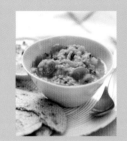 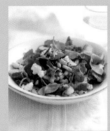 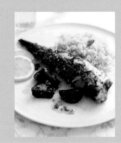 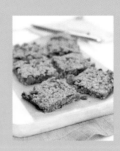 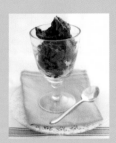

MEAL PLANNERS

The following pages provide an array of daily eating plans, centred around the recipes in this book, that guarantee a healthy, balanced diet and a controlled amount of calories per day. Whether you follow the 1400, 1600, 1800, 2000, or 2500 calories per day planner depends on a number of factors – whether you are male or female, how tall you are, and whether your target is to lose weight or to maintain your healthy weight. For advice on which planner might suit you, consult your doctor or nutritionist.

As well as controlling your calorie intake, these planners are based on the following principles:

Aim to eat roughly 25 per cent of your total daily calories at breakfast, 30 per cent at lunch, 35 per cent at your evening meal, and 10 per cent in snacks (one mid-morning, and one mid-afternoon).

Ensure you have at least one serving of vegetables or fruit at each of your main meals.

To provide enough calcium to keep your bones healthy, aim to have at least 2 servings of dairy a day (1 serving = 200ml milk, 30g cheese, or a pot of low-fat yogurt).

Aim to eat fish at least twice a week, one portion of which should be oily fish, such as mackerel.

1400 CALORIES A DAY

	BREAKFAST	MID-MORNING SNACK	LUNCH	MID-AFTERNOON SNACK	EVENING MEAL
DAY PLAN 1	40g bran flakes or other wholegrain/fibre rich cereal • 15g raisins • 1 tsp sunflower seeds • 150ml semi-skimmed milk	orange	Grilled halloumi and roast tomato salad p.150 • 60g wholemeal roll • 1 kiwi fruit	200ml semi-skimmed milk	Mushroom and coriander rice p.169 • 125g grilled cod • slice of melon
DAY PLAN 2	40g bran flakes or other wholegrain/fibre-rich cereal • 1 small banana • 150ml semi-skimmed milk	apple	Falafel p.101 • mixed green salad with fat-free dressing • pot of low-fat yogurt • pear	reduced-fat wholegrain biscuit	Butternut squash and courgette pasta p.162 • Sugar-free peach sorbet p.320 • 50g blueberries
DAY PLAN 3	2 Apple and oat pancakes p.58 • 3 tbsp low-fat yogurt • fruit	1 rye cracker spread with 20g low-fat soft cheese	Carrot and ginger soup p.75 • 60g wholemeal roll • small banana	200ml semi-skimmed milk	Tuna with black-eyed bean and avocado salsa p.204 • Sugar-free peach sorbet p.320
DAY PLAN 4	1 boiled egg • 2 small slices of wholemeal toast thinly spread with margarine	orange	Mulligatawny p.91 • pot of low-fat yogurt	2 rye crackers topped with salsa	Lamb with aubergine purée p.258 • sugar snap peas • 200g new potatoes • fruit salad
DAY PLAN 5	1 slice of Fruit and seed soda bread p.340 topped with mashed banana	pear	Yellow split peas with peppers and pea shoots p.96 • fruit salad	1 rye cracker with 30g low-fat soft cheese	Butternut squash and spinach curry p.184 • 150g cooked brown rice • 2 tbsp plain low-fat natural yogurt • 80g raspberries
DAY PLAN 6	1 slice Seven-grain bread p.336 with thin scrape of margarine and low-sugar jam	200ml semi-skimmed milk	Mushroom, leek, and red pepper filo pie p.181 • green salad with fat-free dressing • pot of low-fat yogurt • 2 plums	40g dried apricots	Spaghetti with tomatoes and goat's cheese p.161 • slice of fresh pineapple
DAY PLAN 7	Rainbow muesli p.56 • 200ml semi-skimmed milk	apple	Shredded pork and spring onion wrap p.98 • large orange	reduced-fat digestive biscuit	Vegetable curry p.177 • 1 Chapatti p.338 • pot of low-fat yogurt • peach

Suitable for some women as part of a weight-loss plan. Mix and match the daily menus for a balanced diet.

	BREAKFAST	MID-MORNING SNACK	LUNCH	MID-AFTERNOON SNACK	EVENING MEAL
DAY PLAN 8	1 slice of Fruit and seed soda bread *p.340* topped with mashed banana	200ml semi-skimmed milk	Aduki bean and vegetable soup *p.82* • 2 small plums	2 sticks celery filled with 50g low-fat soft cheese	Mushroom and chilli pilaf *p.170* • 125g roast chicken • fruit salad
DAY PLAN 9	40g bran flakes or other wholegrain/fibre-rich cereal • 15g raisins • 1 tsp sunflower seeds • 150ml semi-skimmed milk	orange	Tortilla *p.114* • mixed salad with fat-free dressing • 1 small mango	1 rye cracker spread with low-fat soft cheese	Spicy udon noodles with tuna *p.120* • Roasted figs with citrus crème fraîche *p.330*
DAY PLAN 10	1 slice Seven-grain bread *p.336* thinly spread with margarine and low-sugar jam	apple	Quinoa tabbouleh *p.127* • pot of low-fat yogurt • 50g blueberries	200ml semi-skimmed milk	Mushroom lasagne *p.164* • mixed salad with fat-free dressing • Lemon cheesecake *p.331* • fresh raspberries
DAY PLAN 11	Rainbow muesli *p.56* • 200ml semi-skimmed milk	40g dried apricots	Oven baked red pepper and tomato frittata *p.113* • mixed salad with fat-free dressing • apple	1 reduced-fat wholegrain biscuit	Pasta with green beans and artichokes *p.163* • pot of low-fat yogurt • peach
DAY PLAN 12	1 poached egg • 2 small slices of wholemeal toast thinly spread with margarine	200ml semi-skimmed milk	Sweet potatoes with a smoky tomato filling *p.107* • pot of low-fat yogurt • 80g strawberries	2 sticks celery filled with 50g low-fat soft cheese	Butternut squash and courgette pasta *p.162* • Sugar-free peach sorbet *p.320* • 50g blueberries
DAY PLAN 13	150g 0% fat Greek yogurt • 40g oatmeal • 50g blueberries, calorie-free sweetener to taste	40g dried apricots	Red lentil dahl with cherry tomatoes *p.197* • Chapatti *p.338* • 2 tbsp riata • orange	1 reduced-fat wholegrain biscuit	Spaghetti with courgettes and toasted almonds *p.155* • Summer pudding *p.314* • 3 tbsp low-fat yogurt
DAY PLAN 14	2 Apple and oat pancakes *p.58* • 3 tbsp low-fat yogurt • fruit	small banana	Curried parsnip soup *p.86* • pot of low-fat yogurt	2 sticks celery filled with 50g low-fat soft cheese	Slow roast pork and lentils *p.261* • Cranberry and pomegranate jelly *p.324*

1600 CALORIES A DAY

	BREAKFAST	MID-MORNING SNACK	LUNCH	MID-AFTERNOON SNACK	EVENING MEAL
DAY PLAN 1	small glass (150ml) unsweetened fruit juice • 2 Apple and oat pancakes p.58 • 1 tbsp low-fat yogurt • fruit	orange	Hot and sour noodle salad with tofu p.118 • slice of melon	200ml semi-skimmed milk	Quick turkey cassoulet p.290 • sugar snap peas • 80g fresh raspberries • 3 tbsp 2% fat Greek yogurt
DAY PLAN 2	small glass (150ml) unsweetened fruit juice • Rainbow muesli p.56 • 200ml semi-skimmed milk	40g dried apricots	Pan fried prawns with lemongrass and ginger p.116 • salad with fat-free dressing • 60g wholemeal roll • pot of low-fat yogurt	1 slice Low-fat ginger tea bread p.339	Beef and bean stew p.249 • 150g new potatoes • Cranberry and pomegranate jelly p.324
DAY PLAN 3	small glass (150ml) unsweetened fruit juice • 2 eggs, scrambled • 1 small slice of wholemeal toast	reduced-fat wholegrain biscuit	Chicken salad with fruit and nuts p.145 • 1 slice (35g) of wholemeal bread thinly spread with margarine • slice of melon	200ml semi-skimmed milk	Pork stir-fry with cashew nuts and greens p.265 • 70g (raw weight) egg noodles • Sugar-free peach sorbet p.320 • 50g raspberries
DAY PLAN 4	small glass (150ml) unsweetened fruit juice • 1 slice Seven-grain bread p.336 thinly spread with margarine and low-sugar jam or marmalade	small pot of low-fat yogurt	Roast root vegetables with romesco sauce p.192 • Cranberry and pomegranate jelly p.324 • satsuma	2 sticks celery filled with 50g low-fat soft cheese	Roast lamb with flageolets p.254 • broccoli • Mango, orange, and passion fruit fool p.319
DAY PLAN 5	small glass (150ml) unsweetened fruit juice •1 slice of Fruit and seed soda bread p.338 topped with mashed banana	200ml semi-skimmed milk	Chickpea, bulgur, and walnut salad p.132 • banana	200ml semi-skimmed milk	Spanish eggs p.97 • 60g wholemeal bread • pot of low-fat yogurt
DAY PLAN 6	small glass (150ml) unsweetened fruit juice • 2 eggs, scrambled • 1 small slice of wholemeal toast	apple	Moroccan chicken and chickpea soup p.89 • pot of low-fat yogurt	200ml semi-skimmed milk	Salmon en papillote p.212 • broccoli • 200g new potatoes • Cranberry and pomegranate jelly p.324
DAY PLAN 7	small glass (150ml) unsweetened fruit juice • 1 slice Seven-grain bread p.336 thinly spread with margarine and low-sugar jam or marmalade	pot of low-fat yogurt	Tabbouleh p.126 • 150g roast chicken (skin removed) • pear	1 Oatcake p.66 with 25g low-fat soft cheese	Pasta puttanesca p.157 • Mango, orange, and passion fruit fool p.319

Suitable for some women as part of a weight-loss or weight-maintaining plan. Mix and match the daily menus for a balanced diet.

	BREAKFAST	MID-MORNING SNACK	LUNCH	MID-AFTERNOON SNACK	EVENING MEAL
DAY PLAN 8	small glass (150ml) unsweetened fruit juice • 40g bran flakes or other wholegrain/fibre-rich cereal • 1 banana • 150ml semi-skimmed milk	40g dried apricots	Three-grain salad p.130 • pear	200ml semi-skimmed milk	Cajun chicken with sweetcorn salsa p.283 • 200g new potatoes • Cranberry and pomegranate jelly p.324
DAY PLAN 9	small glass (150ml) unsweetened fruit juice • 1 slice of Fruit and seed soda bread p.340 topped with mashed banana	reduced-fat wholegrain biscuit	Mexican scrambled eggs p.62 • 1 slice (35g) wholemeal toast, thinly spread with polyunsaturated margarine • 2 satsumas	200ml semi-skimmed milk	Tuna kebabs with salsa verde p.217 • 200g new potatoes • peach
DAY PLAN 10	small glass (150ml) unsweetened fruit juice • Rainbow muesli p.56 • 200ml semi-skimmed milk	40g dried apricots	Chicken liver paté p.71 • 2 slices wholemeal toast • pot of low-fat yogurt • 80g strawberries	2 rye crackers with 40g low-fat soft cheese	Brown rice, red pepper, and artichoke risotto p.167 • salad with fat-free dressing • fresh fruit salad • 4 tbsp 2% fat Greek yogurt
DAY PLAN 11	small glass (150ml) unsweetened fruit juice • 150g 0% fat Greek yogurt • 40g oatmeal • 50g blueberries (calorie-free sweetener to taste)	banana	Pea soup p.76 • 2 Oatcakes p.66 • 50g low-fat cream cheese • pear	pot of low-fat yogurt	Roasted snapper with new potatoes and fennel p.215 • Poached pears with toasted almonds p.317
DAY PLAN 12	small glass (150ml) unsweetened fruit juice • 2 small slices of wholemeal toast topped with 20g crunchy peanut butter and 1 small banana, sliced	200ml semi-skimmed milk	Courgette, feta, bean, and pea salad p.136 • Cranberry and pomegranate jelly p.324 • peach	2 rye crackers 40g low-fat soft cheese	Roasted pork chops with mustard rub p.267 • 200g new potatoes • pot of low-fat yogurt • 100g raspberries
DAY PLAN 13	small glass (150ml) unsweetened fruit juice • 1 boiled egg • 2 slices (70g) of wholemeal toast thinly spread with margarine	banana	Farfalle with fresh tomatoes and avocado p.123 • Cranberry and pomegranate jelly p.324	2 rye crackers topped with 50g low-fat soft cheese	Chicken livers with kale and balsamic vinegar p.274 • 200g new potatoes • pot of low-fat yogurt
DAY PLAN 14	small glass (150ml) unsweetened fruit juice • 2 Apple and oat pancakes p.58 • 3 tbsp low-fat yogurt • fruit	low-fat/low-sugar cereal bar	Crab and avocado salad with vinaigrette p.144 • 1 slice wholemeal bread with thin scrape of margarine • satsuma	200ml semi-skimmed milk	Linguine with spiced aubergine p.158 • mixed salad with fat-free dressing • slice of pineapple

1800 CALORIES A DAY

	BREAKFAST	MID-MORNING SNACK	LUNCH	MID-AFTERNOON SNACK	EVENING MEAL
DAY PLAN 1	small glass (150ml) fruit juice • 2 slices wholemeal toast thinly spread with margarine • reduced-sugar jam or marmalade	pot of low-fat yogurt	Curried parsnip soup p.86 • 60g wholemeal roll • satsuma	banana	Roast pork chops with mustard rub p.267 • 200g boiled new potatoes • Apple and walnut strudel p.326
DAY PLAN 2	small glass (150ml) fruit juice • 1 egg poached • 2 slices wholemeal bread thinly spread with margarine	200ml semi-skimmed milk	Roasted butternut squash soup p.80 • 1 slice of Seven-grain bread p.336 thinly spread with margarine • apple	1 Oatcake p.66 with 30g Red pepper hummus p.68	Quick turkey cassoulet p.290 • 200g boiled new potatoes • Lemon cheesecake p.331
DAY PLAN 3	small glass (150ml) fruit juice • 2 eggs, scrambled • 1 slice wholemeal toast	200ml semi-skimmed milk	Oven baked red pepper and tomato frittata p.113 • green salad with 1 tbsp dressing • pot of low-fat fruit yogurt	1 slice Low-fat ginger tea bread p.339	Ragout of venison with wild mushrooms p.259 • medium jacket potato (200g) • sugar snap peas • Summer pudding p.314 • 3 tbsp fat-free Greek yogurt
DAY PLAN 4	small glass (150ml) fruit juice • 2 slices wholemeal toast topped with mashed banana	200ml semi-skimmed milk	Hot and sour noodle salad with tofu p.118 • pot of low-fat fruit yogurt • 50g raspberries	2 rye crackers with Red pepper hummus p.68	Salmon and sweet potato pie p.220 • cabbage • Lemon cheesecake p.331
DAY PLAN 5	small glass (150ml) fruit juice • Rainbow muesli p.56 • 200ml semi-skimmed milk	banana	Sweet potatoes with a smoky tomato filling p.107 • 125g skinless roast chicken • peach	2 rye crackers • Smoked aubergine dip p.72	Cajun chicken with sweetcorn salsa p.283 • 200g boiled new potatoes • fruit salad
DAY PLAN 6	small glass (150ml) fruit juice • 40g wholegrain cereal • 200ml semi-skimmed milk • 2 tbsp raisins	1 slice Low-fat ginger tea bread p.339	Spiced bulgur wheat with feta and a fruity salsa p.128 • pot of low-fat fruit yogurt	1 Oatcake p.66 with Smoked aubergine dip p.72	Beef and bean stew p.249 • 200g boiled new potatoes • carrots • fruit salad
DAY PLAN 7	small glass (150ml) fruit juice • 40g wholegrain cereal • 200ml semi-skimmed milk • banana	1 slice Low-fat ginger tea bread p.339	Falafel p.101 • mixed green salad with 1 tbsp dressing • pot of low-fat fruit yogurt	2 rye crackers with tomato salsa	Chicken, onion, and peas p.278 • Mango, orange, and passion fruit fool p.319

Suitable for some women as part of a weight-loss or weight-maintaining plan and some men as part of a weight-loss plan. Mix and match the daily menus for a balanced diet.

	BREAKFAST	MID-MORNING SNACK	LUNCH	MID-AFTERNOON SNACK	EVENING MEAL
DAY PLAN 8	small glass (150ml) fruit juice • 2 slices wholemeal toast topped with mashed banana	low-fat fruit yogurt	Aduki bean and vegetable soup p.82 • small (60g) wholemeal roll • apple	2 rye crackers topped with 30g low-fat soft cheese	Slow roast pork and lentils p.261 • French beans • Summer pudding p.314 • 3 tbsp 0% fat Greek yogurt
DAY PLAN 9	small glass (150ml) fruit juice • 2 eggs, scrambled • 1 slice wholemeal toast	low-fat fruit yogurt	Tabbouleh p.126 • 150g roast chicken • fresh fruit salad	200ml semi-skimmed milk	Pasta with clams p.237 • Banana cinnamon and pistachio parcels p.327 • 3 tbsp 0% fat Greek yogurt
DAY PLAN 10	small glass (150ml) fruit juice • Rainbow muesli p.56 • 200ml semi-skimmed milk	1 slice Low-fat ginger tea bread p.339	Squash salad with avocado p.140 • 2 rye crackers with 50g low-fat soft cheese • apple	low-fat fruit yogurt	Linguine with spiced aubergine p.158 • Lemon cheesecake p.331
DAY PLAN 11	small glass (150ml) fruit juice • 2 slices wholemeal toast thinly spread with margarine and reduced-sugar jam or marmalade	banana	Tomato and bean soup p.81 • 1 slice of Rye bread p.337 spread with 25g low-fat soft cheese • pear	low-fat fruit yogurt	Pork mince with mushrooms and pasta p.269 • Poached pears with toasted almonds p.317
DAY PLAN 12	small glass (150ml) fruit juice • 2 eggs, scrambled • 1 slice wholemeal toast	200ml semi-skimmed milk	Chickpea, bulgur, and walnut salad p.132 • 100g roast chicken • apple	1 slice Low-fat ginger tea bread p.339	Wild rice, courgette, fennel, and prawn pan-fry p.230 • Chocolate and orange parfait p.329
DAY PLAN 13	small glass (150ml) fruit juice • 1 egg, poached • 2 slices wholemeal bread thinly spread with margarine	200ml semi-skimmed milk	Three-grain salad p.130 • 100g cooked peeled prawns • orange	low-fat fruit yogurt	Pork stir-fry with cashew nuts and greens p.265 • 150g boiled brown rice • Mango, orange, and passion fruit fool p.319
DAY PLAN 14	small glass (150ml) fruit juice • 2 slices wholemeal toast topped with mashed banana	200ml semi-skimmed milk	Mixed bean and goat's cheese salad p.135 • slice of Rye bread p.337 thinly spread with margarine • plum	2 rye crackers with Smoked aubergine dip p.72	Spicy mackerel and beetroot roast p.208 • 100g boiled brown rice • pot of low-fat fruit yogurt with 80g strawberries

2000 CALORIES A DAY

	BREAKFAST	MID-MORNING SNACK	LUNCH	MID-AFTERNOON SNACK	EVENING MEAL
DAY PLAN 1	small glass (150ml) fruit juice • Banana and pecan porridge p.60	200ml semi-skimmed milk	Shredded pork and spring onion wrap p.98 • fruit salad • pot of low-fat fruit yogurt	1 slice Low-fat ginger tea bread p.339	Haddock and spinach gratin p.225 • 250g boiled new potatoes • sugar snap peas • Lemon cheesecake p.331
DAY PLAN 2	small glass (150ml) fruit juice • Rainbow muesli p.56 • 200ml semi-skimmed milk • 1 slice wholemeal toast thinly spread with margarine and reduced-sugar jam or marmalade	200ml semi-skimmed milk	Moroccan chicken and chickpea soup p.89 • banana • pot of low-fat fruit yogurt	banana	Bulgur wheat with lamb and chickpeas p.252 • French beans • Poached pears with toasted almonds p.317
DAY PLAN 3	small glass (150ml) fruit juice • Parsi eggs p.61 • 1 slice wholemeal toast thinly spread with margarine	banana	Pan-fried prawns with ginger and lemongrass p.116 • wholemeal pitta • tomato salad • pot of low-fat fruit yogurt	2 sticks celery spread with 30g low-fat soft cheese	Griddled steak chunks with herby rice p.242 • Dark chocolate and yogurt ice cream p.322
DAY PLAN 4	small glass (150ml) fruit juice • 2 Apple and oat pancakes p.58 • mixed berries • 150ml 2% fat Greek yogurt	2 Oatcakes p.66 • 30g low-fat soft cheese	Pea soup p.76 • small (60g) wholemeal roll • mixed green salad • 100g roast chicken • 1 tbsp reduced-fat mayo	1 slice Low-fat ginger tea bread p.339	Pork tenderloin stuffed with chillies and tomatoes p.262 • Dark chocolate and yogurt ice cream p.322 • 80g fresh raspberries
DAY PLAN 5	small glass (150ml) fruit juice • Mexican scrambled eggs p.62 • 1 slice wholemeal toast thinly spread with margarine	1 slice Low-fat ginger tea bread p.339	Mixed roast vegetable and mushroom soup p.77 • 1 slice Seven-grain bread p.336 thinly spread with margarine	200ml semi-skimmed milk	Butternut squash and courgette pasta p.162 • mixed green salad • 1 tbsp vinaigrette • Mango, orange, and passion fruit fool p.319
DAY PLAN 6	small glass (150ml) fruit juice • 40g wholegrain cereal • 200ml skimmed milk • sliced banana and blueberries	200ml semi-skimmed milk	Chorizo, chickpea, and mango salad p.147 • pear	1 Oatcake p.66 with low-fat soft cheese	Salmon and sweet potato pie p.220 • French beans • Banana, cinnamon and pistachio parcels p.327
DAY PLAN 7	Breakfast smoothie p.63 • 2 slices wholemeal toast thinly spread with margarine and reduced-sugar jam or marmalade	banana	Red lentil dahl with cherry tomatoes p.197 • 2 Chapattis p.338 • 3 tbsp riata • peach	200ml semi-skimmed milk	Pasta with green beans and artichokes p.163 • Chocolate and orange parfait p.329

Suitable for some women as part of a weight-maintaining plan and for some men as part of a weight-loss plan. Mix and match the daily menus for a balanced diet.

	BREAKFAST	MID-MORNING SNACK	LUNCH	MID-AFTERNOON SNACK	EVENING MEAL
DAY PLAN 8	small glass (150ml) fruit juice • 2 Muesli pancakes with summer berry compote p.57 • 150ml 2% fat Greek yogurt	1 slice Low-fat ginger tea bread p.339	Lentil salad with lemon and almonds p.138 • 100g roast chicken • plum	200ml semi-skimmed milk	Cinnamon and ginger beef with noodles p.247 • Chocolate espresso pots p.321
DAY PLAN 9	small glass (150ml) fruit juice • Banana and pecan porridge p.60	1 slice Low-fat ginger tea bread p.339	Carrot and ginger soup p.75 • 2 Oatcakes p.66 with 3 tbsp Red pepper hummus p.68 • pot of low-fat yogurt	2 rye crackers with Red pepper hummus p.68	Tuna with black-eyed bean and avocado salsa p.204 • 250g boiled new potatoes • Sugar-free peach sorbet p.320 • fresh raspberries
DAY PLAN 10	small glass (150ml) fruit juice • Banana and pecan porridge p.60	pot of low-fat fruit yogurt	Courgette, feta, bean, and pea salad p.136 • 1 wholemeal pitta • Cranberry and pomegranate jelly p.324	1 slice Fruit and seed soda bread p.340	Vegetarian cottage pie p.165 • Summer pudding p.314
DAY PLAN 11	small glass (150ml) fruit juice • 2 Apple and oat pancakes p.58 • mixed berries • 150ml 2% fat Greek yogurt	1 slice Low-fat ginger tea bread p.339	White bean soup p.79 • 1 wholemeal roll • fruit salad	40g ready-to-eat dried apricots	Pea and lemon risotto p.168 • Poached pears with toasted almonds p.317
DAY PLAN 12	small glass (150ml) fruit juice • Parsi eggs p.61 • 1 slice wholemeal toast thinly spread with margarine	200ml semi-skimmed milk	Butternut squash, tomato, and pearl barley salad p.141 • pot of low-fat fruit yogurt • kiwi fruit	banana	Poached chicken with star anise, soy, and brown rice p.275 • Apricot crumble p.325
DAY PLAN 13	small glass (150ml) fruit juice • Mexican scrambled eggs p.62 • 1 slice wholemeal toast thinly spread with margarine	200ml semi-skimmed milk	Moroccan tomatoes, peppers, and herbs p.133 • 1 slice Seven-grain bread p.336 thinly spread with margarine • banana • pot of low-fat fruit yogurt	1 slice Low-fat ginger tea bread p.339	Kedgeree p.228 • Sugar-free peach sorbet p.320 • fresh blueberries
DAY PLAN 14	Breakfast smoothie p.63 • 2 slices wholemeal toast thinly spread with margarine and reduced-sugar jam or marmalade	200ml semi-skimmed milk	Spiced bulgur wheat with feta and a fruity salsa p.128 • pot of low-fat fruit yogurt	banana	Chicken jalfrezi p.289 • steamed spinach • 2 chapatti • riata • Mango, orange, and passion fruit fool p.319

2500 CALORIES A DAY

	BREAKFAST	MID-MORNING SNACK	LUNCH	MID-AFTERNOON SNACK	EVENING MEAL
DAY PLAN 1	small glass (150ml) fruit juice • Parsi eggs p.61 • 2 slices wholemeal toast thinly spread with margarine	200ml semi-skimmed milk • plain reduced-fat biscuit	Mixed bean and goat's cheese salad p.135 • slice of Rye bead p.337 thinly spread with margarine • pot of low-fat yogurt	large banana	Linguine with spiced aubergine p.158 • mixed green salad with 1 tbsp dressing • Chocolate espresso pots p.321
DAY PLAN 2	small glass (150ml) fruit juice • 2 slices Fruit and seed soda bread p.340 topped with mashed banana • pot of low-fat fruit yogurt	large banana	Chicken broth with herby dumplings p.87 • pot of low-fat fruit yogurt	low-fat cereal bar	Spaghetti with tomatoes and goat's cheese p.161 • salad with 1 tbsp dressing • Apple and walnut strudel p.326
DAY PLAN 3	small glass (150ml) fruit juice • Banana and pecan porridge p.60 • 1 slice wholemeal bead thinly spread with margarine and reduced-sugar jam or marmalade	pot of low-fat yogurt	Cinnamon and ginger beef with noodles p.247 • pot of low-fat yogurt • banana	1 slice Fruit and seed soda bread p.340 thinly spread with margarine	Chicken jalfrezi p.289 • steamed spinach • 150g boiled brown basmati rice • small naan bread • riata • Mango, orange, and passion fruit fool p.319
DAY PLAN 4	Breakfast smoothie • 2 slices of wholemeal toast topped with mashed banana	200ml semi-skimmed milk • plain reduced-fat biscuit	Roasted snapper with new potatoes and fennel p.215 • banana with low-fat custard	1 slice Low-fat ginger tea bread p.339 • apple	Puy lentil and vegetable pot p.195 • Chocolate espresso pots p.321 • summer berries
DAY PLAN 5	small glass (150ml) fruit juice • Rainbow muesli p.56 • 200ml semi-skimmed milk • banana	1 slice of wholemeal toast spread with 1 tsp peanut butter	Hot and sour (tom yam) soup p.92 • chicken salad sandwich • pot of low-fat fruit yogurt	200ml semi-skimmed milk • plain reduced-fat biscuit	Bulgur wheat with lamb and chickpeas p.252 • sugar snap peas • Chocolate and orange parfait p.329
DAY PLAN 6	small glass (150ml) fruit juice • Banana and pecan muffin p.343 • pot of low-fat fruit yogurt	1 slice Fruit and seed soda bread p.340 thinly spread with margarine	Carrot and ginger soup p.75 • tuna and sweetcorn sandwich • pot of low-fat yogurt	2 plain reduced-fat biscuits	Salmon burgers p.104 • 250g boiled new potatoes • French beans • Lemon cheesecake p.331
DAY PLAN 7	small glass (150ml) fruit juice • 40g wholegrain cereal • 200ml semi-skimmed milk • fresh blueberries • 1 slice wholemeal toast thinly spread with margarine and reduced sugar jam	200ml semi-skimmed milk • plain reduced-fat biscuit	Curried parsnip soup p.86 • Shredded pork and spring onion wrap p.98	2 rye crackers with Red pepper hummus p.68	Leek and tomato pilaf p.171 • mixed green salad with 1 tbsp dressing • Apple and walnut strudel p.326

Suitable for some men as part of a weight-maintaining plan. Mix and match the daily menus for a balanced diet.

	BREAKFAST	MID-MORNING SNACK	LUNCH	MID-AFTERNOON SNACK	EVENING MEAL
DAY PLAN 8	small glass (150ml) fruit juice • 40g wholegrain cereal • 200ml semi-skimmed milk • fresh blueberries • 1 slice wholemeal toast thinly spread with margarine and reduced-sugar jam	200ml semi-skimmed milk • plain reduced-fat biscuit	Salmon salad with raspberry dressing p.142	2 Oatcakes p.66 with Broad bean dip p.69	Pearl barley, spinach, and lamb pot p.257 • Chocolate and orange parfait p.329
DAY PLAN 9	small glass (150ml) fruit juice • Parsi eggs p.61 • 2 slices wholemeal toast thinly spread with margarine	low-fat cereal bar	Moroccan chicken and chickpea soup p.89 • large wholemeal roll thinly spread with margarine • mixed fruit salad	large banana	Vegetarian moussaka p.178 • large mixed green salad with 1 tbsp dressing • Banana, cinnamon, and pistachio parcels p.327
DAY PLAN 10	small glass (150ml) fruit juice • 2 slices Fruit and seed soda bread p.340 topped with mashed banana • pot of low-fat fruit yogurt	200ml semi-skimmed milk • plain reduced-fat biscuit	Mushroom lasagne p.164 • 250g boiled new potatoes • salad with 1 tbsp dressing • fruit salad	1 slice Low-fat ginger tea bread p.339	Spiced lemony lentils with roast potatoes p.200 • 150g salmon steak, grilled • fresh fruit salad
DAY PLAN 11	small glass (150ml) fruit juice • Banana and pecan porridge p.60 • 1 slice wholemeal bread thinly spread with margarine and reduced sugar-jam or marmalade	200ml semi-skimmed milk • plain reduced-fat biscuit	White bean soup p.79 • egg and cress sandwich • fruit salad	pot of low-fat yogurt • kiwi fruit	Brown rice, red pepper, and artichoke risotto p.167 • Chocolate and orange parfait p.329
DAY PLAN 12	small glass (150ml) fruit juice • Rainbow muesli p.56 • 200ml semi-skimmed milk • banana	low-sugar cereal bar	Mulligatawny p.91 • 2 Oatcakes p.66 with Chicken liver paté p.71 • fresh fruit salad	pot of low-fat fruit yogurt • small banana	Chicken tostada with avocado salsa p.103 • mixed green salad • Carpaccio of oranges with pistachio nuts p.316
DAY PLAN 13	Breakfast smoothie p.63 • 2 slices of wholemeal toast topped with mashed banana	40g ready-to-eat dried apricots • 4 Brazil nuts	Lentil salad with lemon and almonds p.138 • 150g roast chicken • pot of yogurt	low-sugar cereal bar	Spicy udon noodles with tuna p.120 • Apricot crumble p.325 • 4 tbsp 2% fat Greek yogurt
DAY PLAN 14	small glass (150ml) fruit juice • Blueberry and oat muffin p.345 • pot of low-fat fruit yogurt	200ml semi-skimmed milk • plain reduced-fat biscuit	Aduki bean and vegetable soup p.82 • 1 wholemeal pitta • 4 tbsp Red pepper hummus p.68 • pot of low-fat yogurt	pot of low-fat fruit yogurt • peach	Turkish-style stuffed peppers p.174 • 150g roast chicken • Sugar-free peach sorbet p.320 • summer berries

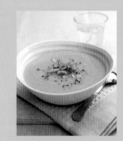 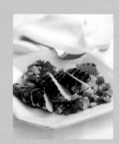 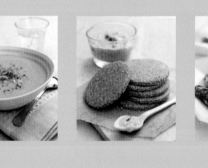 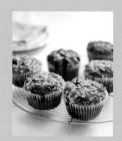 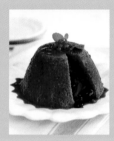

THE RECIPES

The delicious recipes in this book are designed to help you achieve a healthy, balanced diet that includes wholegrain, low-GI carbohydrates, lean protein, dietary fibre, low-fat dairy products, and plenty of vegetables and fruit. They are also lower in salt, fat and sugar. A great diet – whether you have Type 2 diabetes or not.

Where this book goes further is in providing a "Guidelines per serving" chart for each recipe, telling you at a glance whether the recipe is relatively high (3 dots), medium (2 dots), or low (1 dot) in GI, calories, saturated fat, and sugar – the four key dietary areas to watch when you have Type 2 diabetes. So, if you choose a recipe with a relatively high GI, calorie count, saturated fat content, or sugar content, choose dishes that are medium or low in those areas for the rest of the day.

Each recipe also has a "Statistics per serving" breakdown that gives precise details of the number of calories, the number of grams of carbohydrate, sugar, fibre, and fat (total and saturated) in the recipe. So if you really need to crunch the numbers, you can ensure that you are getting the exact balance you need. Many recipes specify only the main part of a meal, allowing you to tailor any accompaniments (such as potatoes or rice) to your own specific needs.

Now, all that's left to do is choose, compare, cook and enjoy!

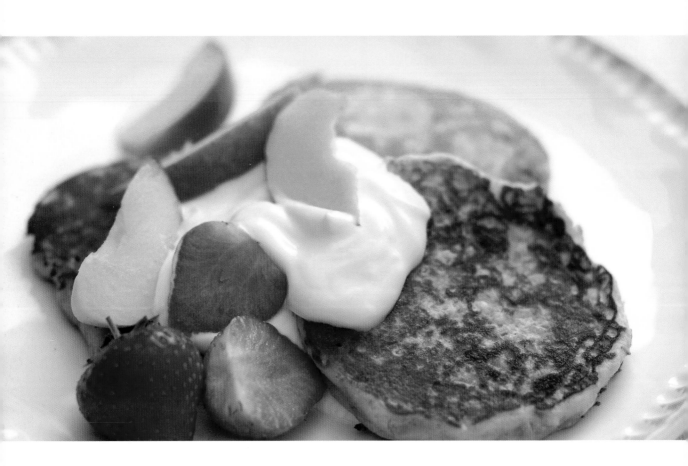

BETTER BREAKFASTS

⬤◯◯ GI

⬤◯◯ CALORIES

⬤◯◯ SATURATED FAT

⬤◯◯ SALT

RAINBOW MUESLI

MAKES 650g   **PREP** 10 MINS
(13 SERVINGS)

This is wonderfully satisfying muesli mix, which will sustain your energy levels throughout the morning. A great breakfast to have on standby in the storecupboard.

100g (3½oz) rye flakes
100g (3½oz) barley flakes
100g (3½oz) porridge oats
100g (3½oz) golden raisins
100g (3½oz) ready-to-eat dried
  apricots, roughly chopped

50g (1¾oz) hazelnuts,
  roughly chopped
50g (1¾oz) pumpkin seeds
50g (1¾oz) sunflower seeds

1 Mix together all the dry ingredients in a bowl and transfer to an airtight container until needed (there are 13 servings).

2 Serve with chilled semi-skimmed milk or a little plain reduced-fat yogurt. For a delicious treat, you could add some seasonal fresh fruit such as blueberries or raspberries.

STATISTICS PER SERVING:

Energy 187kcals/783kJ

Carbohydrate 10g

Sugar 8g

Fibre 3g

Fat 8g
Saturated fat 1g

Salt trace

MUESLI PANCAKES WITH SUMMER BERRY COMPOTE

GUIDELINES PER PANCAKE:

●●○ GI

●○○ CALORIES

●○○ SATURATED FAT

●●○ SALT

MAKES 12 PANCAKES   **PREP** 10 MINS   **COOK** 15-20 MINS
(SERVES 4-6)

The combination of wholegrain cereals, buttermilk, eggs, and fruit helps to provide a balanced and nutritious start to the day.

125g (4½oz) plain wholemeal flour
1 tsp baking powder
75g (2½oz) sugar-free muesli
1 tbsp caster sugar
2 large eggs, separated
284ml carton buttermilk

115g (4oz) fresh blueberries, roughly chopped
2 tbsp sunflower oil, for frying

For the summer berry compote
300g (10oz) mixed summer berries
juice and zest of 1 orange

1 Mix the flour and baking powder in a large bowl, and then stir in the muesli and sugar. Make a well in the centre and beat in the egg yolks and buttermilk to make a thick batter (it should have the consistency of thick cream).

2 Whisk the egg whites until stiff but not dry, and fold into the batter. Stir in the chopped blueberries.

3 Heat a griddle pan or large, heavy, nonstick frying pan over a moderate heat. Add a tiny drop of oil and then when the pan is hot, drop in a tablespoon of the batter and cook for 2–3 minutes, until bubbles start to break on the surface and the pancake is firm enough to flip. Flip it over and cook for 1–2 minutes more, until springy when prodded. Transfer to a warm oven while you cook the rest.

4 To make the compote, place the summer berries in a small saucepan, together with the orange juice and zest. Heat gently, stirring, until the berries are warmed through and have softened slightly. Arrange the pancakes on plates and serve with the compote.

STATISTICS PER PANCAKE:

Energy 117kcals/493kJ

Carbohydrate 14g

Sugar 6g

Fibre 2g

Fat 4g
Saturated fat 0.8g

Salt 0.2g

●●○ GI

●○○ CALORIES

●○○ SATURATED FAT

●●○ SALT

APPLE AND OAT PANCAKES

MAKES 12 PANCAKES   **PREP** 10 MINS   **COOK** 15 MINS
(SERVES 4–6)

These little pancakes are a perfect treat for the weekend. The oats used in the mixture provide soluble fibre and help to slow down the absorption of carbohydrate.

125g (4½oz) plain flour
1 tsp baking powder
75g (2½oz) porridge oats
2–3 tbsp caster sugar
pinch of ground cinnamon

2 eggs, separated
284ml carton buttermilk
2 medium apples
sunflower oil, for frying

1 Sift the flour into a large bowl and mix with the baking powder. Stir in the oats, sugar, and cinnamon. Make a well in the centre and beat in the egg yolks and buttermilk to make a thick batter (it should have the consistency of heavy cream).

2 Core the apples, coarsely grate the flesh, and stir into the batter mixture. Whisk the egg whites until stiff but not dry and fold into the batter.

3 Heat a griddle pan or large heavy-based non-stick frying pan over a moderate heat. Add a tiny drop of oil to the hot pan. When the pan is hot, drop a heaped dessertspoon of the batter into the pan and flatten slightly with the back of the spoon so that the pancakes are about 10cm (4in) in diameter and about 5mm (¼in) thick.

4 Cook for 2 minutes or until bubbles start to break on the surface and the pancakes are firm enough to flip. Flip and cook for 1–2 minutes more, until they feel springy when prodded. Transfer to a warm oven while you cook the rest, adding more oil as necessary. Try these with fresh summer fruits and low-fat Greek yogurt, or with your own favourite topping.

STATISTICS PER PANCAKE:

Energy 100kcals/418kJ

Carbohydrate 14g

Sugar 5.5g

Fibre 1.1g

Fat 2g

Saturated fat 0.5g

Salt 0.17g

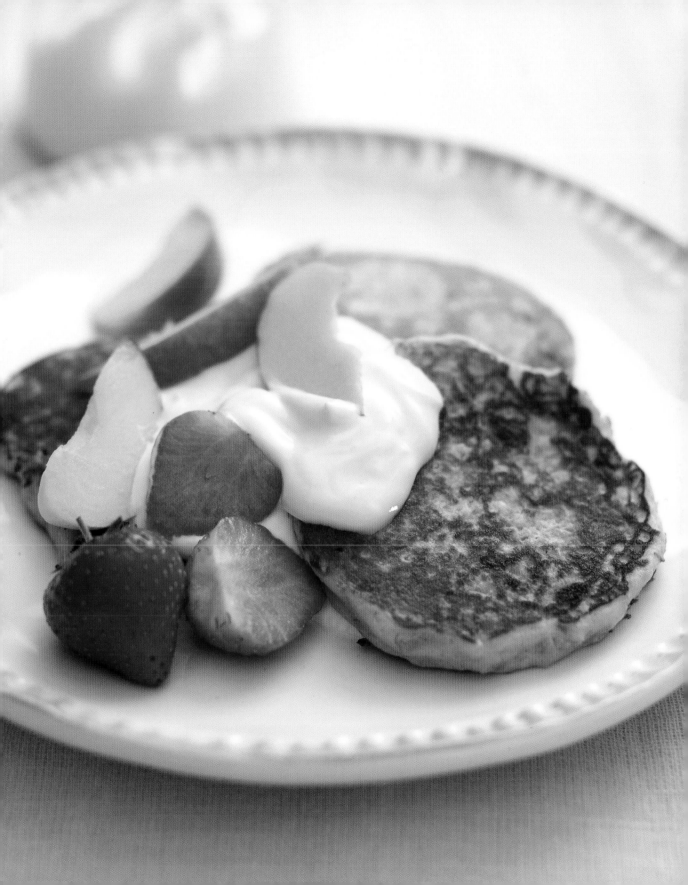

● ○ ○ GI

● ● ○ CALORIES

● ● ○ SATURATED FAT

● ○ ○ SALT

BANANA AND PECAN PORRIDGE

SERVES 2   **PREP** 5 MINS   **COOK** 5-10 MINS
PLUS SOAKING

Oats are rich in slow-release carbohydrates, which help to balance blood sugar levels and keep mid-morning hunger pangs at bay.

60g (2oz) porridge oats
300ml (10fl oz) semi-skimmed milk
generous pinch of ground cinnamon

2 small, very ripe bananas, mashed
15g (½oz) pecan nuts, roughly chopped
4 tbsp Greek yogurt

1 If you have time, soak the oats in the milk overnight. When ready to cook, place the oats, milk, and cinnamon in a nonstick pan.

2 Bring the porridge to the boil, reduce the heat, add the bananas and simmer for 4–5 minutes, stirring occasionally. You may need to add more milk to achieve the consistency you prefer.

3 Spoon the porridge into a bowls and top with the nuts and Greek yogurt. Serve immediately.

COOK'S TIP

If you soak the oats in milk overnight you may find you need more milk in the morning, as some of the liquid will be soaked up by the oats.

STATISTICS PER SERVING:

Energy 366kcals/1,536kJ

Carbohydrate 32g

Sugar 28g

Fibre 4g

Fat 8g

Saturated fat 5g

Salt 0.2g

PARSI EGGS

SERVES 4   **PREP** 10 MINS   **COOK** 30 MINS

This Indian dish has its origins in ancient Persia, and will provide a spicy start to the day – it's a whole new take on scrambled eggs.

GUIDELINES PER SERVING:

●○○ GI

●●○ CALORIES

●●● SATURATED FAT

●○○ SALT

60g (2oz) unsalted butter
4 spring onions, thinly sliced
1 tsp grated fresh root ginger
1 large red or green chilli, deseeded
   and finely chopped
2 tsp mild curry powder

4 tomatoes, deseeded and chopped
8 large eggs
2 tbsp milk
salt and freshly ground black pepper
2 tbsp chopped coriander

1 Melt 30g (1oz) of the butter in a large, nonstick frying pan. Fry the onions, ginger, and chilli over a low heat for 2 minutes, or until softened, stirring often.

2 Add the curry powder and tomatoes and cook for 1 minute. Remove the vegetable mixture from the pan and set aside.

3 Put the rest of the butter in the pan. Beat the eggs and milk, and season with salt and pepper. Pour into the pan, and stir until scrambled and almost set. Add the curried vegetables, stir well, and cook until just set. Scatter the chopped coriander over the top and serve at once.

STATISTICS PER SERVING:

Energy 344kcals/1,440kJ

Carbohydrate 5g

Sugar 4g

Fibre 1.7g

Fat 28g

Saturated fat 12g

Salt 0.5g

⬤◯◯ GI

⬤◯◯ CALORIES

⬤⬤◯ SATURATED FAT

⬤◯◯ SALT

MEXICAN SCRAMBLED EGGS

SERVES 2 **PREP** 5 MINS **COOK** 5 MINS

Eggs are a great source of protein, which helps you to feel full for longer, making this a good choice for breakfast or a light lunch.

2 tbsp vegetable oil
½ red pepper, deseeded and finely diced
4 spring onions, finely chopped
1 small green chilli, deseeded and finely chopped

4 eggs, beaten
salt and freshly ground black pepper
1 tbsp chopped fresh coriander, to serve

1 Heat the oil in a small, heavy frying pan and add the pepper, spring onion, and chilli. Fry for 2–3 minutes.

2 Pour in the eggs and season to taste. Stir, with a wooden spoon, for 1–2 minutes or until the eggs are scrambled to your liking. Sprinkle with the coriander to serve.

STATISTICS PER SERVING:

Energy 292kcals/1,214kJ

Carbohydrate 4g

Sugar 4g

Fibre 4g

Fat 24g

Saturated fat 5g

Salt 0.4g

BREAKFAST SMOOTHIE

GUIDELINES PER SERVING:

● ○ ○ GI

● ● ○ CALORIES

● ○ ○ SATURATED FAT

● ○ ○ SALT

SERVES 2   **PREP** 5 MINS

Smoothies are a great way to boost your intake of fruit, and this sustaining recipe will give you a shot of calcium as well as vitamins and minerals.

2 small, ripe bananas
500ml (16fl oz) semi-skimmed milk
3 tbsp oatmeal

100g (3½oz) fresh raspberries
150ml (7fl oz) fat-free Greek yogurt
½ tsp ground cinnamon

1 Cut the bananas into small chunks and place in a blender along with the remaining ingredients. Blend at high speed for 1–2 minutes or until smooth.

2 Pour into two glasses and drink immediately.

STATISTICS PER SERVING:

Energy 336kcals/1,420kJ

Carbohydrate 52g

Sugar 29g

Fibre 4g

Fat 6g

Saturated fat 3g

Salt 0.3g

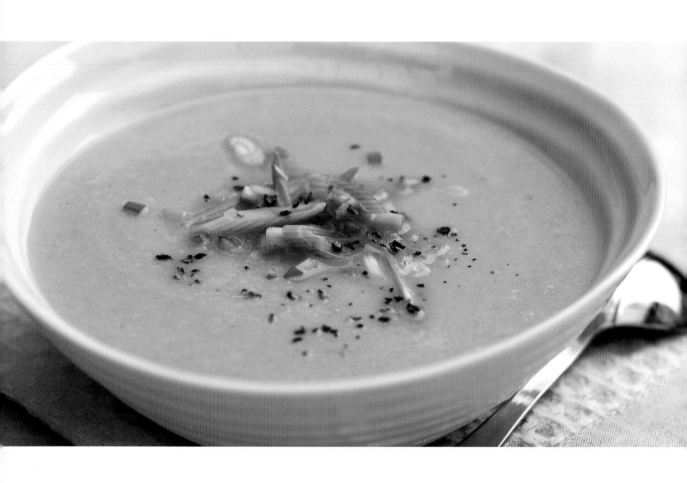

SNACKS AND SOUPS

● ◯ ◯ GI

● ◯ ◯ CALORIES

● ◯ ◯ SATURATED FAT

● ◯ ◯ SALT

SESAME OATCAKES

MAKES 9   **PREP** 5 MINS   **COOK** 10 MINS

These oatcakes make a tasty and low-GI alternative to crackers.

85g (3oz) fine oatmeal
4 tbsp wholemeal flour
1 tbsp sesame seeds

scant ½ tsp salt
pinch of bicarbonate of soda
1 tbsp sesame oil

1 Preheat the oven to 180°C (350°F/Gas 4).

2 Place the oatmeal, flour, sesame seeds, salt, and bicarbonate of soda in a large bowl. Stir in the oil and 75ml (2½fl oz) hot water to make a firm dough.

3 Roll the dough out on a lightly floured surface until about 2mm thick and cut into circles using a 7.5cm (3in) pastry cutter.

4 Bake for 8–10 minutes or until golden and crisp. Store in an airtight container. You could try these with Smoked Aubergine Dip (page 72).

STATISTICS PER OATCAKE:

Energy 72kcals/303kJ

Carbohydrate 11.5g

Sugar 0.1g

Fibre 1g

Fat 2g
Saturated fat 0.2g

Salt 0.2g

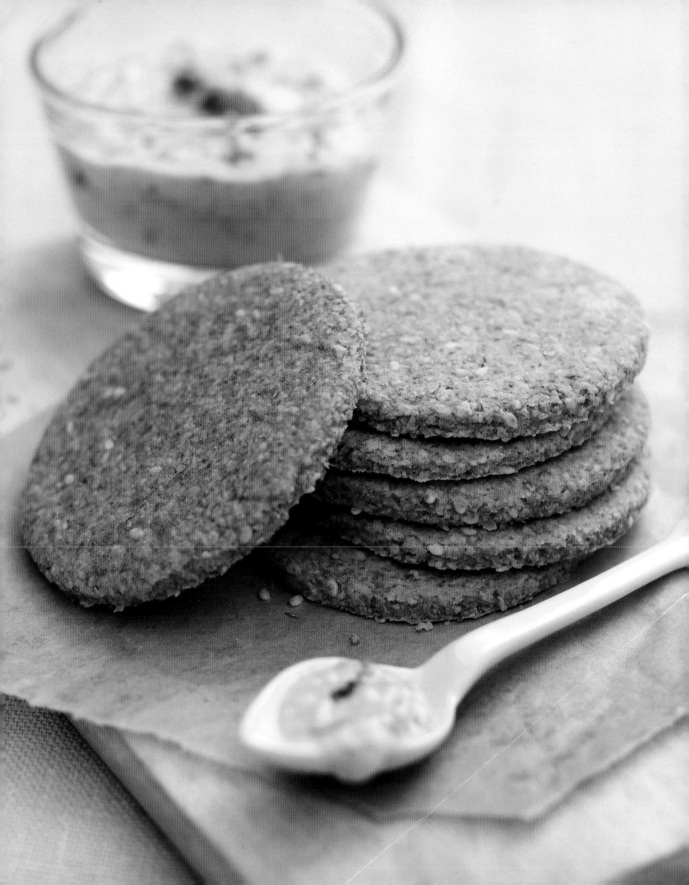

RED PEPPER HUMMUS

SERVES 4   **PREP** 5 MINS   **COOK** 5-10 MINS

Home-made hummus is quick and easy to make and this version contains considerably less fat than the shop-bought variety.

2 large red peppers, halved and
  deseeded
400g can chickpeas, drained
  and rinsed
2 tbsp lemon juice
¼ tsp smoked paprika

3 tbsp olive oil
2 cloves garlic
2 tbsp tahini
2 tbsp natural yogurt
salt and freshly ground black pepper

1 Preheat the grill to high. Place the halved peppers under the grill for 20–25 minutes or until the skin is black. Cover with a clean, wet cloth – or place in a plastic bag – and allow to cool. Peel away and discard the skins and blot the flesh dry with kitchen paper.

2 Place the chickpeas in a small saucepan, cover with water and bring to the boil. Reduce the heat and simmer for 5 minutes.

3 Drain the chickpeas well and place in a food processor or blender with 3 tablespoons of hot water and process for 1–2 minutes. Add the lemon juice, paprika, olive oil, garlic, tahini, and yogurt, season to taste, and process again until smooth. Transfer to a bowl and serve – vegetable crudités or toasted pitta are good accompaniments – or cover and chill until needed.

COOK'S TIP
This dip can be kept in the refrigerator, in a sealed container, for up to three days.

STATISTICS PER SERVING:

Energy 299kcals/951kJ

Carbohydrate 17g

Sugar 7g

Fibre 2g

Fat 13g

Saturated fat 2g

Salt 0.1g

BROAD BEAN PURÉE

SERVES 6   **PREP** 20 MINS   **COOK** 1¼ HOURS

Broad beans are at their best when the pods are picked while they are still young and tender. Try serving this purée with oatcakes, rye crackers, or toast.

250g (9oz) skinless dried broad beans, soaked overnight
3 onions
6 garlic cloves
bunch of coriander, chopped, plus extra to garnish
bunch of flat-leaf parsley, chopped, plus extra to garnish

2 tbsp chopped mint
1 tsp ground cumin
salt and freshly ground black pepper
1–3 tbsp olive oil
juice of 1 lemon

1 Drain the beans and place in a large pan. Pour in enough cold water to cover. Roughly chop 1 onion and 3 garlic cloves, add to the pan and then bring to the boil. Skim off any scum and lower the heat, then cover and simmer for 1 hour, or until the beans are soft.

2 Drain the beans, reserving the cooking liquid. Place the beans in a blender or food processor with the coriander, parsley, mint, and cumin. Add salt and pepper to taste and then blend to a smooth purée, adding enough of the reserved cooking liquid to ensure that the mixture is not too dry. Transfer to a serving dish and keep warm.

3 Slice the remaining onions. Heat 1 tablespoon of the oil in a frying pan, add the onions, and fry, stirring frequently, over a medium-high heat for 10–15 minutes or until they are dark golden and slightly caramelized. Chop the remaining garlic finely, add it to the pan and stir-fry for a further minute.

4 Spread the fried onions and garlic over the top of the purée and drizzle with the lemon juice and remaining oil.

STATISTICS PER SERVING:

Energy 92kcals/385kJ

Carbohydrate 7g

Sugar 0.2g

Fibre 3g

Fat 6g

Saturated fat 0.8g

Salt 0.2g

TAPENADE

SERVES 6   **PREP** 15 MINS

A full-flavoured Mediterranean spread made with capers and olives.

2 large garlic cloves
250g (9oz) Mediterranean black
  olives, pitted
1½ tbsp capers, drained and rinsed
4 anchovy fillets in olive oil, drained
1 tsp thyme leaves

1 tsp chopped rosemary
2 tbsp fresh lemon juice
2 tbsp extra virgin olive oil
1 tsp Dijon mustard
freshly ground black pepper

1 Place the garlic, olives, capers, anchovies, thyme, and rosemary in a food processor or blender, and process until smooth.

2 Add the lemon juice, olive oil, mustard, and black pepper to taste, and blend until a thick paste forms. Transfer to a bowl and chill until ready to use.

COOK'S TIP
Good with crudités and a spread of Mediterranean appetizers, such as olives and stuffed vine leaves.

STATISTICS PER SERVING:

Energy 97kcals/405kJ

Carbohydrate 0.5g

Sugar 0.1g

Fibre 1g

Fat 10g
Saturated fat 1.5g

Salt 1.5g

CHICKEN LIVER PÂTÉ

SERVES 4   **PREP** 10 MINS   **COOK** 15 MINS   **FREEZE** 3 MONTHS

The red wine adds flavour to this spread and cuts through the richness of the liver.

350g (12oz) chicken livers,
  thawed if frozen
50g (1¾oz) butter
¼ tsp dried thyme

150ml (5fl oz) red wine
10 chives, snipped
salt and freshly ground black pepper

1 Rinse the chicken livers and pat them dry with kitchen paper. Trim away any white sinew or greenish portions from the livers with small scissors, then cut each in half.

2 Melt the butter in a large frying pan over a medium heat until it foams. Add the livers and cook, stirring often, for 4 minutes, or until browned.

3 Add the thyme, wine, and chives to the pan. Bring to the boil then reduce the heat and cook, stirring occasionally for 4 minutes, or until the liquid is reduced and the livers are just cooked through.

4 Remove the pan from the heat and leave to cool for 10 minutes. Add salt and pepper to taste, then tip the livers and sauce into a blender, and blend until smooth. Adjust the seasoning if necessary. Spoon the pâté into a serving bowl, pressing it down with the back of the spoon so it is firmly packed. Leave to cool, then chill until needed.

COOK'S TIP
This is good with toasted slices of Seven-grain bread (see page 336).

STATISTICS PER SERVING:

Energy 199kcals/826kJ

Carbohydrate 0g

Sugar 0g

Fibre 0g

Fat 12g

Saturated fat 7g

Salt 0.4g

SMOKED AUBERGINE DIP

SERVES 4   **PREP** 5 MINS   **COOK** 1 HOUR

Grilled aubergines, with their delicious smoky flavour, are the basis for this tasty Middle Eastern dip.

2 aubergines, about 350g (12oz) each
3 tbsp olive oil, plus extra for greasing
3 garlic cloves, crushed
  or finely chopped
1 tbsp lemon juice

2 tsp ground cumin
1 tsp ground coriander
3 tbsp chopped fresh coriander
salt and freshly ground black pepper

1 Preheat the oven to 200°C (400°F/Gas 6). Prick the aubergines all over with a fork and place on a lightly greased baking sheet. Bake for 1 hour, or until the skin is wrinkled and the flesh is soft. Allow the aubergine to cool, then cut in half lengthways and scoop out the flesh with a spoon.

2 Place the aubergine flesh, garlic, lemon juice, cumin, ground coriander, and olive oil in a food processor or blender and blend until smooth. Stir in the coriander and season to taste. Chill until required.

STATISTICS PER SERVING:

Energy 86kcals/361kJ

Carbohydrate 2g

Sugar 1.5g

Fibre 2g

Fat 8g
Saturated fat 1g

Salt 0.1g

CHILLI AND ROSEMARY SPICED NUTS

SERVES 4   **PREP** 5 MINS   **COOK** 20 MINS

A tasty snack, great for serving at drinks parties as a healthier alternative to crisps.

2 tsp chilli powder
2 tbsp fresh rosemary,
  roughly chopped
2 tbsp olive oil
100g (3½oz) mixed whole nuts

1 Preheat the oven to 150°C (300°F/Gas 2). Mix the chilli, rosemary, and oil in a large bowl. Add the nuts and stir until well coated.

2 Place the spiced nuts in an ovenproof dish and transfer to the oven. Cook for 20 minutes, stirring occasionally. Allow to cool slightly and then transfer to kitchen paper to absorb excess oil. Store in an airtight container; the nuts will keep for up to one week.

GUIDELINES PER SERVING:

● ○ ○ GI
● ● ● CALORIES
● ○ ○ SATURATED FAT
● ○ ○ SALT

STATISTICS PER SERVING:

Energy 194kcals/804kJ

Carbohydrate 3g

Sugar 1g

Fibre 1.6g

Fat 18g
Saturated fat 3g

Salt 0.1g

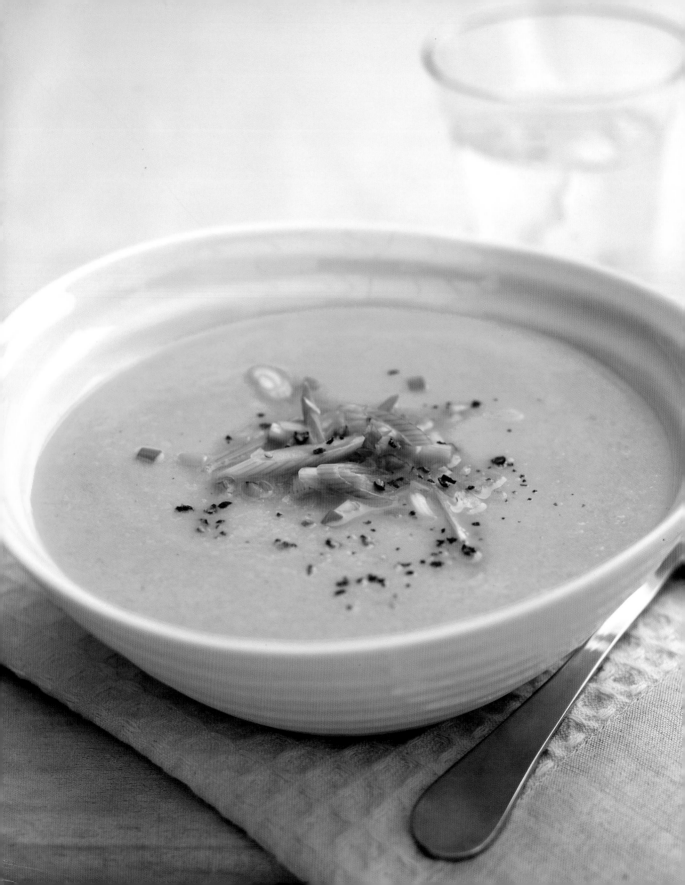

CARROT AND GINGER SOUP

SERVES 4   **PREP** 15 MINS   **COOK** 50 MINS   **FREEZE** 3 MONTHS

Unlike most vegetables, which are most nutritious when eaten raw, cooking carrots increases the availability of betacarotene, which the body can convert into vitamin A.

GUIDELINES PER SERVING:

●●○ GI

●○○ CALORIES

●○○ SATURATED FAT

●●○ SALT

2 tbsp olive oil
1 large onion, peeled and
   finely chopped
1 clove of garlic, peeled and crushed
5cm (2in) piece of fresh root ginger,
   peeled and finely chopped

600g (1lb 5oz) carrots, peeled
   and roughly chopped
750ml (1¼ pints) vegetable stock
zest and juice of 2 large oranges
salt and freshly ground black pepper
spring onions, chopped, to garnish

1 Heat the oil in large non-stick saucepan, add the onion and cook over a medium heat for 3–4 minutes. Add the garlic, ginger, and carrots and continue to cook for a further 5 minutes, stirring occasionally.

2 Add the stock, orange zest and juice, and season to taste with salt and black pepper. Bring to the boil, then reduce the heat, cover, and simmer for 40 minutes or until the carrots are soft.

3 Transfer the soup to a food processor or liquidiser and process until smooth, then return to the pan and reheat gently. If the soup is too thick, you can thin it out with a little extra stock or water. Ladle the soup into bowls, garnish with chopped spring onions, and serve.

STATISTICS PER SERVING:

Energy 200kcals/836kJ

Carbohydrate 25g

Sugar 21g

Fibre 5.5g

Fat 8g

Saturated fat 1.5g

Salt 1.2g

● ● ○ GI

● ○ ○ CALORIES

● ○ ○ SATURATED FAT

● ● ○ SALT

PEA SOUP

SERVES 4   **PREP** 10 MINS   **COOK** 25 MINS   **FREEZE** 3 MONTHS

You can use frozen peas to make this tasty and filling soup in a matter of minutes.

1 tbsp olive oil
1 large onion, finely chopped
2 garlic cloves, peeled and crushed
  or finely chopped
2 celery sticks, finely chopped

1 medium potato, peeled and diced
450g (1lb) frozen peas
1 litre (1¾ pints) vegetable or
  chicken stock
salt and freshly ground black pepper

1 Heat the oil in a large saucepan, add the onion and cook over a medium heat for 2–3 minutes, stirring. Add the garlic, celery, and potato and cook for 1 minute.

2 Add the peas, stock, and seasoning. Bring to the boil then reduce the heat, cover and simmer for 20 minutes.

3 Allow to cool slightly then transfer to a food processor or blender and purée until smooth. Return the soup to the pan, adjust the seasoning and heat until warm.

STATISTICS PER SERVING:

Energy 200kcals/840kJ

Carbohydrate 35g

Sugar 5g

Fibre 7g

Fat 6g

Saturated fat 1g

Salt 1.2g

MIXED ROAST VEGETABLE AND MUSHROOM SOUP

SERVES 4   **PREP** 15 MINS   **COOK** 35–40 MINS   **FREEZE** 3 MONTHS

The roasted vegetables add a wonderfully intense flavour to this dish.

2 red onions, peeled and roughly chopped
4 small courgettes, roughly chopped
2 tbsp olive oil
few stalks of rosemary
salt and freshly ground black pepper
3 medium potatoes, peeled and cubed
4 carrots, peeled and roughly chopped
2 garlic cloves, finely chopped

200g (7oz) chestnut mushrooms, half roughly chopped and half grated
25g (scant 1oz) dried porcini mushrooms, soaked in boiling water to rehydrate
1.2 litres (2 pints) mushroom stock or vegetable stock
handful of flat-leaf parsley, finely chopped

1 Preheat the oven to 200°C (400°F/Gas 6). Cook the potatoes and carrots in a large pan of boiling salted water for about 5 minutes, then drain well. Tip into a roasting tin with the onions and courgettes, add half the oil, and combine with your hands. Add the rosemary stalks, season with salt and pepper, and place in the oven for 15 minutes. Meanwhile, heat the remaining oil in a large saucepan, add the garlic and sweat for a few seconds over a low heat, then add both the chopped and grated chestnut mushrooms and cook for 5 minutes or until they begin to release their juices.

2 Using a slotted spoon, transfer the soaked porcini mushrooms to the pan along with the stock and a little salt and black pepper. Strain the soaking liquid from the mushrooms, to remove any grit, and pour into the pan. Bring to the boil, then reduce the heat and simmer for 5–10 minutes.

3 Tip the roasted vegetables into the pan and cook for a further 5 minutes or until everything is cooked through. Stir through the parsley to serve.

COOK'S TIP
If you prefer, you could blend some of the vegetables to a purée to thicken the soup, but be sure to keep some chunky vegetables and mushrooms for interest.

STATISTICS PER SERVING:

Energy 312kcals/1,311kJ

Carbohydrate 44g

Sugar 15g

Fibre 8g

Fat 9.5g

Saturated fat 2g

Salt 1.5g

● ○ ○ GI

● ○ ○ CALORIES

● ○ ○ SATURATED FAT

● ○ ○ SALT

GAZPACHO

SERVES 4   **PREP** 15 MINS   **FREEZE** 1 MONTH

This chilled, no-cook Spanish soup is always popular when temperatures are hot outside.

1kg (2¼lb) tomatoes
1 small cucumber, peeled and finely chopped, plus extra to serve
1 small red pepper, deseeded and chopped, plus extra to serve
2 garlic cloves, crushed

4 tbsp sherry vinegar
salt and freshly ground black pepper
120ml (4fl oz) extra virgin olive oil, plus extra to serve
1 hard-boiled egg, white and yolk separated and chopped, to serve

1 Bring a kettle of water to the boil. Place the tomatoes in a heatproof bowl, pour over enough boiling water to cover, and leave for 20 seconds, or until the skins split. Drain and cool under cold running water. Gently peel off the skins, cut the tomatoes in half, deseed, and chop the flesh.

2 Put the tomato flesh, cucumber, red pepper, garlic, and sherry vinegar in a food processor or blender. Season to taste with salt and pepper, and process until smooth. Pour in the olive oil and process again. Dilute with a little water if too thick. Transfer the soup to a serving bowl, cover with cling film and chill for at least 1 hour.

3 When ready to serve, finely chop the extra cucumber and red pepper. Place the cucumber, pepper and egg yolk and white in individual bowls and arrange on the table, along with olive oil for drizzling. Ladle the soup into bowls and serve, letting each diner add their own garnish.

COOK'S TIP
The soup can be prepared 2 days in advance, kept covered and chilled.

STATISTICS PER SERVING:

Energy 284kcals/1,176kJ

Carbohydrate 11g

Sugar 11g

Fibre 3.5g

Fat 25g

Saturated fat 4g

Salt 0.2g

WHITE BEAN SOUP

SERVES 4   **PREP** 30 MINS   **COOK** 2 HOURS   **FREEZE** 3 MONTHS
PLUS SOAKING

This thick soup from northern Italy is guaranteed to keep out the winter chills.

GUIDELINES PER SERVING:

● ○ ○ GI

● ● ○ CALORIES

● ● ○ SATURATED FAT

● ● ○ SALT

3 tbsp olive oil
2 onions, finely chopped
2 garlic cloves, crushed
225g (8oz) dried cannellini beans, soaked overnight
1 celery stick, chopped
1 bay leaf
3 or 4 parsley stalks, without leaves

1 tbsp lemon juice
1.2 litres (2 pints) vegetable stock
salt and freshly ground black pepper
3 shallots, thinly sliced
60g (2oz) pancetta, chopped
80g Fontina cheese or Taleggio cheese, chopped into small pieces

1 Heat 2 tbsp of the olive oil in a saucepan, add the onions, and fry over a low heat for 10 minutes, or until softened, stirring occasionally. Add the garlic and cook, stirring, for 1 minute.

2 Drain and rinse the soaked beans and add to the pan with the celery, bay leaf, parsley stalks, lemon juice, and stock. Bring to the boil, cover, and simmer for 1½ hours, or until the beans are soft, stirring occasionally.

3 Remove the bay leaf and liquidize the soup in batches in a blender, or through a hand mill. Rinse out the pan. Return the soup to the pan and season to taste with salt and pepper.

4 Heat the remaining olive oil in a small frying pan, and fry the shallots and pancetta, until golden and crisp, stirring frequently to stop them sticking to the pan.

5 Reheat the soup, adding a little stock or water if it is too thick. Stir the Fontina or Taleggio into the soup. Ladle into individual bowls, and sprinkle each serving with the shallots and pancetta.

STATISTICS PER SERVING:

Energy 383kcals/1,604kJ

Carbohydrate 34g

Sugar 8g

Fibre 12g

Fat 19g

Saturated fat 6g

Salt 1.1g

ROASTED BUTTERNUT SQUASH SOUP

SERVES 4   **PREP** 15 MINS   **COOK** 50 MINS–1 HOUR

Roasting the squash helps to intensify the flavour and gives this soup a wonderfully sweet flavour.

1 medium butternut squash, peeled and diced (about 800g/1¾lb prepared weight)

2 medium red onions, peeled and thickly sliced

4 garlic cloves, unpeeled

4 tbsp olive oil

pinch of dried chilli flakes

1 litres (1¾ pints) vegetable stock

salt and freshly ground black pepper

1 Preheat the oven to 200°C (400°F/Gas 6). Place the squash, onions, and garlic in a large roasting tin. Drizzle over the oil and stir to ensure the vegetables are well coated. Sprinkle over the chilli flakes, then place in the oven for 45–50 minutes or until the squash is soft.

2 Gently squeeze the garlic cloves from their skins and transfer to a liquidizer or blender along with the other roasted vegetables. Add the stock and process until smooth.

3 Transfer the soup to a large saucepan and gently heat through. Season to taste and serve.

STATISTICS PER SERVING:

Energy 239kcals/1,001kJ

Carbohydrate 23g

Sugar 12g

Fibre 4g

Fat 13g

Saturated fat 2g

Salt 1.2g

TOMATO AND BEAN SOUP

SERVES 4   **PREP** 10 MINS   **COOK** 20 MINS

A flavoursome Mediterranean-style soup.

1 tbsp olive oil
1 onion, finely chopped
salt and freshly ground black pepper
2 garlic cloves, finely chopped
1 tsp fennel seeds
6 tomatoes, skinned and quartered
1 tbsp tomato purée

400g can of chopped tomatoes
400g can of borlotti beans, drained
  and rinsed
400g can of cannellini beans, drained
  and rinsed
500ml (16fl oz) vegetable stock
chopped parsley, to serve

1 Heat the olive oil in a large pan, add the onion, and cook over a low heat for 7–8 minutes until it softens and turns transparent. Season with a pinch of salt and some black pepper. Stir in the garlic and the fennel seeds.

2 Add the fresh tomatoes and break them up with the back of a spoon. Stir in the tomato purée and canned tomatoes.

3 Tip in the beans, add the stock and bring to the boil. Reduce the heat to a simmer and cook, uncovered, for about 20 minutes, topping up with more stock if needed. Taste and season as necessary. Stir through a little chopped parsley and serve.

STATISTICS PER SERVING:

Energy 286kcals/1,202kJ

Carbohydrate 40g

Sugar 12g

Fibre 4g

Fat 4g
Saturated fat 0.5g

Salt 0.6g

ADUKI BEAN AND VEGETABLE SOUP

SERVES 4   **PREP** 10 MINS   **COOK** 35 MINS   **FREEZE** 3 MONTHS

A wholesome mix of goodness, these red beans have a meaty texture to them.

1 tbsp olive oil
1 red onion, finely chopped
2 cloves of garlic, finely chopped
3 celery stalks, finely diced
3 carrots, peeled and finely diced
1 bay leaf

1 tbsp yeast extract (Marmite)
2 x 410g cans aduki beans,
  drained and rinsed
750ml (1^1/$_4$ pints) vegetable stock
freshly ground black pepper

1 Heat the oil in a large saucepan, then add the onion and cook on a low heat for 2–3 minutes or until soft. Stir in the garlic, celery, carrot, and bay leaf and continue to cook for a further 10 minutes until the vegetables begin to soften.

2 Stir through the yeast extract, add the beans and the stock, and bring to the boil. Reduce the heat and simmer gently for 20 minutes, adding more stock if needed.

3 Remove the bay leaf and season to taste with black pepper (you are unlikely to need salt, as the yeast extract can be salty). Spoon into bowls and serve. Chunky pieces of fresh Seven Grain Bread (see page 336) or other wholemeal bread make a good accompaniment.

STATISTICS PER SERVING:

Energy 388kcals/1,632kJ

Carbohydrate 41g

Sugar 10g

Fibre 11g

Fat 6.5g

Saturated fat 2g

Salt 0.5g

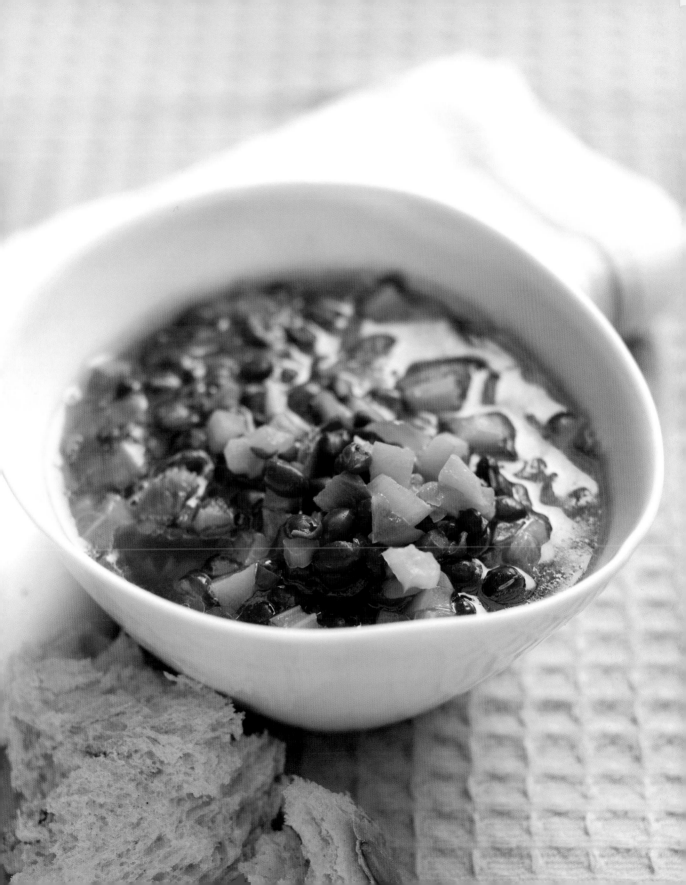

● ○ ○ GI

● ● ○ CALORIES

● ○ ○ SATURATED FAT

● ○ ○ SALT

CHICKPEA AND SQUASH SOUP

SERVES 4   **PREP** 10 MINS   **COOK** 30 MINS   **FREEZE** 3 MONTHS

A delicious thick soup, livened up with cinnamon.

1 tbsp olive oil
1 onion, finely chopped
salt and freshly ground black pepper
2 garlic cloves, finely chopped
2 sage leaves, finely chopped
few sprigs of thyme, leaves only,
  chopped
1 butternut squash, peeled and
  cut into 2.5cm (1in) cubes

1 cinnamon stick
pinch of chilli flakes
900ml (1½ pints) mushroom stock
  or vegetable stock
2 x 400g cans of chickpeas,
  drained and rinsed

1 Heat the olive oil in a large pan, add the onion and cook over a low heat for 5 minutes or until it softens and turns transparent. Season with a pinch of salt and some black pepper. Add the garlic and cook for a few seconds, then add the fresh herbs and the squash and cook, stirring, for 10 minutes or until the squash begins to colour slightly. Add the cinnamon stick and chilli flakes and pour in a little stock. Bring to the boil, then pour in the remaining stock.

2 Tip in the chickpeas, bring to a simmer then cook over a low heat, partially covered, for 15–20 minutes or until the squash is soft.

3 Remove the cinnamon stick, then ladle the soup into a liquidizer and whiz until smooth. If the soup is too thick, add some boiling water. Taste and adjust the seasoning, reheat if necessary, and serve.

COOK'S TIP

Mushroom stock can be found in Italian delis, either ground or as cubes. It is well worth getting hold of, as it imparts a wonderful flavour into soups and casseroles.

STATISTICS PER SERVING:

Energy 314kcals/1,321kJ

Carbohydrate 48g

Sugar 14g

Fibre 5g

Fat 4g

Saturated fat 0.5g

Salt 0.4g

LENTIL AND TOMATO SOUP

SERVES 4   **PREP** 15 MINS   **COOK** 40 MINS   **FREEZE** 3 MONTHS

Plenty of vegetables are packed into this flavourful soup.

2 tbsp olive oil
1 onion, peeled and finely chopped
2 garlic cloves, peeled and crushed
  or finely chopped
1 red pepper, deseeded and diced
1 large carrot, peeled and finely diced
2 celery sticks, chopped
125g (4½oz) red lentils, rinsed

400g can chopped tomatoes
2 tbsp tomato purée
600ml (1 pint) well-flavoured chicken
  stock or vegetable stock
60g (2oz) chorizo, diced
salt and freshly ground black pepper
3 tbsp chopped fresh coriander

1 Heat the oil in a large saucepan, add the onion and cook over a medium heat for 2–3 minutes or until beginning to soften. Add the garlic, red pepper, carrot, and celery and continue to cook, stirring occasionally, for a further 5 minutes.

2 Add the lentils, tomatoes, tomato purée, stock, and chorizo. Season with salt and black pepper, stir, and bring the mixture to the boil.

3 Reduce the heat, cover, and simmer for 30 minutes or until the lentils are soft. Just before serving, stir through the chopped coriander.

STATISTICS PER SERVING:

Energy 273kcals/1,147kJ

Carbohydrate 30g

Sugar 11g

Fibre 4.5g

Fat 10g

Saturated fat 2.5g

Salt 1.1g

⬤⬤◯ GI

⬤⬤◯ CALORIES

⬤⬤◯ SATURATED FAT

⬤⬤◯ SALT

CURRIED PARSNIP SOUP

SERVES 4   **PREP** 15 MINS   **COOK** 55 MINS   **FREEZE** 3 MONTHS
AFTER STEP 3

A mildly spiced soup that is perfect for a chilly winter's day. Parsnips are at their best in winter, and will boost your vitamin C, fibre, and folate intake.

2 tbsp vegetable oil
1 large onion, finely chopped
1 garlic clove, crushed or
  finely chopped
1 tbsp mild curry paste
750g (1lb 10oz) parsnips, cored
  and diced

1.2 litres (2 pints) chicken
  or vegetable stock
salt and freshly ground black pepper
200ml (7fl oz) Greek yogurt
3 tbsp chopped fresh coriander,
  to garnish

1 Heat the oil in a large saucepan, add the onion and cook over a moderate heat, stirring occasionally, for 5 minutes. Add the garlic and cook for 1 minute.

2 Stir in the curry paste and parsnips and cook, stirring, for 5 minutes.

3 Add the stock and season to taste. Bring to the boil and then reduce the heat, cover, and simmer for about 30 minutes. Allow the soup to cool slightly, then transfer the mixture to a food processor or blender and whiz until smooth.

4 Return the soup to the pan, stir in the yogurt and then gently reheat, taking care to not let it boil. Ladle into bowls and garnish with coriander before serving.

STATISTICS PER SERVING:

Energy 318kcals/1,331kJ

Carbohydrate 31g

Sugar 15g

Fibre 9g

Fat 16g

Saturated fat 5g

Salt 1.8g

CHICKEN BROTH
WITH HERBY DUMPLINGS

SERVES 4   **PREP** 5 MINS   **COOK** 45 MINS   **FREEZE** 3 MONTHS
(BROTH ONLY)

A substantial broth for cold, rainy nights when you want
to treat yourself to some comfort food.

GUIDELINES PER SERVING:

● ● ○ GI

● ● ○ CALORIES

● ● ● SATURATED FAT

● ● ● SALT

900ml (1½ pints) chicken stock,
   plus 500ml (16fl oz) extra
2 skinless chicken breasts
200g (7oz) baby button mushrooms,
   any larger ones halved
50g (1¾oz) flat-leaf parsley,
   finely chopped
salt and freshly ground black pepper
15g (½oz) fresh Parmesan, grated, to
   serve

For the dumplings
100g (3½oz) vegetable suet
6 sage leaves, finely chopped
50g (1¾oz) fresh thyme leaves
175g (6oz) fresh white breadcrumbs
3 eggs

1 First, make the broth. Pour 900ml (1½ pints) chicken stock into a large
pan and bring to the boil. Add the chicken, reduce the heat until the stock is
simmering, partially cover the pan, and cook for about 20 minutes or until
the chicken is done. Remove the chicken with a slotted spoon and set aside.

2 While the chicken is cooking, prepare the dumplings. Tip the suet, herbs,
breadcrumbs, and eggs into a bowl, season, and mix well. Form into a
dough – add a little water if necessary to get the dough to start clinging
together in lumps. Shape into balls the size of a walnut, and put on a plate.

3 Top up the broth with the remaining stock, bring to the boil, part-cover,
and simmer for 10 minutes. Add the dumplings and mushrooms and poach
for 10 minutes. Slice or tear the chicken and return it to pan with the
parsley. Heat through. Season and serve sprinkled with a little Parmesan.

COOK'S TIP
To save time, prepare the dumplings 30 minutes ahead and keep them in the
refrigerator until needed.

STATISTICS PER SERVING:

Energy 527kcals/2,204kJ

Carbohydrate 28g

Sugar 1g

Fibre 1.5g

Fat 31.5g

Saturated fat 14g

Salt 2g

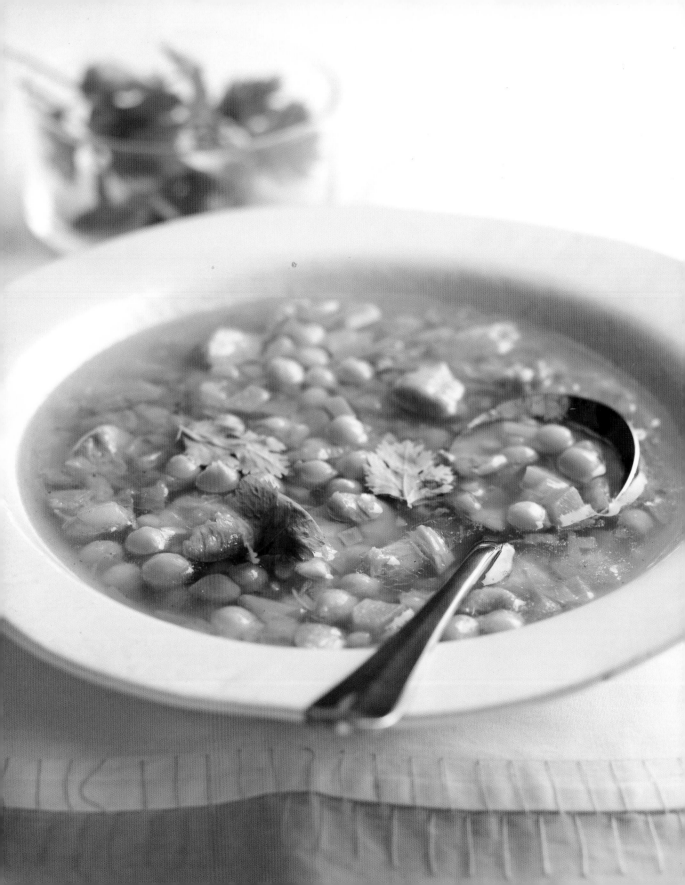

MOROCCAN CHICKEN AND CHICKPEA SOUP

GUIDELINES PER SERVING:

⬤◯◯ GI

⬤⬤◯ CALORIES

⬤⬤⬤ SATURATED FAT

⬤◯◯ SALT

SERVES 4   **PREP** 15 MINS   **COOK** 30 MINS

A hearty soup that is perfect for a light lunch.

2 tbsp olive oil
500g (1lb 2oz) skinless chicken thighs,
  chopped into bite-sized pieces
1 large onion, roughly chopped
2 garlic cloves, crushed
2 large carrots, diced
2 tsp harissa paste

1 litre (1¾ pints) chicken stock
1 cinnamon stick
400g can chickpeas, rinsed and
  drained
salt and freshly ground black pepper
4 tbsp fresh coriander, to garnish

1 Heat 1 tablespoon of the oil in a large saucepan, add the chicken and cook over a high heat for 2–3 minutes or until beginning to brown (you may need to do this in batches). Remove from the pan and set aside.

2 Heat the remaining oil, tip in the onion and cook for 1–2 minutes. Add the garlic, carrots, and harissa paste. Cook for 1–2 minutes.

3 Return the chicken to the pan, and add the stock and cinnamon stick. Bring to the boil, reduce the heat and simmer for 30 minutes.

4 Add the chickpeas and continue to cook for 1–2 minutes. Remove and discard the cinnamon stick, then season to taste with salt and black pepper. Ladle the soup into bowls and garnish with the coriander.

STATISTICS PER SERVING:

Energy 344kcals/1,440kJ

Carbohydrate 5g

Sugar 4g

Fibre 1.7g

Fat 28g

Saturated fat 12g

Salt 0.5g

● ○ ○ **GI**

● ● ○ **CALORIES**

● ○ ○ **SATURATED FAT**

● ● ● **SALT**

RED LENTIL AND BACON SOUP

SERVES 4   **PREP** 10 MINS   **COOK** 40 MINS   **FREEZE** 1 MONTH

A warming meal in one; the apricots add a hint of sweetness to the earthy lentils.

1 tbsp olive oil
1 onion, finely chopped
4 slices back bacon, fat removed
  and roughly chopped
50g (1¾oz) dried apricots, finely
  chopped

275g (9½oz) red lentils, rinsed
salt and freshly ground black pepper
300ml (10fl oz) passata
1.7 litre (3 pints) vegetable stock

1 Heat the oil in a large pan, add the onion and cook over a low heat for 7–8 minutes until it softens and turns transparent. Add the bacon and cook for a further 5 minutes until the bacon begins to colour. Stir through the apricots and lentils and season with a pinch of salt and some black pepper.

2 Stir through the passata, increase the heat slightly and add a little of the stock. Bring to the boil, then reduce the heat to a simmer and add more stock, 600ml (1 pint) or so at a time, stirring and bringing to a simmer each time. Cook over a low heat for 25–30 minutes until the lentils are cooked and the sauce thickens. Taste, adjust the seasoning if required, and serve.

COOK'S TIP
This soup is best left to sit awhile before serving. In fact, the flavours are even better when it is eaten the day after cooking; keep it in the refrigerator overnight and reheat gently before serving.

STATISTICS PER SERVING:

Energy 437kcals/1,842kJ

Carbohydrate 54g

Sugar 9g

Fibre 6g

Fat 11g

Saturated fat 3g

Salt 3g

MULLIGATAWNY

SERVES 6   **PREP** 15 MINS   **COOK** 40 MINS   **FREEZE** 3 MONTHS

A spicy, hot, filling soup for cold days.

2 tbsp olive oil
1 large onion, finely chopped
1 carrot, peeled and finely chopped
1 potato, peeled and finely chopped
1 cooking apple, peeled, cored and
  finely chopped
500g (1lb 2oz) finely diced lean beef
1 heaped tsp curry powder
2.5cm (1in) piece of fresh root ginger,
  peeled and grated

2 green birds-eye chillies,
  deseeded and finely chopped
4 garlic cloves, finely chopped
125g (4½oz) dried red lentils
2 litres (3½ pints) chicken stock
large handful of fresh coriander,
  finely chopped
salt and freshly ground black pepper

GUIDELINES PER SERVING:

● ○ ○ GI

● ● ○ CALORIES

● ○ ○ SATURATED FAT

● ● ○ SALT

1 Heat the olive oil in a large pan, add the onion, carrot, potato, and apple and cook gently for a couple of minutes, then stir in the beef and curry powder and cook until the beef is no longer pink.

2 Add the ginger, chillies, and garlic and cook for 1 minute. Stir in the lentils so they are well coated in the spices then pour in the stock and bring to the boil. Reduce to a simmer and cook for 30 minutes or until the lentils are soft.

3 Stir through the coriander, season with salt and black pepper and cook for a further 5 minutes. You could serve this with chapattis alongside (see page 338).

COOK'S TIP
Traditionally this soup is blended; do so before serving if you wish.

STATISTICS PER SERVING:

Energy 324kcals/1,365kJ

Carbohydrate 27g

Sugar 7g

Fibre 3g

Fat 10g

Saturated fat 3g

Salt 1.8g

HOT AND SOUR (TOM YAM) SOUP

SERVES 4   **PREP** 5 MINS   **COOK** 15 MINS

A classic Thai broth, which is full of flavour and yet low in fat. This soup is perfect for a quick and healthy lunch, and its piquant ingredients are a treat for the tastebuds.

1.2 litres (2 pints) chicken
  or vegetable stock
4 kaffir lime leaves
4 slices of fresh ginger
1 red chilli, deseeded and sliced
1 stalk lemongrass, bruised
100g (3½oz) shiitake mushrooms,
  sliced

100g (3½oz) rice noodles
200g (7oz) peeled prawns, raw
4 spring onions, finely shredded
1 tsp Thai fish sauce
juice of 2 limes
1 tbsp chopped fresh coriander

1 Put the stock, lime leaves, ginger, chilli, and lemongrass in a large saucepan. Cover and bring to the boil. Add the mushrooms and simmer for 10 minutes. Break the noodles into short lengths and drop them into the soup. Simmer for 3 minutes.

2 Add the prawns and spring onions, and simmer for 2 minutes or until the prawns turn pink. Add the fish sauce and lime juice. Remove the lemongrass and adjust the seasoning. Sprinkle with the fresh coriander and serve.

STATISTICS PER SERVING:

Energy 196kcals/820kJ

Carbohydrate 23g

Sugar 1.5g

Fibre 0.7g

Fat 3g

Saturated fat 0.7g

Salt 2g

BEEF BROTH

SERVES 4   **PREP** 15 MINS   **COOK** 2 HOURS 10 MINS   **FREEZE** 1 MONTH

Slow-cooked beef, left to simmer until tender, infuses this broth with rich juices to make a wholesome and satisfying soup that is a meal in itself.

GUIDELINES PER SERVING:

●● ○ GI

● ○ ○ CALORIES

● ○ ○ SATURATED FAT

● ○ ○ SALT

500g (1lb 2oz) lean beef, diced
bouquet garni of bay leaf, parsley,
  and thyme
salt and freshly ground black pepper
1 tbsp olive oil

2 onions, diced
2 carrots, diced
2 small potatoes, peeled and diced
2 leeks, trimmed and chopped

1 Pour 2 litres (3½ pints) of water into a large pan, bring to the boil, and season well with salt and black pepper. Add the beef and bouquet garni to the pan, return to the boil and skim off any scum that rises to the surface, then reduce to a simmer. Cook, partially covered, over a very low heat for 1½ hours.

2 While the beef is cooking, heat the olive oil in a large frying pan, and add the onions, carrots, and potatoes. Cook for about 5 minutes. Add the leeks and cook for a further 5 minutes.

3 Tip the vegetable mixture into the pan with the beef, stir, season well, and cook gently for a further 30 minutes or until the vegetables are soft. Remove the bouquet garni, and serve.

STATISTICS PER SERVING:

Energy 283kcals/1,191kJ

Carbohydrate 22g

Sugar 8g

Fibre 4g

Fat 8.5g
Saturated fat 2.5g

Salt 0.3g

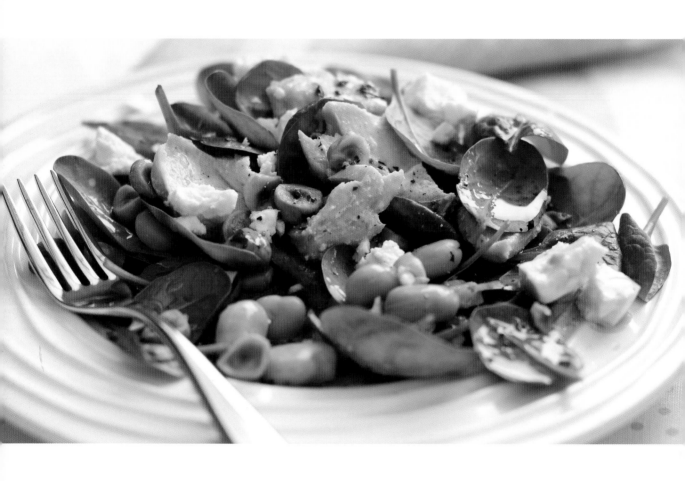

LIGHT LUNCHES AND SALADS

● ○ ○ GI

● ● ○ CALORIES

● ○ ○ SATURATED FAT

● ● ○ SALT

YELLOW SPLIT PEAS WITH PEPPERS AND PEA SHOOTS

SERVES 2 **PREP** 15 MINS **COOK** 35 MINS

Like all pulses, split peas provide good amounts of protein and dietary fibre. They are also a low-GI food. Here they are served as a tasty open sandwich

1 tbsp olive oil
1 small red onion, finely chopped
1 clove garlic, crushed or finely chopped
2cm (¾in) piece fresh ginger, finely chopped
85g (3oz) yellow split peas

300ml (10fl oz) vegetable stock
1 red pepper, halved
2 slices pumpernickel or toasted rye bread (about 50g/1¾oz per slice)
25g (scant 1oz) pea shoots (if unavailable, use rocket or watercress)

1 Heat the oil in a small saucepan and then scatter in the onion, garlic, and ginger. Cook, stirring, for 1–2 minutes. Add the split peas and stock, bring to the boil, then cover and reduce the heat. Simmer for 30–35 minutes or until the split peas are very soft. Add a little more stock or water if needed.

2 While the split peas are cooking, prepare the red pepper: place the two halves, skin-side up, under a hot grill for 15–20 minutes or until the skin is charred and black. Cover with a clean, damp tea towel – or place in a plastic freezer bag – and allow to cool for 10 minutes. Remove the skin and seeds from the pepper. Blot the pepper dry with kitchen paper, then slice it into thick strips.

3 Place the pumpernickel bread on serving plates, spoon the split peas over it, top with the strips of red pepper, and finish with the pea shoots.

COOK'S TIP
Pea shoots are the leaves of the garden pea plant, and are high in vitamin C. They make an interesting alternative to traditional salad leaves – look out for them in the supermarket.

STATISTICS PER SERVING:

Energy 348kcals/1,472kJ

Carbohydrate 53g

Sugar 5g

Fibre 6g

Fat 9g

Saturated fat 1.5g

Salt 1.5g

SPANISH EGGS

SERVES 2   **PREP** 10 MINS   **COOK** 35 MINS

Eggs are one of the few dietary sources of vitamin D and also contain good amounts of protein and B-vitamins, making this dish a great choice for a quick, healthy lunch.

1 tbsp olive oil
1 large red onion, diced
2 garlic cloves, crushed
  or finely chopped
½ red chilli, deseeded and
  finely chopped
1 small red pepper, deseeded
  and diced

400g can cherry tomatoes
2 tbsp tomato purée
½ tsp smoked paprika
150ml (5fl oz) red wine
salt and freshly ground black pepper
4 large eggs
2 tbsp chopped fresh coriander,
  to garnish

1 Heat the oil in a nonstick frying pan. Add the onion and sauté over a medium heat for 2–3 minutes, then add the garlic, chilli, and red pepper. Continue to cook, stirring occasionally, for 3 minutes.

2 Add the tomatoes, tomato purée, paprika, and red wine. Season to taste. Cook, uncovered, over a medium heat for 15–20 minutes or until the mixture begins to thicken.

3 Using the back of a tablespoon, make 4 egg-shaped hollows in the tomato mixture and crack an egg into each hollow. Put a lid on the pan and cook over a low heat for 8–10 minutes, or until the eggs are done to your liking.

4 Sprinkle with the coriander and serve.

STATISTICS PER SERVING:

Energy 370kcals/1,542kJ

Carbohydrate 19g

Sugar 16g

Fibre 4g

Fat 19g

Saturated fat 4.5g

Salt 0.7g

● ● ○ GI

● ● ○ CALORIES

● ○ ○ SATURATED FAT

● ● ○ SALT

SHREDDED PORK AND SPRING ONION WRAP

SERVES 4   **PREP** 10 MINS   **COOK** 2 HOURS

Succulent shredded pork with a Cajun-style coating.

350g (12oz) pork tenderloin, trimmed
  of fat and sinew
2 bunches spring onions,
  sliced lengthways
4–8 Turkish flatbreads

For the marinade
1 medium onion, peeled and
  quartered

1 tsp freshly ground black pepper
½ tsp salt
1 scotch bonnet chilli, deseeded
1 tsp allspice
½ tsp paprika
2 ripe peaches, stoned and quartered
2 cloves garlic, peeled and
  roughly chopped

1 Preheat the oven to 150°C (300°F/Gas 2). Put the marinade ingredients into a blender and whiz to a smooth paste. Deeply slash the pork and liberally rub all over with the marinade. Place the pork in a roasting tin and cover with any remaining marinade. Cover loosely with foil and roast for 2 hours, basting occasionally.

2 Shred the pork using two forks and toss in any remaining cooking juices. Arrange on flatbreads, each with a liberal handful of spring onions, roll or fold, and serve.

STATISTICS PER SERVING:

Energy 388kcals/1,440kJ

Carbohydrate 50g

Sugar 11g

Fibre 4g

Fat 6g

Saturated fat 2g

Salt 1.5g

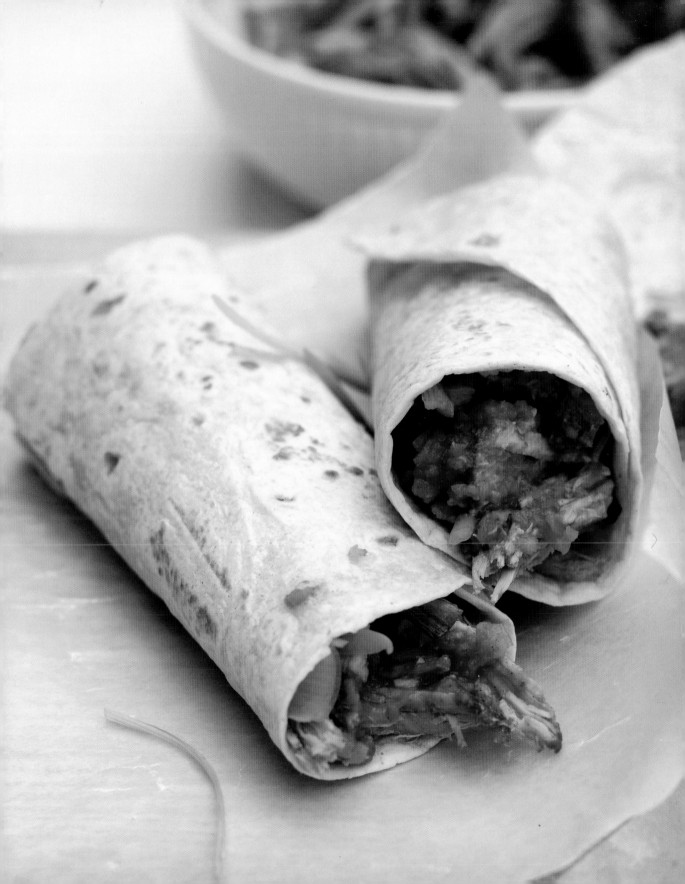

● ○ ○ GI

● ○ ○ CALORIES

● ○ ○ SATURATED FAT

● ○ ○ SALT

MIXED BEAN BURGER

SERVES 4   **PREP** 10 MINS   **COOK** 15 MINS   **FREEZE** 3 MONTHS
PLUS CHILLING

Vegetarian burgers with a hint of Indian spice.

1 red onion, roughly chopped
2 garlic cloves, finely chopped
1 green chilli, deseeded and
  roughly chopped
pinch of garam masala
handful of fresh coriander

2 x 400g cans of mixed beans, drained
125g (4½oz) mushrooms, grated
salt and freshly ground black pepper
2 tbsp fresh breadcrumbs
1–2 eggs, lightly beaten
2 tbsp sunflower oil

1 Place the onion, garlic, chilli, garam masala, coriander, beans, and mushrooms in a food processor and whiz until well combined, but do not overblend and let it become mushy.

2 Season well with salt and black pepper then tip in the breadcrumbs and a little of the egg and pulse until it all binds together but is neither too wet nor too dry – add a little more egg if needed. Shape into 8 patties, arrange on a plate and transfer to the refrigerator for 20 minutes to firm up.

3 Heat the oil in a non-stick frying pan and cook a few burgers at a time for 6–7 minutes or until the underside starts to brown. Turn over the burgers using a fish slice and cook the other side for the same amount of time, adding more oil if needed. You could serve these in wholemeal bread rolls, each with a small quantity of tomato salad.

STATISTICS PER SERVING:

Energy 250kcals/1,061kJ

Carbohydrate 37g

Sugar 4g

Fibre 12g

Fat 5g
Saturated fat 1g

Salt 0.3g

FALAFEL

SERVES 4   **PREP** 25 MINS   **COOK** 15 MINS
PLUS SOAKING
PLUS CHLLING

Based on chickpeas, these tasty and substantial bites are a
Middle Eastern classic.

GUIDELINES PER SERVING:

●○○ GI

●○○ CALORIES

●○○ SATURATED FAT

●●○ SALT

225g (8oz) dried chickpeas, soaked
  overnight in cold water
1 tbsp tahini
1 garlic clove, crushed
1 tsp salt
1 tsp ground cumin

1 tsp turmeric
1 tsp ground coriander
½ tsp cayenne pepper
2 tbsp finely chopped parsley
juice of 1 small lemon
vegetable oil, for frying

1 Drain the soaked chickpeas and place them in a food processor with the
rest of the ingredients. Process until finely chopped but not puréed.

2 Transfer the mixture to a bowl and set it aside for at least 30 minutes (and
up to 8 hours), covered in the refrigerator.

3 Wet your hands and shape the mixture into 12 balls. Press the tops down
slightly to flatten.

4 Heat 5cm (2in) of oil in a deep pan or wok. Fry the balls in batches for
3–4 minutes, or until lightly golden. Drain on kitchen paper and serve.
A simple green salad makes a good accompaniment.

STATISTICS PER SERVING:

Energy 277kcals/1,161kJ

Carbohydrate 30g

Sugar 1.5g

Fibre 6g

Fat 13.5g

Saturated fat 1.5g

Salt 1g

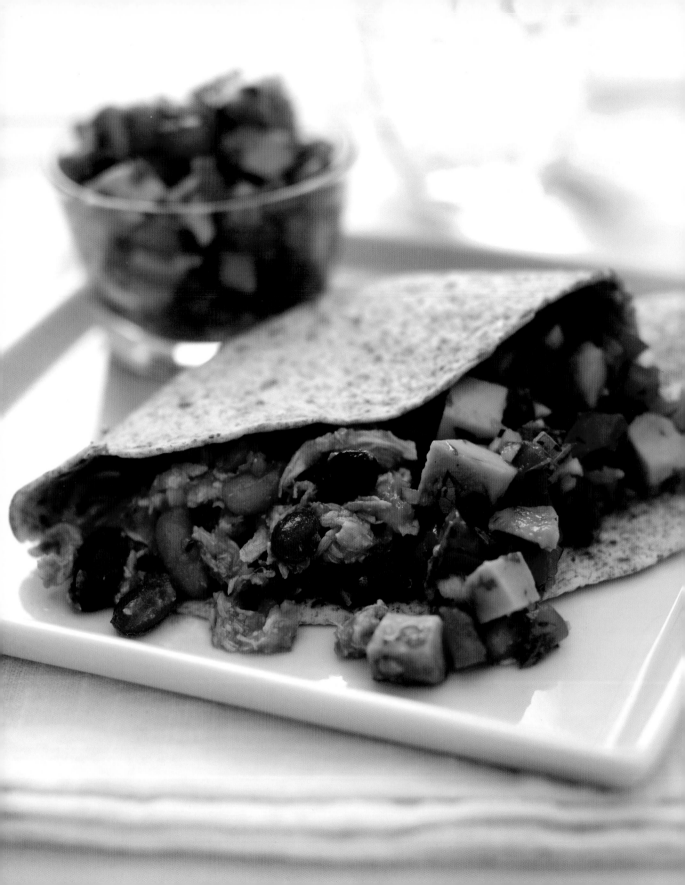

CHICKEN TOSTADA WITH AVOCADO SALSA

GUIDELINES PER SERVING:

GI

CALORIES

SATURATED FAT

SALT

SERVES 4   **PREP** 15 MINS   **COOK** 50 MINS

A tasty and filling lunch or supper dish that is full of flavour and high in dietary fibre.

6 tomatoes, skinned, quartered, and seeds removed
1 large red onion, peeled and sliced into thin wedges
1 small red pepper, deseeded and roughly chopped
3 cloves of garlic, unpeeled
1 red chilli, deseeded
3 tbsp olive oil
salt and freshly ground black pepper
400g (14oz) cooked chicken, shredded

415g can mixed beans, rinsed and drained
8 wholemeal flour tortillas

For the salsa
6 tomatoes, seeds removed and flesh diced
2 small ripe avocado, peeled, stones removed, and flesh diced
1 small red onion, finely chopped
3 tbsp chopped fresh coriander
juice of 1 lime

1 Preheat the oven to 200°C (400°F/Gas 6). Place the tomatoes, onions, red pepper, garlic, and chilli in a roasting tin, drizzle with oil, and bake for 20–30 minutes or until soft and slightly charred. Squeeze the garlic cloves from their skins and place in a food processor along with the other cooked vegetables and process until smooth. Season to taste with salt and black pepper.

2 Place the drained mixed beans in a large saucepan and cook over a low heat for 2 minutes. Add the vegetable sauce, stir in the chicken, and cook for a further 2 minutes, stirring occasionally.

3 To make the salsa, mix together the tomatoes, avocado, onion, coriander, and lime juice in a bowl, and season to taste.

4 Heat the tortillas according to the packet instructions. To serve, spoon a little of the chicken mixture into each tortilla, fold, and serve with the salsa.

STATISTICS PER SERVING:

Energy 745kcals/3,140kJ

Carbohydrate 90g

Sugar 17g

Fibre 13g

Fat 24g
Saturated fat 3.5g

Salt 1g

● ○ ○ GI

● ● ○ CALORIES

● ● ○ SATURATED FAT

● ● ○ SALT

SALMON BURGERS

SERVES 6   **PREP** 10 MINS   **COOK** 10 MINS   **FREEZE** 1 MONTH
PLUS CHILLING

These tasty burgers are heavy on the fish and have no added potato – a luxurious version of the humble fishcake.

700g (1lb 9oz) salmon fillets, skinned
  and cut into chunks
125g (4oz) breadcrumbs
bunch of spring onions, trimmed
  and roughly chopped

2 tsp capers, drained and rinsed
50g (1¾oz) flat-leaf parsley
salt and freshly ground black pepper
1 egg
2 tbsp sunflower oil

1 Put the salmon, breadcrumbs, spring onions, capers, and parsley into a food processor or blender. Process until well combined. Season with salt and black pepper, and then pulse to mix.

2 Add the egg to the food processor and pulse again so that the mixture is evenly combined. Divide the mixture into six and, one at a time, roll each lump into a ball and then pat flat to shape into a burger. Put the burgers on a plate and place in the refrigerator to firm up for 20 minutes.

3 Heat the oil in a large, nonstick frying pan and add the burgers. Cook for 3–4 minutes, or until the underside begins to turn golden, then flip them over and cook the other side for the same length of time.

COOK'S TIP
You can cook the burgers in the oven if you wish. Preheat the oven to 200°C (400°F/Gas 6), place the burgers in a lightly oiled roasting tin and cook for 15–20 minutes or until golden and cooked through.

STATISTICS PER SERVING:

Energy 506kcals/2,118kJ

Carbohydrate 26g

Sugar 3g

Fibre 1g

Fat 27g

Saturated fat 4g

Salt 1g

PRAWN CAKES WITH MANGO SALSA

GUIDELINES PER CAKE:

●○○ GI
●○○ CALORIES
●○○ SATURATED FAT
●○○ SALT

MAKES 9   **PREP** 10 MINS   **COOK** 20 MINS   **FREEZE** 1 MONTH
PLUS CHILLING   (PRAWN CAKES)

Small bites with bags of flavour, complemented by a fresh and juicy mango salsa.

2.5cm (2in) piece of fresh root ginger, roughly chopped
2 garlic cloves
1 red chilli, halved and deseeded
1 stalk lemongrass, trimmed and tough outer leaves removed
salt and freshly ground black pepper
250g (9oz) cooked prawns

1 small egg, beaten
1–2 tbsp sunflower oil

For the mango salsa
1 mango, diced
3 spring onions, finely diced
1 tbsp finely chopped fresh coriander
1 tsp rice vinegar

1 First, make the mango salsa. Put all the ingredients in a bowl and mix, then set aside for the flavours to develop.

2 Put the ginger, garlic, chilli, and lemongrass in a food processor or blender and whizz until finely chopped. Add a pinch of salt and some black pepper and process again. Add the prawns and pulse until the prawns are chopped but not mushy, then taste the mixture and adjust the seasoning if needed. Add a little of the egg and process so the mixture binds together; add more of the egg if needed.

3 Using your hands to scoop up the mixture, roll it into nine balls and pat them flat into cakes. Sit them on a plate and place in the refrigerator for 30 minutes to firm up a little. The mixture will be wet and quite delicate.

4 When ready to cook, heat the oil in a nonstick frying pan and fry the cakes for a minute or so until the underside begins to crisp a little. Then, using a spatula, carefully turn the cakes over and cook the other side for a couple of minutes or until golden. Serve with the mango salsa.

STATISTICS PER CAKE:

Energy 57kcals/283kJ

Carbohydrate 4g

Sugar 3g

Fibre 0.6g

Fat 2g

Saturated fat 0.4g

Salt 0.4g

● ● ○ GI

● ○ ○ CALORIES

● ○ ○ SATURATED FAT

● ○ ○ SALT

POTATO AND THYME RÖSTI WITH MUSHROOMS

SERVES 4   **PREP** 15 MINS   **COOK** 25 MINS

This traditional Swiss favourite pleases everyone.

550g (1¼lb) potatoes (use large
  waxy ones), unpeeled
salt and freshly ground black pepper
few stalks of fresh thyme, leaves only
1 onion, finely chopped

2 tbsp sunflower oil
150g (5½oz) chestnut mushrooms,
  sliced
2 garlic cloves, finely chopped

1 Cook the potatoes in a large pan of salted water for 10–15 minutes until just beginning to soften. Remove with a slotted spoon and set aside until cool enough to handle. Grate the potatoes into a bowl and season with plenty of salt and black pepper. Add the thyme and onion, and stir gently.

2 Put 1 tablespoon of the oil into a medium-sized, nonstick frying pan and add the potato mixture, pressing it down so that it becomes a cake – it should be about 1cm (½in) thick. Cook over a low heat for 10–12 minutes until the underside begins to turn golden and form a crust. Invert the cake onto a large plate and return it to the pan to cook the other side until golden. (Alternatively, if the handle of the pan is heatproof, you could finish it off in an oven preheated to a medium heat.)

3 Meanwhile, heat the remaining oil in another frying pan, add the mushrooms and cook for 5 minutes or until they begin to release their juices. Add the garlic and cook for a further couple of minutes, then season to taste. Using a spatula, slide the rösti out of the pan and onto a serving plate. Top with the mushrooms and slice the rösti to serve.

COOK'S TIP
You can use grated raw potato if you prefer, but do make sure you squeeze out all the water or else the rösti will become wet. You will also need to use a lower heat and cook it for longer, otherwise the inside will not cook.

STATISTICS PER SERVING:

Energy 166kcals/699kJ

Carbohydrate 26g

Sugar 2g

Fibre 2.6g

Fat 6g

Saturated fat 0.7g

Salt trace

SWEET POTATOES WITH A SMOKY TOMATO FILLING

GUIDELINES PER SERVING:

● ○ ○ GI

● ○ ○ CALORIES

● ○ ○ SATURATED FAT

● ○ ○ SALT

SERVES 2   **PREP** 5 MINS   **COOK** 40 MINS

A tasty and filling light lunch, which is low in fat and salt.

4 sweet potatoes, unpeeled
2 tbsp olive oil
1 small red onion, finely chopped
1 small red pepper, deseeded and
 diced
½ red chilli, deseeded and
 finely chopped

225g (8oz) cherry tomatoes, halved
150g (5oz) sweetcorn, defrosted
 if frozen
½ tsp smoked sweet paprika
salt and freshly ground black pepper

1 Preheat the oven to 180°C (350°F/Gas 4). Pierce the sweet potatoes in several places and put in the oven for 40 minutes or until cooked.

2 Meanwhile, heat the oil in a frying pan, add the onion and cook for 1–2 minutes. Stir in the red pepper and chilli; cook for a further 1–2 minutes or until the pepper is starting to soften. Add the cherry tomatoes, sweetcorn, and paprika. Season to taste with salt and black pepper, and cook for a further 1–2 minutes.

3 Slice the potatoes in half and spoon the tomato mixture over them.

STATISTICS PER SERVING:

Energy 289kcals/1,226kJ

Carbohydrate 55g

Sugar 17g

Fibre 7g

Fat 7g

Saturated fat 1g

Salt 0.2g

● ● ○ GI

● ● ○ CALORIES

● ○ ○ SATURATED FAT

● ○ ○ SALT

SWEET POTATO CAKES

SERVES 4   **PREP** 10 MINS   **COOK** 20 MINS   **FREEZE** 1 MONTH

Spring onion adds a crunchy texture to these cakes.

500g (1lb 2oz) cooked sweet potato, mashed
5cm (2in) piece of fresh ginger, peeled and grated
bunch of spring onions, finely chopped

pinch of freshly grated nutmeg
2 eggs, lightly beaten
flour for dusting
3–4 tbsp polenta
vegetable oil for shallow frying
lime wedges, to serve

1 Add the sweet potato to a large bowl then add the ginger, spring onions, and nutmeg then add a little of the egg, a drop at time, reserving plenty for coating, until the mixture binds together.

2 Season well with salt and black pepper, then scoop up a handful of the mixture, roll into a ball, then flatten out into a cake. Repeat until all the mixture is used.

3 Dust the cakes in flour, dip in the reserved egg, then lightly coat with polenta. Heat the oil in a non-stick frying pan and add the cakes a couple at a time. Cook for 2–3 minutes or until the underside turns golden, then carefully flip and cook for a further 2–3 minutes or until evenly golden brown. Serve with lime wedges for squeezing over.

COOK'S TIP
To cook the sweet potatoes, you could bake or microwave them, then scoop out the insides and mash with a fork. Alternatively, peel them, cut into chunks, boil, and drain before mashing.

STATISTICS PER SERVING:

Energy 272kcals/1,140kJ

Carbohydrate 36g

Sugar 16g

Fibre 3.5g

Fat 12g

Saturated fat 2g

Salt 0.2g

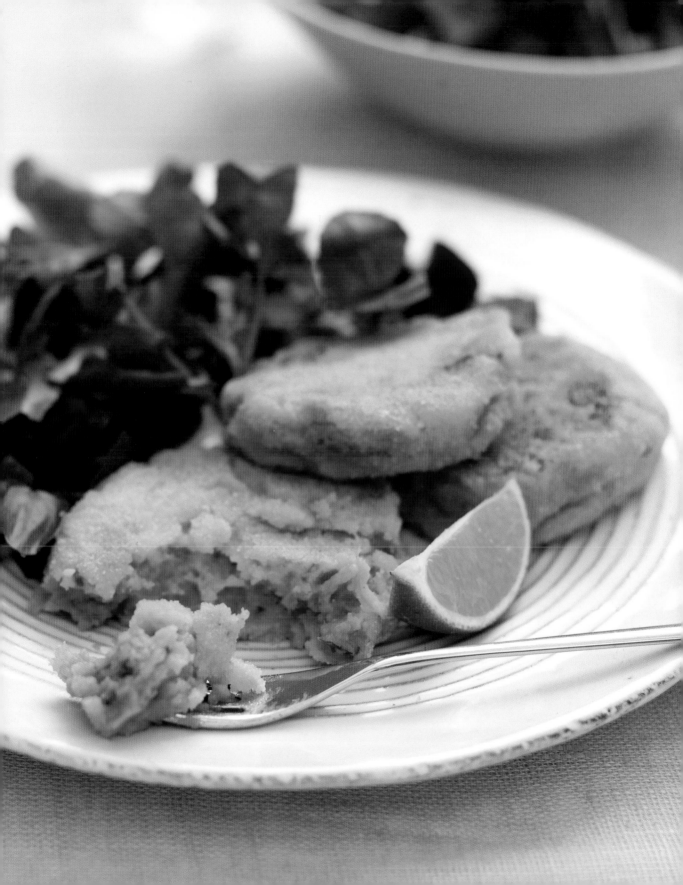

● ○ ○ GI

● ○ ○ CALORIES

● ○ ○ SATURATED FAT

● ● ○ SALT

FETA AND COURGETTE CAKES

SERVES 4   **PREP** 15 MINS   **COOK** 10 MINS   **FREEZE** 1 MONTH
PLUS DRAINING
PLUS CHILLING

These moreish light and tasty cakes are perfect for a spring lunch.

550g (1¼lb) courgettes, grated
salt, for sprinkling
125g (4½oz) feta cheese, crumbled
freshly ground black pepper

pinch of paprika
1 egg, lightly beaten
1 tbsp flour, plus extra for dusting
2 tbsp olive oil

1 Put the courgettes in a colander, sprinkle with salt and leave to drain for 20 minutes (you need as much water as possible to drain away), then squeeze out any remaining moisture.

2 Tip the courgettes into a bowl. Add the feta, season with black pepper and paprika, and stir. Add the egg and flour, and stir until well combined.

3 Scoop up the courgette and feta mixture, a tablespoon at a time, and pat it into cakes. Place these on a plate of flour and turn once to coat lightly, then put in the refrigerator for 20 minutes to firm up.

4 Heat a little of the olive oil in a frying pan and cook the cakes, two at a time – adding the rest of the oil as required – for a couple of minutes each side, or until golden and crispy.

COOK'S TIP
For ease, you could grate the courgettes using a food processor.

STATISTICS PER SERVING:

Energy 160kcals/657kJ

Carbohydrate 5g

Sugar 2.5g

Fibre 1.5g

Fat 10g

Saturated fat 3g

Salt 1g

CAPONATA

SERVES 4   **PREP** 15 MINS   **COOK** 30 MINS   **FREEZE** 1 MONTH

Caponata has wonderful, contrasting sweet and sour tastes, and can be eaten hot or cold.

GUIDELINES PER SERVING:

● ○ ○ GI

● ○ ○ CALORIES

● ○ ○ SATURATED FAT

● ○ ○ SALT

3 tbsp olive oil
2 aubergines, cut into bite-sized
  chunks
1 onion, finely chopped
3 celery sticks, roughly chopped
salt and freshly ground black pepper
400g can chopped tomatoes

handful of green olives, pitted
  and chopped
2 tbsp capers, drained and rinsed
2 tbsp red wine vinegar
1 tbsp fresh basil, torn
25g (scant 1oz) pine nuts, toasted

1 Heat 2 tablespoons of the oil in a large pan and add the aubergine. Cook – working in batches if necessary – for 6–8 minutes, or until it starts to turn golden brown, adding more oil if needed. Remove with a slotted spoon and set aside.

2 Add the remaining oil to the same pan and heat for a minute. Add the onion and celery, and season with salt and black pepper. Cook for 5 minutes or until the onion begins to soften, then add the tomatoes, olives, and capers. Simmer gently for 15 minutes, partially covered.

3 Add the vinegar and increase the heat to bring the mixture to the boil. Cook for a minute or so until the smell of the vinegar disappears, then stir in the cooked aubergine and the basil. Stir in most of the pine nuts, saving a few for decoration. Spoon into a serving dish and scatter with the reserved pine nuts.

COOK'S TIP
Choose young aubergines if possible, as older ones tend to be more bitter and may need degorging (sprinkling with salt to draw out moisture and bitterness).

STATISTICS PER SERVING:

Energy 189kcals/787kJ

Carbohydrate 11g

Sugar 9g

Fibre 6g

Fat 15g

Saturated fat 2g

Salt 0.8g

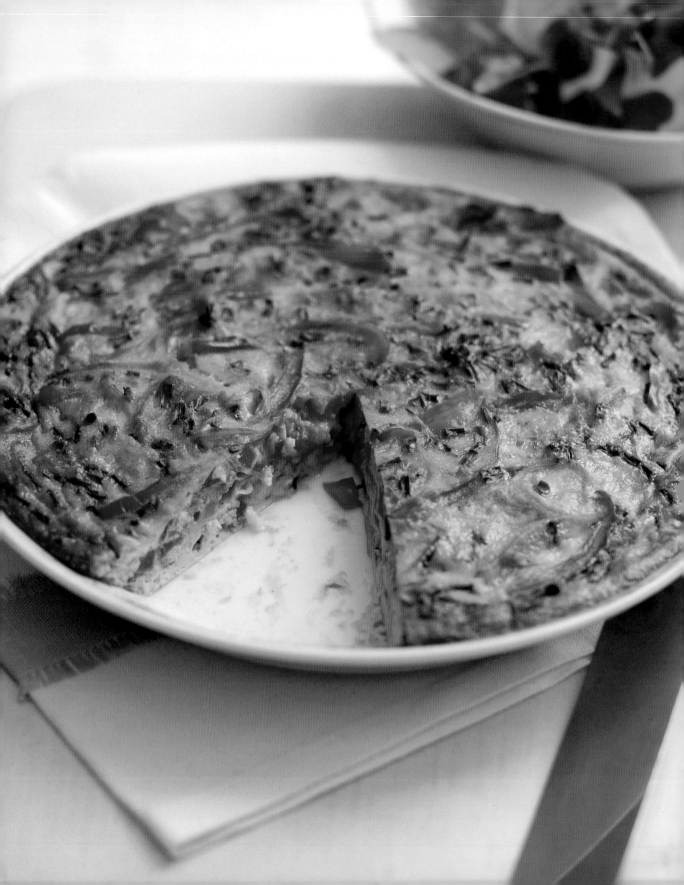

OVEN-BAKED RED PEPPER AND TOMATO FRITTATA

SERVES 2   **PREP** 15 MINS   **COOK** 30 MINS

An easy way to cook this simple vegetable and egg dish.

1 tbsp olive oil
1 onion, finely chopped
2 red peppers, deseeded and finely
  chopped or sliced
salt and freshly ground black pepper
pinch of paprika

4 tomatoes, skinned, deseeded,
  and flesh chopped
25g (scant 1oz) bunch of chives,
  finely chopped
4 large eggs, lightly beaten

1 Preheat the oven to 180°C (350°F/Gas 4). Heat the oil in a medium non-stick frying pan, add the onion and red peppers, and cook for 5–8 minutes until soft. Season with salt and pepper, add the paprika, and stir.

2 Transfer the cooked vegetables to a heatproof dish and stir in the tomatoes and chives. Add the eggs and mix gently, then place in the oven for 20–30 minutes until risen and golden.

3 Allow to cool for a few minutes before serving. A simple green salad makes a good accompaniment.

COOK'S TIP
Swap herbs to suit the seasons and add a pinch of chilli flakes to heat things up.

STATISTICS PER SERVING:

Energy 336kcals/1,402kJ

Carbohydrate 22g

Sugar 19g

Fibre 0.5g

Fat 20g

Saturated fat 5g

Salt 0.3g

- ●○○ GI
- ●●○ CALORIES
- ●●○ SATURATED FAT
- ●○○ SALT

TORTILLA

SERVES 4   **PREP** 15 MINS   **COOK** 45 MINS

This variation of a traditional thick Spanish omelette includes broccoli and peas as well as potatoes.

115g (4oz) fresh or frozen peas
115g (4oz) broccoli florets
4 tbsp olive oil
350g (12oz) floury potatoes, such as
  King Edward, peeled and cut into
  2cm (¾in) cubes

2 small red onions, finely chopped
6 eggs, beaten
salt and freshly ground
  black pepper

1 Bring a large saucepan of lightly salted water to the boil over a high heat. Add the peas and boil for 5 minutes, or until just tender. Use a slotted spoon to transfer the peas to a bowl of cold water. Return the pan to the boil, add the broccoli and boil for 4 minutes or until just tender. Remove the florets and add to the peas to cool, then drain both vegetables well, and set aside.

2 Heat 3 tbsp of the oil in a non-stick frying pan over a medium heat. Add the potatoes and onions, and cook for 10–15 minutes, stirring often, or until the potatoes are tender.

3 Beat the eggs in a large bowl, and season with salt and pepper, then use a slotted spoon to transfer the potatoes and onions to the eggs. Add the peas and broccoli and gently stir. Discard the excess oil from the pan and remove any crispy bits stuck to the bottom.

4 Heat the remaining oil in the pan over a high heat. Add the egg mixture, immediately reduce the heat to low, and smooth the surface. Leave to cook for 20–25 minutes, or until the top of the omelette begins to set and the base is golden brown.

5 Carefully slide the tortilla on to a plate, place a second plate on top and invert so that the cooked side is on top. Slide the tortilla back into the pan and cook for 5 minutes, until both sides are golden brown and set. Remove from the heat and leave to set for at least 5 minutes. Serve warm or cooled, cut into wedges.

STATISTICS PER SERVING:

Energy 333kcals/1,388kJ

Carbohydrate 20g

Sugar 3g

Fibre 4g

Fat 22g

Saturated fat 4g

Salt 0.4g

PEAS WITH HAM

SERVES 4   **PREP** 5 MINS   **COOK** 15 MINS

Guisantes con jamón is a classic tapas dish with delicious sweet and savoury flavours.

GUIDELINES PER SERVING:

● ○ ○   GI

● ○ ○   CALORIES

● ○ ○   SATURATED FAT

● ● ○   SALT

2 tbsp olive oil
1 onion, finely diced
200g (7oz) Serrano ham, diced
200ml carton sieved tomatoes
1 tsp sweet paprika

500g (1lb 2oz) peas
1 garlic clove, crushed
1 tbsp finely chopped parsley
150ml (5fl oz) dry white wine
salt and freshly ground black pepper

1 Heat the oil in a frying pan and add the onion. Fry for 5 minutes, stirring frequently, until soft.

2 Increase the heat, add the ham and fry until it begins to brown, then add the tomatoes and sweet paprika. Bring to boiling point, reduce the heat, and simmer for 3 minutes, stirring frequently. Stir in the peas.

3 Mix together the garlic and chopped parsley, then stir in the wine. Pour this mixture into the pan, and season to taste with salt and pepper. Simmer for 5 minutes, then transfer to a heated serving dish and serve hot.

STATISTICS PER SERVING:

Energy 301kcals/1,253kJ

Carbohydrate 20g

Sugar 4g

Fibre 6.5g

Fat 12g
Saturated fat 3.5g

Salt 1.5g

PAN FRIED PRAWNS WITH LEMONGRASS AND GINGER

SERVES 2   **PREP** 10 MINS   **COOK** 5 MINS

A quick and simple dish with Thai-inspired flavours.

1 stalk of lemongrass, trimmed,
   tough outer skin removed, and
   finely chopped
5cm (2in) piece of fresh ginger,
   peeled and finely chopped
2 tsp fish sauce
pinch of palm sugar or
   Demerara sugar
1 tsp dried chilli flakes

juice of 1 lime
250g (9oz) large raw prawns,
   shelled, tails intact
2 tsp sunflower oil
handful of fresh coriander leaves,
   finely chopped
1 tbsp dry roasted peanuts,
   finely chopped
lime or lemon wedges, to serve

1 Mix together the lemongrass, ginger, fish sauce, sugar, chilli flakes, and lime juice, then add the prawns and stir to coat.

2 Heat the sunflower oil in a wok, then use a slotted spoon to transfer the prawns to the hot oil and stir fry for 3–5 minutes until the prawns turn pink, then transfer them to a serving dish.

3 Pour the marinade mixture into the wok, heat, and allow to bubble for 1–2 minutes, then pour it over the prawns. Sprinkle with the coriander and peanuts and serve with wedges of lime or lemon to squeeze over. A simple tomato salad makes a good accompaniment for this dish.

STATISTICS PER SERVING:

Energy 171kcals/717kJ

Carbohydrate 2g

Sugar 1.7g

Fibre 0.5g

Fat 7g

Saturated fat 1.2g

Salt 1.5g

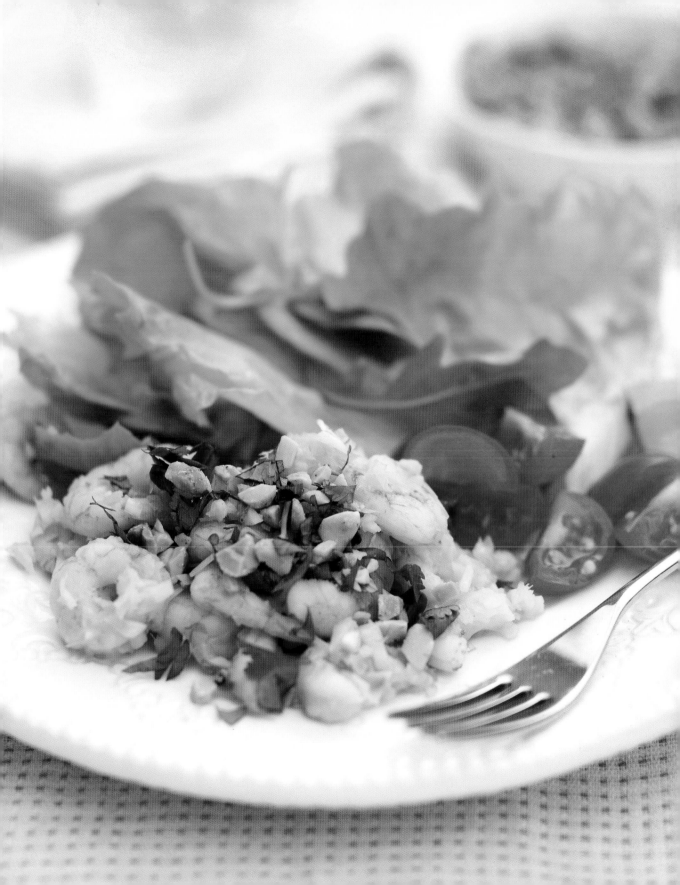

⬤◯◯ GI

⬤⬤◯ CALORIES

⬤◯◯ SATURATED FAT

⬤⬤◯ SALT

HOT AND SOUR NOODLE SALAD WITH TOFU

SERVES 4   **PREP** 25 MINS   **COOK** 20 MINS

An easy, oriental-style salad. Tofu, which is made from soya beans, is a good source of protein and calcium.

2 tbsp sunflower oil
200g (7oz) firm tofu, cut into
   1cm x 3cm (½in x 1¼in) cubes
1 tbsp soy sauce
250g (9oz) medium rice noodles
2 red peppers, deseeded and cut
   into strips
1 white cabbage, shredded
1 red chilli, deseeded and cut
   into strips
2 tbsp fresh coriander leaves, roughly
   chopped

3 spring onions, trimmed and
   finely chopped

For the dressing
3 tbsp rice vinegar
1 tbsp soy sauce
2.5cm (1in) piece of fresh ginger,
   finely chopped
juice of 1 lime
salt and freshly ground black pepper

1 First, make the dressing. Put all the ingredients in a small bowl and whisk together. Season with a little salt and black pepper to taste. Set aside.

2 Put 1 tablespoon of the oil in a wok and, when hot, add half of the tofu and half of the soy sauce (it is easiest to cook the tofu in batches). Stir-fry for 5–10 minutes (depending on the type of tofu being used) until golden all over. Add the remaining 1 tablespoon of oil and fry the rest of the tofu, with the other half of the soy sauce, in the same way. Set aside on a plate covered with kitchen paper.

3 Put the rice noodles in a large bowl and cover with boiling water. Leave for a few minutes, or according to the instructions on the packet, until soft. Drain well.

4 Put the peppers, cabbage, and chilli in a large, shallow serving dish. Top with the drained noodles, and then add the dressing and toss to coat. Arrange the tofu on top and sprinkle with the coriander and spring onions.

STATISTICS PER SERVING:

Energy 381kcals/1,590kJ

Carbohydrate 63g

Sugar 10g

Fibre 3g

Fat 9g

Saturated fat 1g

Salt 1.4g

NOODLES WITH MUSHROOMS AND SESAME SEEDS

SERVES 4   **PREP** 5 MINS   **COOK** 20 MINS

These rich-tasting Japanese noodles work perfectly with woody mushrooms and crisp sugarsnap peas.

GUIDELINES PER SERVING:

● ● ○ GI
● ○ ○ CALORIES
● ○ ○ SATURATED FAT
● ● ○ SALT

1 tbsp sunflower oil
1 onion, sliced
3 garlic cloves, sliced
200g (7oz) sugarsnap peas
salt and freshly ground black pepper
250g (9oz) chestnut mushrooms, quartered

120ml (4fl oz) vegetable stock
175g (6oz) soba wheat noodles with buckwheat
2 tbsp sesame seeds
2 tbsp fresh basil leaves, torn

1 Heat the oil in a wok, add the onion and cook for about 5 minutes until soft and translucent. Add the garlic and stir for a few seconds, then add the sugarsnap peas and stir-fry for a further 5 minutes, moving the ingredients all the time so that the garlic doesn't burn. Season well with salt and black pepper.

2 Add the mushrooms, stir to coat, and cook for a few minutes until they begin to soften. Pour in the stock, a little at a time, and bring to the boil. Reduce to a simmer and cook for a couple of minutes.

3 Meanwhile, cook the noodles in a pan of salted boiling water for 5–7 minutes, then drain well.

4 Stir the noodles into the mushrooms. Sprinkle with sesame seeds and stir in the basil leaves.

STATISTICS PER SERVING:

Energy 270kcals/1,123kJ

Carbohydrate 41g

Sugar 4g

Fibre 2.5g

Fat 8g

Saturated fat 1g

Salt 1g

● ● ○ GI

● ● ○ CALORIES

● ○ ○ SATURATED FAT

● ● ○ SALT

SPICY UDON NOODLES WITH TUNA

SERVES 4 **PREP** 15 MINS **COOK** 15 MINS
PLUS MARINATING

Thick juicy noodles tossed with hot and sweet fresh tuna.

1 tsp wasabi paste
2–3 tbsp dark soy sauce
1–2 tsp runny honey
4 tuna steaks
2 tsp sunflower oil
2 garlic cloves, finely sliced

5cm (2in) piece of fresh root ginger, finely sliced
600g (1lb 5oz) thick udon noodles
handful of coriander leaves
lime wedges, to serve

1 First make the marinade: mix together the wasabi paste, 2 tablespoons of soy sauce, and the honey in a bowl. Add the tuna, turning each steak to coat, and leave to marinate for 15 minutes. Heat a griddle pan, add the tuna steaks (reserving the marinade) two at a time, and cook undisturbed for 2–3 minutes. Turn the steaks over using tongs (they should lift quite easily) and cook on the other side for the same time. The steaks should still be a little pink inside. Remove from the heat and set aside.

2 Heat the sunflower oil in a wok, add the garlic and ginger and keep stirring to prevent burning. Pour in the reserved marinade and allow it to bubble, then add the noodles and stir for a couple of minutes until softened.

3 Slice the tuna into strips, add to the wok, and mix together with the other ingredients. Season with a little extra soy sauce if desired, sprinkle over the coriander, and serve with lime wedges.

COOK'S TIP
Wasabi is Japanese horseradish and is very hot, so use sparingly. You can buy it as powder and add water instead of as a ready-made paste, but be warned that this makes a hotter wasabi.

STATISTICS PER SERVING:

Energy 443kcals/181kJ

Carbohydrate 45g

Sugar 1g

Fibre 2g

Fat 10g

Saturated fat 2g

Salt 1.5g

OYSTER MUSHROOMS WITH PUMPKIN AND MISO

SERVES 4   **PREP** 10 MINS   **COOK** 25 MINS

A rich mixture of sweet vegetables, livened up with the addition of pickled ginger.

1 tbsp sunflower oil
½ small pumpkin, peeled and cut
  into bite-sized pieces
salt and freshly ground black pepper
3 garlic cloves, sliced
1 large tbsp pickled ginger
125g (4½oz) oyster mushrooms,
  large ones halved

1 tbsp sweet white miso
450ml (15fl oz) vegetable stock
600g (1lb 5oz) thick ready-to-wok
  udon noodles
few stalks of spring onions, finely
  sliced, to serve

1 Heat the oil in a wok, add the pumpkin, stir and cook for 5–8 minutes, then add some salt and black pepper. Stir through the garlic and pickled ginger and cook for a few seconds, then add the mushrooms.

2 Add the miso and a little of the stock to the wok and bring to the boil. Reduce to a simmer and add the remaining stock a little at a time, then simmer until the pumpkin is cooked.

3 Add the noodles to the wok, stir through to coat and cook following the packet instructions. Serve sprinkled with sliced spring onion.

GUIDELINES PER SERVING:

●●○ GI
●○○ CALORIES
●○○ SATURATED FAT
●●○ SALT

STATISTICS PER SERVING:

Energy 273kcals/1,141kJ

Carbohydrate 49g

Sugar 3g

Fibre 2g

Fat 5g
Saturated fat 0.5g

Salt 1g

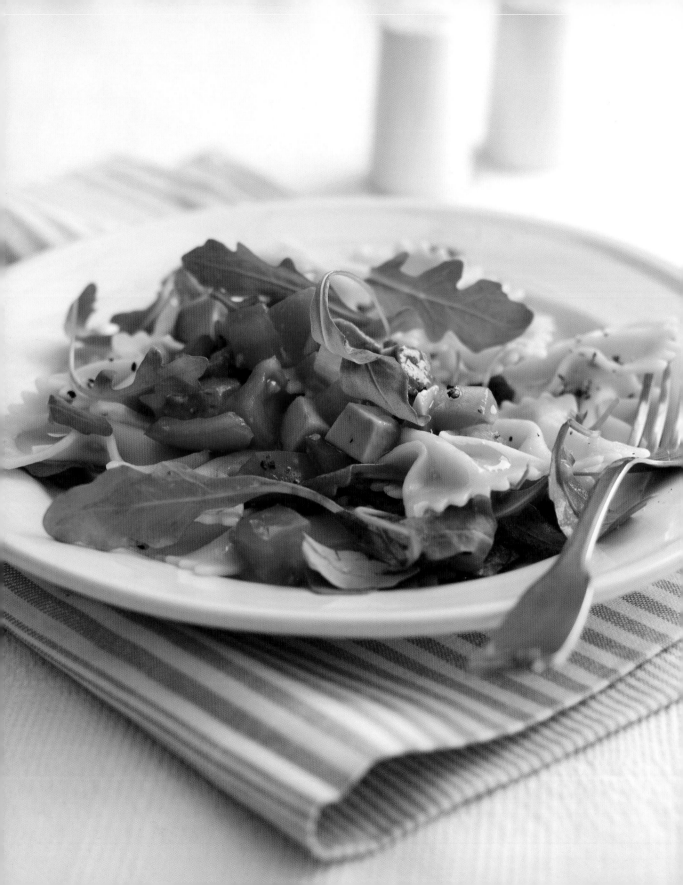

FARFALLE WITH FRESH TOMATOES AND AVOCADO

SERVES 4   **PREP** 10 MINS   **COOK** 15 MINS

A really simple dish – a fresh-tasting no-cook sauce tossed with pasta bows.

5 tomatoes, diced
1 avocado, halved, stoned
  and diced
juice of 1 lemon

salt and freshly ground black pepper
3 tbsp olive oil
350g (12oz) dried farfalle bows
75g (2½oz) wild rocket leaves

1 Place the tomatoes in a bowl with the avocado and lemon juice and season well with salt and pepper. Gently stir to combine, then add the olive oil and stir again. Set aside to allow the flavours to develop.

2 Meanwhile, cook the pasta in a large pan of boiling salted water for 10–12 minutes or according to packet instructions. Drain, return to the pan, and stir in the tomato mixture. Add the rocket leaves and serve straight away.

GUIDELINES PER SERVING:

◕ GI
◕ CALORIES
◔ SATURATED FAT
◔ SALT

STATISTICS PER SERVING:

Energy 387kcals/1,628kJ

Carbohydrate 52g

Sugar 5.5g

Fibre 4.5g

Fat 17g

Saturated fat 3g

Salt trace

LEMON, GARLIC AND PARSLEY LINGUINE

SERVES 4   **PREP** 5 MINS   **COOK** 10 MINS

An instant meal when there is little in the fridge: you just need fresh parsley, garlic, olive oil, and lemon to transform pasta into something special.

350g (12oz) linguine
3 tbsp olive oil
2 garlic cloves, finely chopped
juice of 1 lemon and zest of ½ lemon

handful of fresh flat-leaf parsley, finely chopped
pinch of chilli flakes (optional)
salt and freshly ground black pepper

1 Add the linguine to a large pan of salted boiling water and cook for 8–10 minutes or according to the instructions on the packet. Drain, then return to the pan with a little of the cooking water and toss together.

2 While the pasta is cooking, heat the oil in a frying pan, add the garlic and cook on a very low heat, being very careful not to burn the garlic. Cook for about 1 minute, then add the lemon zest and juice and cook for a couple more minutes.

3 Stir in the parsley and chilli flakes, if using. Season with salt and black pepper and then add the mixture to the pasta and toss to coat. A tomato and basil salad would work well with this dish.

STATISTICS PER SERVING:

Energy 350kcals/1,477kJ

Carbohydrate 65g

Sugar 3g

Fibre 2.5g

Fat 7g

Saturated fat 1g

Salt trace

AVOCADO AND BROWN RICE SALAD

SERVES 4   **PREP** 15 MINS   **COOK** 35 MINS

The creamy texture of avocado complements brown rice; this salad also provides vitamins B6 and E, and heart-friendly essential fats.

175g (6oz) brown basmati rice
300g (10oz) skinless roast chicken, diced
2 ripe avocados, peeled, stoned and diced
6 spring onions, finely sliced
250g (9oz) cherry tomatoes, cut in half

pinch of dried chilli flakes (optional)
salt and freshly ground black pepper

For the dressing
3 tbsp olive oil
1 tbsp balsamic vinegar
1 small garlic clove, crushed

1 Cook the rice in a pan of boiling water according to the instructions on the packet. Once the rice is cooked, drain well and allow to cool.

2 To make the dressing, combine the oil, vinegar, and garlic.

3 Transfer the rice to a serving bowl, stir in the chicken, avocado, spring onions, tomatoes, and chilli flakes, if using. Pour the dressing over the salad and serve immediately.

GUIDELINES PER SERVING:

GI
CALORIES
SATURATED FAT
SALT

STATISTICS PER SERVING:

Energy 511kcals/2,126kJ

Carbohydrate 40g

Sugar 4g

Fibre 3.5g

Fat 26g
Saturated fat 5g

Salt 0.2g

●●○ GI

●○○ CALORIES

●○○ SATURATED FAT

●○○ SALT

TABBOULEH

SERVES 4   **PREP** 20 MINS

This Lebanese speciality of parsley, mint, tomatoes, and bulgur is refreshing all year round.

115g (4oz) bulgur wheat
juice of 2 lemons
75ml (2½fl oz) extra virgin olive oil
freshly ground black pepper
225g (8oz) flat-leaf parsley, coarse
  stalks discarded

75g (2½oz) mint leaves, coarse
  stalks discarded
4 spring onions, finely chopped
2 large tomatoes, deseeded
  and diced
1 head of Little Gem lettuce

1 Put the bulgur wheat in a large bowl, pour over cold water to just cover, and leave to stand for 15 minutes, or until the wheat has absorbed all the water and the grains have swollen.

2 Add the lemon juice and olive oil to the wheat, season to taste with pepper, and stir to mix.

3 Just before serving, finely chop the parsley and mint. Mix the parsley, mint, spring onions, and tomatoes into the wheat.

4 Arrange the lettuce leaves on a serving plate and spoon the salad into the leaves to serve.

STATISTICS PER SERVING:

Energy 241kcals/1,000kJ

Carbohydrate 25g

Sugar 3g

Fibre 1g

Fat 14.5g

Saturated fat 2g

Salt trace

QUINOA TABBOULEH

SERVES 4   **PREP** 10 MINS   **COOK** 20 MINS

In this healthy salad, the quinoa has a creamy, nutty taste with a slight crunch once it is cooked.

200g (7oz) quinoa
½ tsp salt
juice of 1 large lemon
125ml (9fl oz) olive oil
1 large cucumber, peeled, deseeded and chopped
1 large red onion, chopped

45g (1½oz) chopped parsley
45g (1½oz) chopped mint
115g (4oz) reduced-fat feta cheese, crumbled
100g (3½oz) Kalamata olives, pitted
salt and freshly ground black pepper

1 Rinse the quinoa thoroughly in a fine mesh strainer. Drain and place it in a heavy pan. Heat, stirring constantly until the grains separate and begin to brown.

2 Add 600ml (1 pint) water and the salt and bring to the boil, stirring. Reduce the heat and cook for 15 minutes, or until the liquid is absorbed. Transfer to a bowl and set aside to cool.

3 Whisk together the lemon juice and 1 tbsp of the oil in a small bowl. Set aside.

4 Place the remaining oil, cucumber, onion, parsley, and mint in a separate, larger bowl. Add the quinoa and the lemon and oil dressing and toss. Sprinkle with the feta cheese and olives. Season to taste with salt and pepper.

STATISTICS PER SERVING:

Energy 260kcals/1,096kJ

Carbohydrate 32g

Sugar 6g

Fibre 1.5g

Fat 9g
Saturated fat 2.5g

Salt 1.3g

● ● ○ GI

● ● ○ CALORIES

● ○ ○ SATURATED FAT

● ○ ○ SALT

SPICED BULGUR WHEAT WITH FETA AND A FRUITY SALSA

SERVES 4   **PREP** 15 MINS   **COOK** 10 MINS

A tasty grain mixed with salty feta and fresh beans.

280g (10oz) bulgur wheat
300ml (10fl oz) hot vegetable stock
150g (5½oz) fine green beans,
  chopped into 1cm (½in) pieces
salt and freshly ground black pepper
125g (4½oz) reduced fat Feta
  cheese, crumbled

For the salsa
½ fresh pineapple, diced
1 mango, diced
juice of ½–1 lime
1 red chilli, deseeded and
  finely chopped

1 First, make the salsa: mix all the ingredients together in a small bowl and leave to sit for a while to allow the flavours to develop.

2 Tip the bulgur wheat into a large heatproof bowl and pour over the stock; it should just cover it – if not, add a little extra hot water. Allow to sit for 8–10 minutes then fluff up with a fork, separating the grains.

3 Add the beans to a pan of salted boiling water and cook for 3–5 minutes until they just soften but still have a bite to them. Drain and stir into the bulgur wheat. Season well with salt and pepper, then stir in the Feta. Add a spoonful of the fruity salsa on the side and serve. You can enjoy this on its own, with a few salad leaves, or for a more substantial meal you could add a piece of grilled chicken.

COOK'S TIP
Bulgur wheat needs lot of flavour added to it, otherwise it can be bland, so make sure you use a well-flavoured stock.

STATISTICS PER SERVING:

Energy 370kcals/1,547kJ

Carbohydrate 70g

Sugar 16g

Fibre 2.5g

Fat 4g

Saturated fat 2g

Salt 0.5g

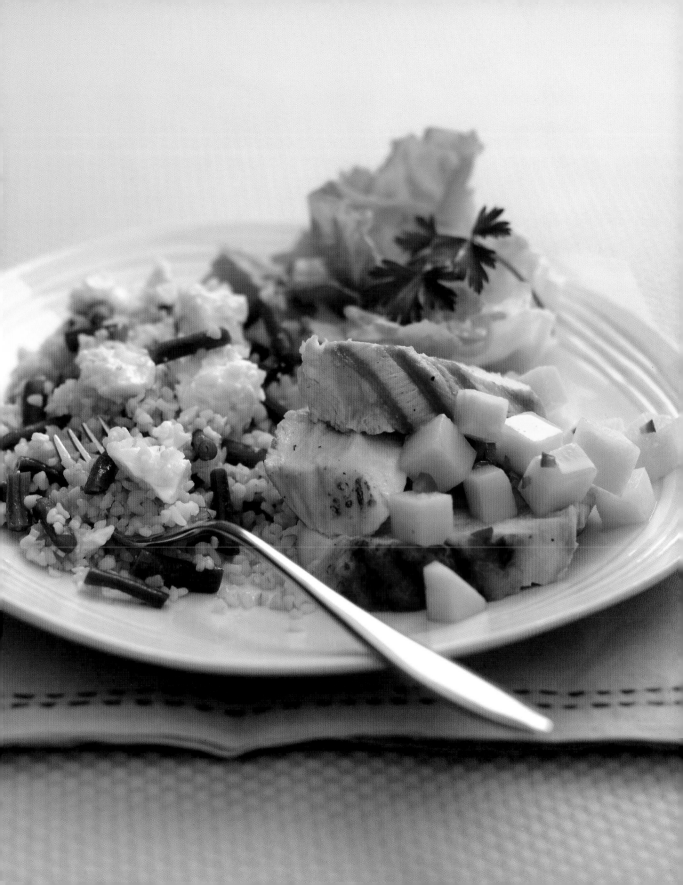

THREE-GRAIN SALAD

SERVES 6   **PREP** 5 MINS   **COOK** 35 MINS

A real good-for-you, wholesome salad mix. The mixture of grains is rich in B-vitamins, minerals, and fibre.

150g (5½oz) brown rice
125g (4½oz) bulgur wheat
125g (4½oz) couscous
4 tomatoes, diced
½ cucumber, peeled and diced

50g (1¾oz) fresh mint, finely chopped
50g (1¾oz) fresh parsley, finely chopped
30g (1oz) raisins
salt and freshly ground black pepper

1 Cook the rice in a pan of salted water for about 35 minutes until tender, or follow the instructions on the packet. Drain and set aside to cool.

2 Tip the bulgur wheat into a bowl and pour boiling water over it until it is just covered. Leave to stand for 5 minutes while you prepare the couscous in another bowl in the same way; leave this also for 5 minutes. Fluff up both the grains with a fork and then mix them together with the rice.

3 Stir the tomatoes, cucumber, herbs, and raisins into the grain mixture. Taste and then season if needed.

STATISTICS PER SERVING:

Energy 381kcals/1,385kJ

Carbohydrate 73g

Sugar 6g

Fibre 2g

Fat 2g

Saturated fat 0.5g

Salt trace

BULGUR WHEAT WITH AUBERGINE AND POMEGRANATE

GUIDELINES PER SERVING:

● ● ○ GI

● ● ○ CALORIES

● ○ ○ SATURATED FAT

● ○ ○ SALT

SERVES 4   **PREP** 5 MINS   **COOK** 25 MINS

A nutritious dish, full of colour and texture. The nuts and seeds add a crunch as well as a vitamin and mineral boost.

2 tbsp olive oil
2 aubergines, chopped into
  bite-sized pieces
pinch of paprika
275g (9½oz) bulgur wheat

300ml (10fl oz) hot vegetable stock
salt and freshly ground black pepper
75g (3oz) hazelnuts, toasted
75g (3oz) pomegranate seeds

1 Put half the oil in a large frying pan set over a low heat, and toss the aubergines in the oil. Cook on a fairly high heat for 10–15 minutes or until the aubergine starts to turn golden, adding the remaining oil when needed (you may need to add extra oil as the aubergine will soak it up quickly). Add the paprika, toss, and cook for a few more minutes. Remove from the heat and set aside.

2 Put the bulgur wheat into a large bowl and pour the stock over it so that it is just covered; use extra stock if needed. Cover with cling film and leave for 8–10 minutes, then fluff up with a fork to separate the grains.

3 Stir the bulgur wheat into the pan with the aubergine and mix well. Taste and season as required. Stir in the hazelnuts and sprinkle with the pomegranate seeds.

COOK'S TIP

Buy pomegranate seeds in a vacuum pack as they are far easier to use than having to extract them from a fresh pomegranate. However, if you prefer to use a fresh fruit, keep the juice and use it in a salad dressing.

STATISTICS PER SERVING:

Energy 454kcals/1,891kJ

Carbohydrate 59g

Sugar 5g

Fibre 4g

Fat 20g

Saturated fat 2g

Salt 0.4g

● ○ ○ GI

● ● ○ CALORIES

● ○ ○ SATURATED FAT

● ○ ○ SALT

CHICKPEA, BULGUR, AND WALNUT SALAD

SERVES 4 **PREP** 10 MINS

A hearty and filling salad with nuts, fruits, and grains.

125g (4½oz) bulgur wheat
salt and freshly ground black pepper
400g can of chickpeas, drained
  and rinsed
1 sweet crisp apple, cored,
  and diced

handful of walnuts, roughly chopped
25g (scant 1oz) dried cranberries
juice of 1 lemon
½ tsp paprika
2–3 tbsp olive oil

1 Put the bulgur wheat in a bowl and pour over enough hot water to cover. Set aside and leave to stand for about 5 minutes, then fluff up the grains with a with fork. Season with salt and black pepper.

2 Put the chickpeas in another bowl, then add the apple, walnuts, and cranberries and stir to combine.

3 Tip in the bulgur wheat and lemon juice, sprinkle over the paprika, and stir. Drizzle over a little olive oil and serve.

COOK'S TIP
You could gently warm the chickpeas in a pan, still in their water, as it softens them and helps to bring out their flavour.

STATISTICS PER SERVING:

Energy 331kcals/1,379kJ

Carbohydrate 40g

Sugar 4g

Fibre 5g

Fat 11g
Saturated fat 1g

Salt trace

MOROCCAN TOMATOES, PEPPERS, AND HERBS

● ○ ○ GI

● ○ ○ CALORIES

● ○ ○ SATURATED FAT

● ○ ○ SALT

SERVES 4   **PREP** 15 MINS   **COOK** 30 MINS

A colourful vegetarian dish scented with herbs and spices.

2 onions, sliced
400g (14oz) cherry tomatoes, halved
2 red peppers, deseeded and
  roughly chopped
2 green peppers, deseeded
  and roughly chopped
pinch of dried oregano
pinch of chilli flakes

pinch of ground cinnamon
salt and freshly ground black pepper
2 tbsp olive oil
juice of 1 lemon
handful of fresh flat-leaf
  parsley, finely chopped
handful of fresh mint, finely chopped

1 Preheat the oven to 180°C (350°F/Gas 4). Put the onions, tomatoes, and peppers in a roasting tin and sprinkle over the oregano, chilli flakes, and cinnamon. Season with salt and black pepper. Add 1 tablespoon of the oil and toss together using your hands to coat the vegetables evenly. Roast for 30 minutes or until they are soft and just beginning to char.

2 Remove the vegetables from the oven, drizzle over the remaining olive oil, squeeze over the lemon juice and add the parsley and mint. Toss it all together and serve.

COOK'S TIP
You could use different herbs such as coriander or dill, if you prefer.

STATISTICS PER SERVING:

Energy 142kcals/593kJ

Carbohydrate 18.5g

Sugar 15g

Fibre 4.5g

Fat 7g

Saturated fat 1g

Salt trace

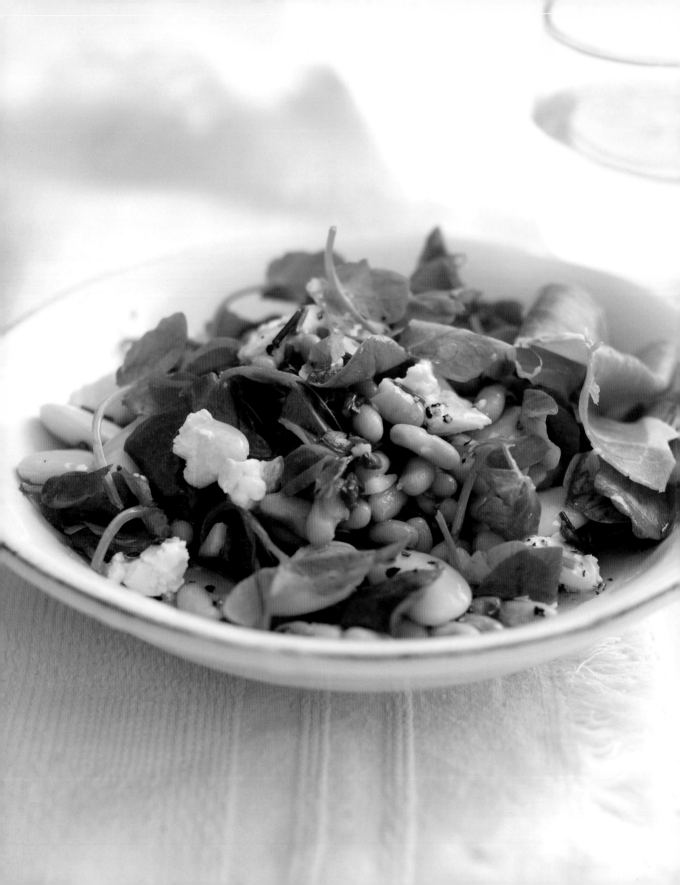

MIXED BEAN AND GOAT'S CHEESE SALAD

GUIDELINES PER SERVING:

⬤◯◯ GI

⬤◯◯ CALORIES

⬤⬤◯ SATURATED FAT

⬤◯◯ SALT

SERVES 4   **PREP** 10 MINS

The mealy beans complement the rich cheese.

400g tin of butter beans,
  drained and rinsed
400g tin of flageolet beans,
  drained and rinsed
25g (scant 1oz) bunch of chives,
  finely chopped
2 tsp white wine vinegar
1 tbsp of fruity olive oil plus
  extra to serve

1 tbsp of fresh thyme leaves
pinch of chilli flakes
salt and freshly ground black pepper
50g packet of pea shoots
lemon juice, to season (optional)
100g (3½oz) semi-hard goat's cheese,
  broken up into pieces

1 Put the beans in a large bowl and add the chives, vinegar, olive oil, thyme, and chilli flakes and stir to combine. Season well with salt and black pepper.

2 Stir through the pea shoots, taste and add a squeeze of lemon if you wish. Transfer to a shallow serving dish and top with the goat's cheese, a drizzle of olive oil and a twist of freshly ground black pepper. If you are a meat eater, you might try a little Serrano ham as an accompaniment.

COOK'S TIP

If you prefer, you could use a soft goat's cheese and toss it with the beans; it will become almost like a thick, creamy dressing. You can also substitute rocket for the pea shoots.

STATISTICS PER SERVING:

Energy 280kcals/1,170kJ

Carbohydrate 30g

Sugar 3g

Fibre 8.5g

Fat 11g

Saturated fat 5g

Salt 0.2g

COURGETTE, FETA, BEAN, AND PEA SALAD

SERVES 4   **PREP** 5 MINS   **COOK** 10 MINS

A fresh and light salad to serve as a main meal or side dish. Containing protein from plant and dairy sources, this quick salad ticks several nutritional boxes .

300g (10oz) frozen peas
1 tbsp olive oil
3 small courgettes, diced
salt and freshly ground black pepper
2 garlic cloves, finely chopped
150g (5½oz) feta cheese, crumbled
400g can borlotti beans, drained
  and rinsed

½ red onion, finely chopped
2 heads baby gem lettuce,
  sliced lengthways

For the dressing
3 tbsp extra virgin olive oil
1 tbsp raspberry vinegar
1 tbsp fresh rosemary, finely chopped

1 Put the peas in a bowl and pour in enough boiling water to just cover them. Leave for 3 minutes, drain, then refresh with cold water, drain again and set aside.

2 Heat the olive oil in a large frying pan, tip in the courgettes and fry for 3 minutes or until beginning to soften and turn a light golden colour. Season with salt and black pepper, then stir in the garlic and cook for a few seconds. Remove from the heat, transfer to a bowl and leave to cool.

3 Add the feta, borlotti beans, and onion to the peas. Stir, then add the courgettes and lettuce and mix to combine.

4 Finally, make the dressing: mix the olive oil, vinegar, and rosemary in a jug and season. Drizzle the dressing over the salad just before serving, tossing it gently so that it is all coated.

COOK'S TIP
Small courgettes will be sweetest, but if not available, use two large ones instead.

STATISTICS PER SERVING:

Energy 360kcals/1,498kJ

Carbohydrate 26g

Sugar 5g

Fibre 10g

Fat 20g

Saturated fat 7g

Salt 1.3g

EDAMAME, GREEN BEAN, AND SUGARSNAP SALAD

GUIDELINES PER SERVING:

● ○ ○ GI
● ○ ○ CALORIES
● ○ ○ SATURATED FAT
● ○ ○ SALT

SERVES 4   **PREP** 10 MINS   **COOK** 5 MINS

Edamame beans (fresh soya beans) are usually bought frozen and are useful to have in reserve in the freezer. You can use them in a salad or add them to a casserole.

200g (7oz) frozen edamame beans
  (soya beans)
200g (7oz) green beans, trimmed
200g (7oz) sugarsnap peas
225g (8oz) cherry tomatoes,
  sliced in half

3 spring onions, finely chopped
2 tbsp chopped fresh coriander
3 tbsp rice wine vinegar
3 tbsp sweet chilli dipping sauce

1 Place the edamame beans in a large pan of boiling water for 3 minutes. Add the green beans and sugarsnap peas, and cook for 2 minutes. Refresh under cold running water and then drain well.

2 Place the beans and sugarsnap peas in a large bowl. Add the cherry tomatoes, spring onions, and coriander.

3 Whisk together the vinegar and sweet chilli sauce. Drizzle it over the vegetables, toss well and serve.

STATISTICS PER SERVING:

Energy 142kcals/595kJ

Carbohydrate 18g

Sugar 11g

Fibre 5g

Fat 4g
Saturated fat 0.7g

Salt 0.3g

○○○ GI

●○○ CALORIES

●○○ SATURATED FAT

●○○ SALT

LENTIL SALAD WITH LEMON AND ALMONDS

SERVES 6   **PREP** 10 MINS
PLUS STANDING   **COOK** 15-20 MINS

Puy lentils have a crisp taste when combined with the refreshing flavours of fragrant coriander and preserved lemon.

400g (14oz) Puy (French) green lentils
2 preserved lemons, rinsed and cut
  into small dice
2 tbsp chopped coriander
2 spring onions, thinly sliced

3 tbsp red wine vinegar
100ml (3½fl oz) extra virgin olive oil
salt and freshly ground black pepper
4 tbsp flaked almonds, toasted
coriander leaves, to garnish

1 Bring a large pan of water to the boil and add the lentils. Return to the boil, reduce the heat, cover, and simmer for 15–20 minutes, or until the lentils are just tender. Drain, then rinse quickly in cold water and drain well.

2 Place the lentils into a large bowl and stir in the diced lemons, chopped coriander, and half the spring onions. Whisk together the wine vinegar and oil, season to taste with salt and pepper, and stir into the lentils.

3 Cover the salad and leave to stand for 20 minutes to allow the flavours to develop.

4 Mix the almonds with the remaining spring onion and the coriander leaves, then scatter over the salad and toss lightly to serve.

COOK'S TIP
Leftovers can be mixed with cooked leftover wild rice to make a tasty accompaniment to Middle Eastern dishes.

STATISTICS PER SERVING:

Energy 364kcals/1,527kJ

Carbohydrate 33g

Sugar 1g

Fibre 6g

Fat 19g

Saturated fat 2.5g

Salt trace

CARROT AND ORANGE SALAD

GUIDELINES PER SERVING:

● ● ○ GI

● ○ ○ CALORIES

● ○ ○ SATURATED FAT

● ○ ○ SALT

SERVES 4   **PREP** 20 MINS

This light, colourful salad is excellent as a refreshing summer lunch.

2 large carrots
2 large navel oranges
1 fennel bulb
85g (3oz) watercress

For the dressing
3 tbsp light olive oil
3 tbsp grapeseed oil or sunflower oil

1 tbsp lemon juice
3 tbsp orange juice
1 tsp clear honey
salt and freshly ground black pepper
2 tsp sesame seeds, lightly toasted

1 Trim and peel the carrots using a vegetable peeler to make thin strips.

2 Cut away the peel and pith from the oranges and divide into segments. Do this over a bowl to catch any juice, and use this in the dressing. Trim the fennel and thinly slice. Remove any yellow leaves or tough stalks from the watercress.

3 Put the carrot, orange, fennel, and watercress into a serving bowl. Whisk together the dressing ingredients and pour over. Toss lightly so all the ingredients are coated in the dressing, and serve.

STATISTICS PER SERVING:

Energy 231kcals/957kJ

Carbohydrate 14g

Sugar 13g

Fibre 4g

Fat 18.5g

Saturated fat 2.5g

Salt trace

● ○ ○   GI

● ● ○   CALORIES

● ● ○   SATURATED FAT

● ○ ○   SALT

SQUASH SALAD WITH AVOCADO

SERVES 4   **PREP** 15 MINS   **COOK** 25 MINS

A wonderful combination of sweet squash, peppery leaves, and hot chilli.

1 butternut squash, chopped
  into chunks
1 tbsp olive oil
salt and freshly ground
  black pepper
1–2 tsp chilli flakes
250g (9oz) wild rocket leaves
250g (9oz) spinach leaves
2 ripe avocados, peeled, stoned,
  and sliced

2 tomatoes, skinned and finely
  chopped
1 tbsp flat-leaf parsley

For the dressing
3 tbsp olive oil
1 tbsp lemon juice
zest of ½ lemon
½ tsp mayonnaise

1 Preheat the oven to 200°C (400°F/Gas 6). First, make the dressing: put all the ingredients in a small bowl or jug and whisk to combine. Season to taste with salt and pepper and set aside.

2 Put the butternut squash in a large roasting tin, drizzle with the olive oil and mix well with your hands. Season with salt and pepper, and sprinkle with the chilli flakes. Roast in the oven for 20–30 minutes or until soft and beginning to char. Remove from the oven and allow to cool slightly (this will prevent the spinach from wilting).

3 Tip the rocket and spinach leaves into a large serving bowl and add the avocado pieces. Top with the squash and toss gently to combine, then scatter the chopped tomatoes on top. When ready to serve, whisk the dressing and drizzle it over the salad. Finish with a sprinkling of parsley.

COOK'S TIP
Squeeze a little lemon juice over the avocados to prevent them from discolouring.

STATISTICS PER SERVING:

Energy 345kcals/1,434kJ

Carbohydrate 19g

Sugar 11g

Fibre 8g

Fat 27g

Saturated fat 5g

Salt 0.3g

BUTTERNUT SQUASH, TOMATO, AND PEARL BARLEY SALAD

GUIDELINES PER SERVING:

⬤⬤◯ GI

⬤⬤◯ CALORIES

⬤◯◯ SATURATED FAT

⬤◯◯ SALT

SERVES 2   **PREP** 20 MINS   **COOK** 40 MINS

Barley is a low-GI food and its deliciously chewy texture works well in salads.

½ small butternut squash, cut into
  1cm (½in) cubes (about 300g/10oz
  prepared weight)
2 tbsp olive oil
salt and freshly ground black pepper
pinch of chilli flakes

85g (3oz) pearl barley
500ml (16fl oz) vegetable stock
4 plum tomatoes
3 spring onions, finely sliced
75g (2½oz) rocket

1 Preheat the oven to 200°C (400°F/Gas 6). Place the squash in a roasting tin and drizzle 1 tablespoon of the oil over it. Season with salt and black pepper and scatter the chilli flakes on top. Put in the oven and cook for 30–40 minutes until the squash is soft and starting to brown around the edges.

2 Place the barley in a small saucepan and pour in the stock. Bring to the boil and then reduce the heat, cover, and simmer for 20–30 minutes. Add a little more stock or water if needed.

3 Slice the tomatoes into quarters and remove the seeds. Pat the flesh dry with kitchen paper and place the segments in a clean roasting tin. Drizzle with the remaining oil and cook in the oven for 20–30 minutes until soft and beginning to brown.

4 Allow the barley to cool for 10 minutes, then stir in the squash, tomatoes, spring onions, and rocket.

STATISTICS PER SERVING:

Energy 345kcals/1,442kJ

Carbohydrate 28g

Sugar 14g

Fibre 2g

Fat 11g
Saturated fat 2g

Salt 0.4g

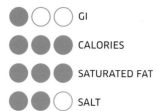

SALMON SALAD WITH RASPBERRY DRESSING

SERVES 4   **PREP** 10 MINS   **COOK** 25 MINS

The fruity dressing adds a spot of glamour to this dish and cuts through the rich salmon.

4 salmon fillets, about 400g
  (14oz) in total
1 tbsp olive oil
few stalks of fresh thyme,
  leaves only
salt and freshly ground black pepper
75g (2½oz) broad beans, fresh (out of
  their pods) or frozen
250g (9oz) baby spinach leaves

25g (scant 1oz) hazelnuts, toasted
  and roughly chopped
75g (2½oz) reduced-fat Feta cheese,
  crumbled

For the dressing
3 tbsp olive oil
1 tbsp raspberry vinegar

1 Preheat the oven to 180°C (350°F/Gas 4). To make the dressing, mix the olive oil and raspberry vinegar together, season well with salt and pepper, and leave for the flavours to develop.

2 Arrange the salmon fillets in a roasting tin, drizzle over the olive oil, and scatter the thyme leaves over. Season with salt and pepper and bake in the oven for 15 minutes until the fish is cooked and flakes easily. Remove from the oven and set aside to cool.

3 Cook the broad beans in a pan of boiling salted water for 8 minutes or until tender, then drain, refresh with cold water, and drain again. Arrange the spinach leaves on a platter, flake over the fish and add the broad beans. Sprinkle over the hazelnuts and Feta and drizzle with the dressing when ready to serve.

COOK'S TIP
You can toast hazelnuts in a small frying pan over a medium-high heat: cook for 5 minutes, moving them around regularly to prevent burning. Alternatively, roast them in a hot oven for 5 minutes, again keeping a close eye on them.

STATISTICS PER SERVING:

Energy 752kcals/3,118kJ

Carbohydrate 6g

Sugar 3g

Fibre 6g

Fat 56g

Saturated fat 10g

Salt 1.1g

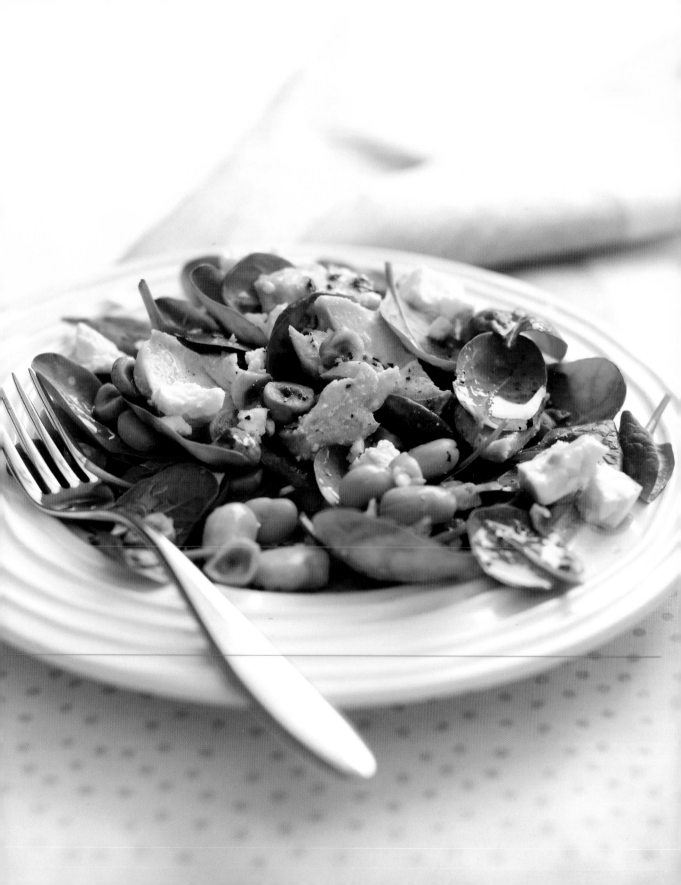

● ○ ○ GI

● ● ○ CALORIES

● ● ○ SATURATED FAT

● ● ○ SALT

CRAB AND AVOCADO SALAD WITH VINAIGRETTE

SERVES 4   **PREP** 5 MINS

Fresh white crabmeat is a treat: here it is pepped up with chilli and herbs and served with dressed salad leaves.

300g (10oz) fresh white crabmeat
2 ripe avocados, peeled, stoned,
  and diced
25g (scant 1oz) chives, finely chopped
25g (scant 1oz) dill, finely chopped
25g (scant 1oz) parsley, finely chopped
½ red chilli, deseeded and finely
  chopped
salt and freshly ground black pepper

100g (3½oz) mixed salad leaves
4 lemon wedges, to serve

For the dressing
3 tbsp olive oil
1 tbsp cider vinegar
½ tsp paprika
2 tsp capers, finely chopped
½ tsp mayonnaise

1 Put the crabmeat and avocado in a bowl along with the herbs and the chilli, stir well, and season with salt and black pepper.

2 Mix together all the dressing ingredients. Taste the dressing and season if necessary.

3 Lay the salad leaves on a serving plate or individual plates and top with the crabmeat mixture. Drizzle with the dressing and serve with the lemon wedges.

STATISTICS PER SERVING:

Energy 323kcals/1,334kJ

Carbohydrate 2g

Sugar 0.5g

Fibre 2.5g

Fat 28g

Saturated fat 5g

Salt 1g

COOK'S TIP
Prepare the crab mixture and dressing ahead and keep them in refrigerator, covered, until needed. Don't prepare the crab mixture more than 1–2 hours ahead. To prevent the avocado from discolouring, toss it in a little lemon juice.

CHICKEN SALAD WITH FRUIT AND NUTS

SERVES 4   **PREP** 10 MINS

A protein-rich, fruity salad with a creamy, lightly curried dressing – low in saturated fat and utterly delicious.

350g (12oz) ready-cooked chicken, thickly shredded
1 small, crisp lettuce (such as iceberg or romaine), shredded
25g (scant 1oz) salted peanuts
25g (scant 1oz) cashew nuts
½ fresh pineapple, peeled, cored, and cut into segments
1 mango, stoned and cut into bite-sized pieces

For the dressing
3–4 tbsp reduced-fat Greek-style yogurt
pinch of mild curry powder (add more according to your liking), plus extra to garnish
juice of ½ lime
salt and freshly ground black pepper

1 First, make the dressing. Mix the ingredients together in a small bowl or jug and season with salt and black pepper. Set aside.

2 Put the chicken, lettuce, and nuts in a large bowl and toss gently to combine. Pour the dressing over the salad and mix well to coat.

3 When ready to serve, combine the pineapple and mango with the salad and add a pinch of black pepper. Transfer to a serving bowl and sprinkle with a little curry powder.

COOK'S TIP
Greek yogurt is also available in a fat-free version. The reduced-fat and fat-free types are thinner than full-fat yogurt, so you sometimes need to use a little more of them.

GUIDELINES PER SERVING:

GI
CALORIES
SATURATED FAT
SALT

STATISTICS PER SERVING:

Energy 312kcals/1,310kJ

Carbohydrate 20g

Sugar 18g

Fibre 3.5g

Fat 14g
Saturated fat 3g

Salt 0.2g

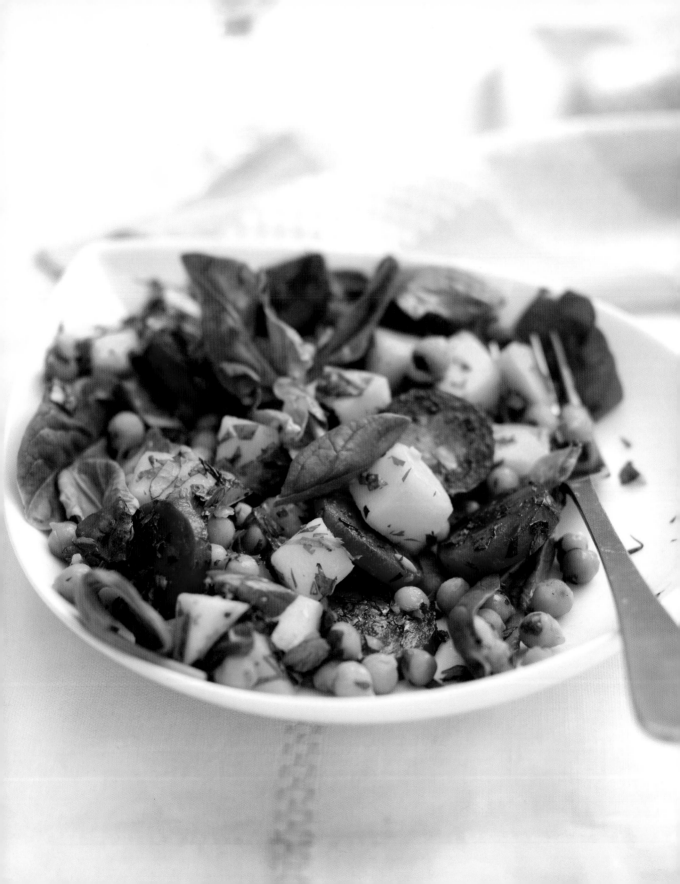

CHORIZO, CHICKPEA, AND MANGO SALAD

SERVES 2   **PREP** 15 MINS   **COOK** 15 MINS

A hearty, main meal salad with great variety of flavour.

GUIDELINES PER SERVING:

●○○ GI
●●● CALORIES
●●● SATURATED FAT
●●○ SALT

1 tbsp olive oil
150g (5½oz) chorizo,
  roughly chopped
400g can of chickpeas,
  drained and rinsed
3 cloves of garlic, finely chopped
handful of flat-leaf parsley,
  finely chopped
1 tbsp dry sherry

2 ripe mangos, stoned,
  and flesh diced
small handful of fresh basil,
  roughly chopped
small handful of fresh mint leaves,
  roughly chopped
small handful of fresh coriander
  leaves, roughly chopped
250g (9oz) baby spinach leaves

1 Heat the olive oil in a frying pan, add the chorizo and chickpeas and cook over a low heat for 1 minute, then add the garlic and parsley and cook for a further minute. Add the sherry and cook for 10 minutes, stirring occasionally.

2 Put the mango and remaining herbs in a bowl and toss together, then add the chickpea mixture and combine well. Spoon onto a bed of spinach to serve.

COOK'S TIP
Choose a full-flavoured, spicy chorizo; it will marry well with the chickpeas.

STATISTICS PER SERVING:

Energy 504kcals/2,106kJ

Carbohydrate 31g

Sugar 5.5g

Fibre 2.5g

Fat 24g
Saturated fat 8g

Salt 1.5g

WATERCRESS, BRESAOLA AND WALNUTS

SERVES 4   **PREP** 7 MINS

The sharpness of watercress is delicious with bresaola, an air-dried beef. The fruity dressing complements both.

2 bunches of really fresh watercress,
  stalks trimmed
8 slices bresaola
1 fennel bulb, trimmed and
  finely shredded
20g (¾oz) walnuts, roughly chopped

For the dressing
3 tbsp extra virgin olive oil
1 tbsp white wine vinegar
juice of 1 orange
1 tsp horseradish sauce (hot
  or creamed)
salt and freshly ground black pepper

1 First, make the dressing. Put all the ingredients in a small bowl or jug and whisk until combined. Season well with salt and black pepper and set aside.

2 Scatter the watercress in a large, shallow serving bowl and top with the bresaola.

3 Add the fennel, toss to combine and sprinkle the walnuts on top. When ready to serve, drizzle with some of the dressing – you may not need it all.

COOK'S TIP
Make sure you buy good-quality bresaola, preferably from a delicatessen.

STATISTICS PER SERVING:

Energy 140kcals/569kJ

Carbohydrate 1g

Sugar 0.9g

Fibre 2g

Fat 11g

Saturated fat 2g

Salt 0.7g

SPINACH, FETA AND DATE SALAD

SERVES 2   **PREP** 10 MINS

A refreshing, tangy salad with an interesting mix of sweet and sour flavours.

GUIDELINES PER SERVING:

GI

CALORIES

SATURATED FAT

SALT

150g (5½oz) baby spinach leaves
50g (1¾oz) fresh dates, stoned and
  chopped
50g (1¾oz) pine nuts, toasted
125g (4½oz) reduced-fat feta cheese,
  crumbled or cut into small cubes
salt and freshly ground black pepper
2 preserved lemons, halved, pith
  removed and skin finely chopped

For the dressing
1 tbsp olive oil
splash of white wine vinegar
salt and freshly ground black pepper
½ tsp Dijon mustard
few stalks of fresh dill, finely chopped

1 First, make the dressing: mix together the oil and vinegar and season with salt and black pepper, then stir in the mustard and the dill. Taste and adjust as needed, then set aside.

2 Tip the spinach leaves into a bowl and add the dates, pine nuts, and feta. Season if desired (if you are using a salty feta you may not need to add salt).

3 When ready to serve, whisk the dressing, pour into an empty salad bowl, and swirl until the dressing coats the bowl. Add the leaf and feta mixture and very gently toss with your hands to lightly coat the leaves. Sprinkle with the chopped lemon and serve.

COOK'S TIP
Buy medjool dates if you can, these are larger and sweeter than other varieties.

STATISTICS PER SERVING:

Energy 352kcals/1,459kJ

Carbohydrate 10g

Sugar 10g

Fibre 3g

Fat 27g
Saturated fat 5g

Salt 1g

GRILLED HALLOUMI AND ROAST TOMATO SALAD

SERVES 4   **PREP** 5 MINS   **COOK** 15 MINS

A perfect balance of rich and fresh flavours.

200g cherry tomatoes, halved
3 tbsp olive oil
salt and freshly ground black pepper
250g (9oz) halloumi, cut into
 5mm- (¼in-) thick slices
3 cloves of garlic, finely chopped

small handful of flat leaf parsley,
 finely chopped
½ tsp paprika
small handful of fresh basil,
 roughly chopped
250g (9oz) fresh baby spinach leaves

1 Preheat the oven to 180°C (350°F/Gas 4). Place the tomatoes in a small roasting tin, drizzle with 1 tablespoon of the oil and season with salt and pepper. Toss together using your hands, then roast in the oven for 15 minutes with the tomatoes sitting skin side down.

2 While they are cooking, put the halloumi, garlic, parsley, paprika, and the remaining oil into a bowl and combine well. Heat a griddle pan until hot then carefully add a slice of halloumi, letting it drain before adding it to the pan. Repeat, adding the halloumi slices one by one until they are all in the griddle pan. When you have added the last one, go back to the first one and begin turning them over to cook on the other side. They should be golden brown. When you have turned them all, go back to the first one and begin removing them from the griddle pan.

3 Put the halloumi slices back into the bowl with the garlic, herb, and spice mix and stir gently. Add the cooked tomatoes to the mix along with the basil and stir to combine so everything is well coated. Add the spinach leaves, toss together, and serve straight away on a shallow platter.

STATISTICS PER SERVING:

Energy 293kcals/1,221kJ

Carbohydrate 3.5g

Sugar 2.5g

Fibre 1.5g

Fat 24g

Saturated fat 12g

Salt 1.7g

COOK'S TIP
It is important to serve this straight away, as the hot mixture will begin to wilt the spinach. Alternatively, you could allow the mixture to cool completely before adding the spinach.

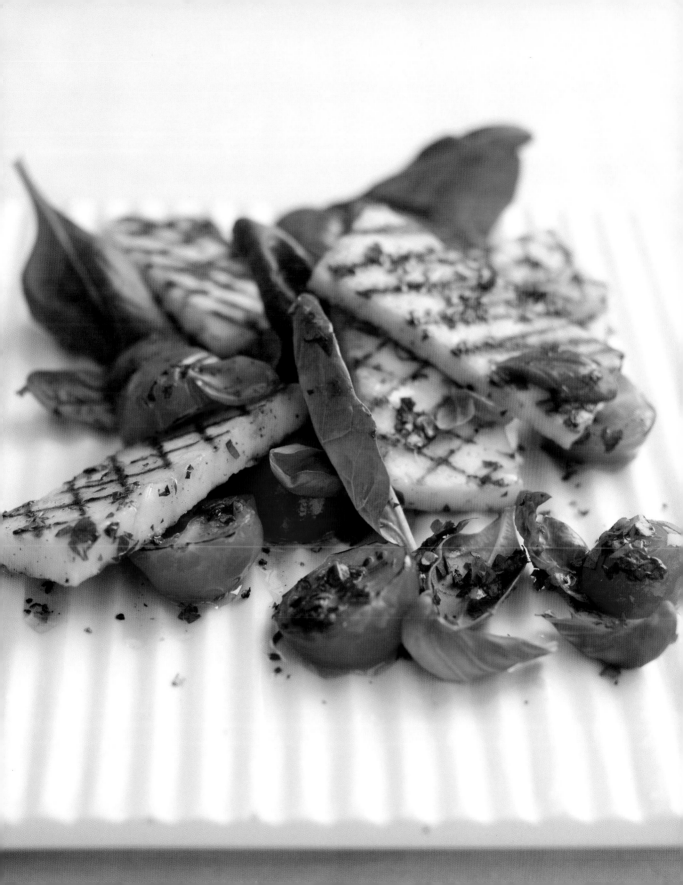

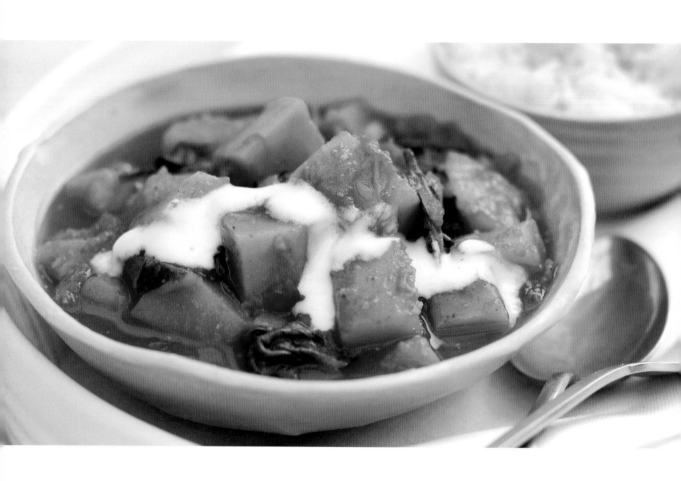

SIMPLE SUPPERS
– VEGETARIAN

UDON NOODLES WITH SWEET AND SOUR TOFU

SERVES 4   **PREP** 5 MINS   **COOK** 10 MINS

Pickled ginger gives noodles and tofu an unusual twist, complemented by a tangy sweet and sour sauce.

2 tbsp sunflower oil
1 tbsp pickled ginger
250g (9oz) firm tofu, cut into cubes
salt and freshly ground black pepper
300g (10oz) udon noodles

For the sweet and sour sauce
1 tbsp sunflower oil
3 garlic cloves, finely chopped

5cm (2in) piece of fresh root ginger, cut into fine strips
pinch of brown sugar
10 cherry tomatoes, halved
4 spring onions, finely chopped
1 tbsp dark soy sauce
1 tbsp rice vinegar
1 tbsp Chinese cooking wine

1 First, make the sauce. Pour 1 tablespoon of sunflower oil into a wok, then add the garlic and fresh ginger and cook for 1 minute. Tip in the sugar and stir for a few seconds, then add the tomatoes and spring onions. Keep stirring for a few more minutes, until the tomatoes start to break down (you can squash them with the back of a fork).

2 Add the soy sauce, vinegar, and cooking wine. Bring to the boil, reduce to a simmer and cook for a couple of minutes.

3 Fry the tofu in 2 tablespoons of sunflower oil until golden. Stir the tofu and pickled ginger into the sweet and sour sauce. Taste, and season with salt and black pepper if required.

4 To finish, stir in the noodles and wait until they soften (about 2 minutes), then serve.

STATISTICS PER SERVING:

Energy 281kcals/1,173kJ

Carbohydrate 30g

Sugar 3g

Fibre 0.5g

Fat 13.5g

Saturated fat 2g

Salt 1g

SPAGHETTI WITH COURGETTES AND TOASTED ALMONDS

SERVES 4   **PREP** 10 MINS   **COOK** 15 MINS

Lemony courgettes add a real zing to this quick pasta dish, which is sprinkled with crunchy toasted almonds.

300g (10oz) spaghetti
2 tbsp olive oil
2 courgettes, diced
2 courgettes, grated
salt and freshly ground black pepper

2 garlic cloves, finely chopped
juice of 1 lemon
pinch of dried oregano
25g (scant 1oz) flaked almonds,
  toasted (see Cook's Tip)

1 Cook the pasta in a large pan of salted boiling water for 8–10 minutes, or according to the instructions on the packet.

2 Meanwhile, heat the olive oil in a large frying pan. Add all the courgettes, together with a pinch of salt and some black pepper. Cook for 5–8 minutes until soft and just beginning to turn golden at the edges. Stir in the garlic and cook for a few more seconds, then add the lemon juice and oregano and simmer for about 5 minutes.

3 Drain the pasta, reserving some of the cooking water, then return it to the pan with a little of the water. Add the courgette mixture and toss well. Transfer to a serving dish, or dishes, and top with the toasted almonds.

COOK'S TIP
To toast the almonds, tip them onto a baking tray and place it in the oven, which has been preheated to 200°C (400°F/Gas 6). Cook for 3–5 minutes until golden, turning them halfway through cooking. Alternatively, cook them in a small frying pan for a few minutes until golden, stirring occasionally so they don't burn.

STATISTICS PER SERVING:

Energy 362kcals/1,528kJ

Carbohydrate 58g

Sugar 4g

Fibre 3.5g

Fat 11g
Saturated fat 1g

Salt trace

● ● ○ GI

● ● ○ CALORIES

● ○ ○ SATURATED FAT

● ○ ○ SALT

PASTA WITH ROASTED FENNEL

SERVES 4   **PREP** 10 MINS   **COOK** 30 MINS

Roasted fennel, partnered by sweet cherry tomatoes, adds a stylish flair to spaghetti or linguine.

2 fennel bulbs, trimmed and
  sliced lengthways
250g (9oz) cherry tomatoes, halved
2 tbsp olive oil
salt and freshly ground black pepper

1 red onion, finely chopped
2 garlic cloves, finely chopped
350g (12oz) spaghetti or linguine
1 tbsp flat-leaf parsley,
  finely chopped

1 Preheat the oven to 200°C (400°F/Gas 6). Put the fennel in a pan of salted boiling water, bring back to the boil and cook for about 5 minutes until softened, then drain well.

2 Turn the fennel into a roasting tin, add the tomatoes, drizzle with half the olive oil and sprinkle with salt and black pepper. Combine thoroughly, using your hands. Roast in the oven for about 20 minutes or until soft and beginning to char very slightly.

3 Put a pan of salted water on to boil for the pasta. Meanwhile, heat the remaining oil in a frying pan, add the onion and cook for about 5 minutes until soft. Stir in the garlic and cook for a few more seconds, then remove the pan from the heat and set aside.

4 Cook the pasta in the boiling water for 8–10 minutes or according to the instructions on the packet. Drain, reserving some of the cooking water, then return the pasta to the pan with a little of the water. Toss together with the onion mixture, fennel, and tomatoes. Transfer to a serving dish (or dishes) and sprinkle with the parsley to serve.

COOK'S TIP
You don't have to boil the fennel first, but it does soften it and stops it from becoming too brittle when roasted.

STATISTICS PER SERVING:

Energy 382kcals/1,617kJ

Carbohydrate 71g

Sugar 6g

Fibre 5g

Fat 7.5g
Saturated fat 1g

Salt trace

PASTA PUTTANESCA

SERVES 4   **PREP** 15 MINS   **COOK** 20 MINS

A rich, elegant and satisfying sauce makes this pasta dish perfect for entertaining.

GUIDELINES PER SERVING:

● ● ○ GI

● ● ○ CALORIES

● ○ ○ SATURATED FAT

● ○ ○ SALT

1 tbsp olive oil
1 red onion, finely chopped
2 garlic cloves, finely chopped
4 salted anchovy fillets, chopped
1 red chilli, deseeded and
  finely chopped

2 tbsp black olives, chopped
3 tsp capers (rinsed, if salty), chopped
6 tomatoes, diced
300g (10oz) spaghetti
1 tbsp flat-leaf parsley, finely
  chopped, to garnish

1 Heat the oil in a large frying pan, add the onion and cook for a few minutes until beginning to soften. Add the garlic and cook for a few more seconds. Stir in the anchovy fillets and chilli, and cook until the anchovies have melted.

2 Stir in the olives, capers, and tomatoes. Simmer over a low heat for about 15 minutes, partially covered. (If the sauce becomes too dry whilst simmering, loosen it with a little of the pasta cooking water.)

3 Meanwhile, cook the pasta in a pan of salted boiling water for 8–10 minutes or according to the instructions on the packet. Drain, reserving some of the cooking water, then return it to the pan with a little of the water and toss with half the sauce. Transfer the pasta to a serving dish (or dishes) and top with the remaining sauce. Sprinkle with the parsley.

STATISTICS PER SERVING:

Energy 333kcals/1,412kJ

Carbohydrate 62g

Sugar 8g

Fibre 4g

Fat 6g

Saturated fat 1g

Salt 0.8g

● ● ○ GI

● ○ ○ CALORIES

● ○ ○ SATURATED FAT

● ○ ○ SALT

LINGUINE WITH SPICED AUBERGINE

SERVES 4   **PREP** 15 MINS   **COOK** 25 MINS

A fiery sauce for this elegant pasta.

6 tbsp olive oil
2 onions, peeled and finely chopped
2 aubergines, one cut into 1cm
  (½in) dice, the other grated
4 cloves of garlic, peeled and chopped

½ tsp chilli flakes
500ml (16fl oz) passata
1 tsp dried oregano
salt and freshly ground black pepper
400g (14oz) linguine

1 Pour the olive oil into a large frying pan and heat, add the onion and cook over a low heat for 3 minutes until soft, then add the diced aubergine and cook for 3 minutes more. Add the grated aubergine, garlic, and chilli flakes and cook for a further 3 minutes. Pour in the passata, add the oregano, and season well with salt and pepper. Bring to a simmer and allow to cook, uncovered, for 15 minutes.

2 Meanwhile add the pasta to a large pan of boiling salted water and cook for 8–10 minutes or according to pack instructions. Drain and return to the pan.

3 Add half the aubergine mixture to the pasta and toss, then transfer to a large serving dish, or individual dishes, and top with the remaining sauce.

STATISTICS PER SERVING:

Energy 518kcals/2,186kJ

Carbohydrate 90g

Sugar 7g

Fibre 2g

Fat 13g
Saturated fat 2g

Salt trace

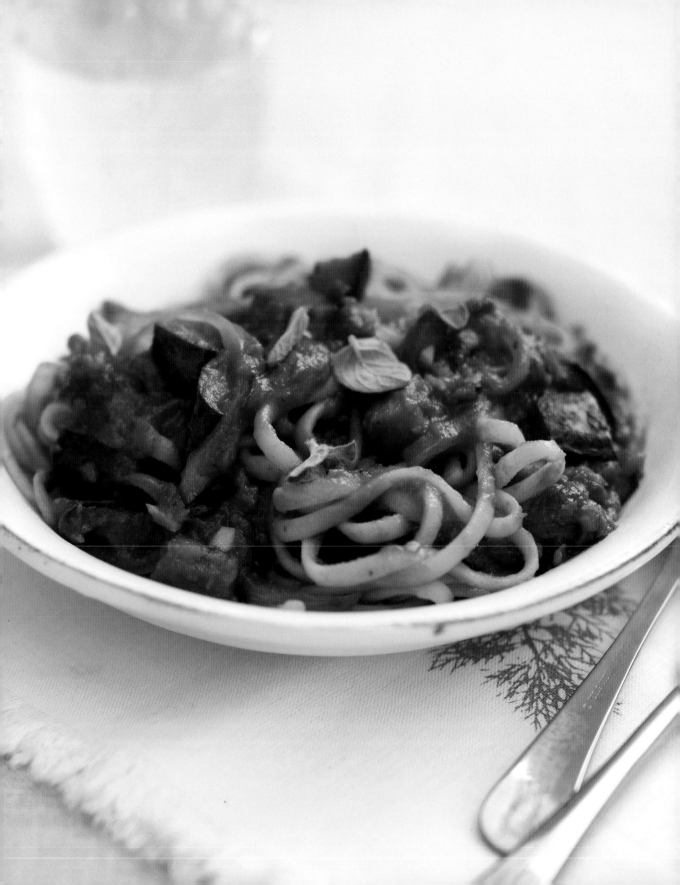

● ● ○ GI

● ● ○ CALORIES

● ○ ○ SATURATED FAT

● ○ ○ SALT

COURGETTE AND FRESH TOMATO PENNE

SERVES 4   **PREP** 5 MINS   **COOK** 15 MINS

A fresh summer sauce with uncooked tomatoes and basil is a simple, yet truly tasty crowning glory for pasta. Enjoy it at its best when the vegetables are in season.

1 tbsp olive oil
3 courgettes, diced
salt and freshly ground black pepper
3 garlic cloves, finely chopped

4 tomatoes, diced
1 tbsp fresh basil, chopped
350g (12oz) penne pasta

1 Heat the olive oil in a large frying pan, add the courgettes and cook for about 5 minutes until tender. Season with salt and black pepper, stir in the garlic and cook for 2 minutes, then remove from the heat.

2 Add the tomatoes and basil, and stir to combine. Allow to cool a little.

3 Cook the pasta in a pan of salted boiling water for 10–12 minutes or according to the instructions on the packet. Drain, reserving some of the cooking water, then return it to the pan with a little of the water. Add the courgette and tomato mixture and stir. Season again, if needed. You can serve this dish hot or cold

COOK'S TIP
This is best made with plump, juicy tomatoes when they are in season and full of flavour.

STATISTICS PER SERVING:

Energy 360kcals/1,528kJ

Carbohydrate 70g

Sugar 6g

Fibre 4g

Fat 5g
Saturated fat 0.8g

Salt trace

SPAGHETTI WITH TOMATOES AND GOAT'S CHEESE

GUIDELINES PER SERVING:

⬤⬤⚪ GI

⬤⬤⚪ CALORIES

⬤⬤⬤ SATURATED FAT

⬤⬤⚪ SALT

SERVES 4   **PREP** 10 MINS   **COOK** 10 MINS
PLUS STANDING

Fresh cherry tomatoes are the basis for an instant cheesy topping that doesn't need cooking: just heap it on plates of steaming spaghetti.

20 cherry tomatoes, halved
1 tbsp capers, rinsed and dried
3 tbsp fruity extra virgin olive oil
2 garlic cloves, finely chopped
150g (5½oz) semi-hard goat's cheese, broken or sliced into chunks

1 tsp dried oregano
1 tbsp fresh basil, chopped
salt and freshly ground black pepper
350g (12oz) spaghetti

1 Put all the ingredients except for the spaghetti in a bowl. Season well with salt and black pepper, and set aside for about 20 minutes for the flavours to mingle and develop.

2 When ready to serve, cook the spaghetti in a pan of salted boiling water for 8–10 minutes or according to the instructions on the packet. Drain, then return to the pan with a little of the cooking water.

3 Add the tomato mixture to the spaghetti and toss well to coat. Serve immediately.

STATISTICS PER SERVING:

Energy 498kcals/2,099kJ

Carbohydrate 66g

Sugar 5g

Fibre 3g

Fat 19g

Saturated fat 8g

Salt 0.6g

BUTTERNUT SQUASH AND COURGETTE PASTA

SERVES 4   **PREP** 15 MINS   **COOK** 30 MINS

Sweet butternut squash makes an excellent sauce for spaghetti and is a good source of vitamins A and C.

2 tbsp olive oil
½ butternut squash (about
   350g/12oz), cut into
   1cm (½in) dice
salt and freshly ground black pepper
2 courgettes, cut into 1cm (½in) dice

3 garlic cloves, finely chopped
1 tbsp fresh thyme stalks,
   leaves only
400g can chopped tomatoes
350g (12oz) spaghetti

1 Heat the oil in large frying pan, add the squash and season with salt and black pepper. Cook for 5 minutes, then add the courgettes and cook for 5–10 minutes until soft and beginning to turn golden (you may need to add a little more oil).

2 Stir in the garlic and thyme, cook for a minute, then add the tomatoes and simmer for about 10–15 minutes. Taste and then season if needed.

3 Meanwhile, put the pasta in a large pan of salted boiling water and cook for 8–10 minutes or according to the instructions on the packet. Drain, reserving some of the cooking water, then return the pasta to the pan with a little of the water. Combine with the sauce and put onto plates.

STATISTICS PER SERVING:

Energy 410kcals/1,738kJ

Carbohydrate 77g

Sugar 10.5g

Fibre 5g

Fat 7.5g

Saturated fat 1g

Salt 0.2g

COOK'S TIP
Chop up the remaining squash, put it in a plastic freezer bag and seal, then store in the freezer. It will keep for up to three months.

PASTA WITH GREEN BEANS AND ARTICHOKES

GUIDELINES PER SERVING:

●●○ GI
●●○ CALORIES
●○○ SATURATED FAT
●○○ SALT

SERVES 4   **PREP** 5 MINS   **COOK** 15 MINS

Green vegetables tossed with basil and pasta make a speedy supper that can be on the table in no time.

200g (7oz) green beans, trimmed
1 tbsp basil leaves
25g (scant 1oz) pine nuts

250g jar artichokes in oil, drained and roughly chopped (reserve the oil)
350g (12oz) trofi or penne pasta

1 Drop the green beans into a pan of salted boiling water and cook for 3–4 minutes, then drain and refresh in cold water (this will help them to keep their colour and stop them from cooking any longer). Set aside.

2 Put the basil and pine nuts in a food processor or blender and whiz until chopped, then drizzle in a little of the oil from the artichokes and whiz again to form a paste.

3 Cook the pasta in a pan of salted boiling water for 8–10 minutes or according to the instructions on the packet. Drain, reserving some of the cooking water, and then return the pasta to the pan with a little of the water. Toss the pasta with the basil paste, green beans, and artichokes.

STATISTICS PER SERVING:

Energy 419kcals/1,774kJ

Carbohydrate 70g

Sugar 3g

Fibre 4g

Fat 12g

Saturated fat 0.5g

Salt trace

MUSHROOM LASAGNE

SERVES 4   **PREP** 20 MINS   **COOK** 45 MINS   **FREEZE** 3 MONTHS

A meatless lasagne made with robust mushrooms and flavour-packed leeks.

1 tbsp olive oil
2 leeks, trimmed and finely chopped
400g (14oz) white and chestnut
  mushrooms, half of them chopped,
  half grated
3 garlic cloves, finely chopped
1 tbsp plain flour
300ml (10fl oz) semi-skimmed milk

salt and freshly ground black pepper
pinch of dried oregano
100g (3½oz) fresh Parmesan cheese,
  grated
6 tomatoes, deseeded and diced
10 lasagne sheets (no need for
  precooked ones)

1 Preheat the oven to 200°C (400°F/Gas 6). Heat the olive oil in a large pan, add the leeks and cook for 5–8 minutes until soft. Add all the mushrooms plus the garlic, and cook for a further 5–8 minutes until the mushrooms begin to release their juices.

2 Stir in the flour and combine it well with the juices in the pan. Remove from the heat, add a little of the milk and stir until smooth. Return to the heat and add the remaining milk, little by little, until you have a smooth sauce. Season well with salt and black pepper, then add the oregano and Parmesan. Stir in the tomatoes.

3 Coat the bottom of an ovenproof baking dish with some of the sauce, then a layer of lasagne; continue adding alternate layers, ending with some sauce as the topping. Put the dish in the oven to bake for 15–20 minutes, or until the sauce is golden and bubbling.

COOK'S TIP
Lasagne is a great reheat-and-eat dish, so make it ahead to save time later.

STATISTICS PER SERVING:

Energy 312kcals/1,316kJ

Carbohydrate 35g

Sugar 10g

Fibre 4.5g

Fat 13g

Saturated fat 6g

Salt 0.7g

VEGETARIAN COTTAGE PIE

GUIDELINES PER SERVING:

● ● ○ GI

● ● ○ CALORIES

● ○ ○ SATURATED FAT

● ● ○ SALT

SERVES 4   **PREP** 15 MINS   **COOK** 30–35 MINS   **FREEZE** 3 MONTHS

Canned lentils are a fantastic low-GI ingredient to have on standby in your storecupboard.

2 tbsp olive oil
2 leeks, trimmed and finely chopped
3 sticks celery, finely chopped
2 large carrots, diced
1 red pepper, deseeded and diced
125g (4½oz) chestnut mushrooms, roughly chopped
2 cloves garlic, crushed
300ml (10fl oz) vegetable stock
2 tsp soy sauce
pinch of dried chilli flakes
salt and freshly ground black pepper
2 x 400g cans brown lentils, drained and rinsed

1 tbsp sunflower or pumpkin seeds, or a mixture of the two

For the mash
450g (1lb) white potatoes, peeled and cut into even-sized chunks
600g (1lb 5oz) sweet potatoes, peeled and cut into even-sized chunks
150ml (5fl oz) warmed semi-skimmed milk
25g (scant 1oz) polyunsaturated margarine

1 Preheat the oven to 200°C (400°F/Gas 6). Heat the oil in a large, deep, heavy, nonstick frying pan. Add the leeks, celery, carrots, red pepper, mushrooms, and garlic and cook, stirring, for 5 minutes.

2 Add the stock, soy sauce, and chilli flakes. Season to taste with salt and black pepper. Bring to the boil, then reduce the heat, cover and simmer for 15 minutes, adding more stock if necessary. Remove from the heat and stir in the lentils.

3 To make the mash, boil the potatoes and sweet potatoes in a large pan of salted water for 15–20 minutes or until tender. Drain well, then return to the pan and add the milk and margarine. Mash well and season to taste.

4 Pour the vegetable and lentil mixture into a large ovenproof dish. Spread the mashed potato evenly over the top and smooth the surface. Scatter with the seeds and transfer to the oven. Bake for 20–25 minutes or until the top is golden.

STATISTICS PER SERVING:

Energy 594kcals/2,506kJ

Carbohydrate 90g

Sugar 18g

Fibre 15g

Fat 17g

Saturated fat 2g

Salt 1.2g

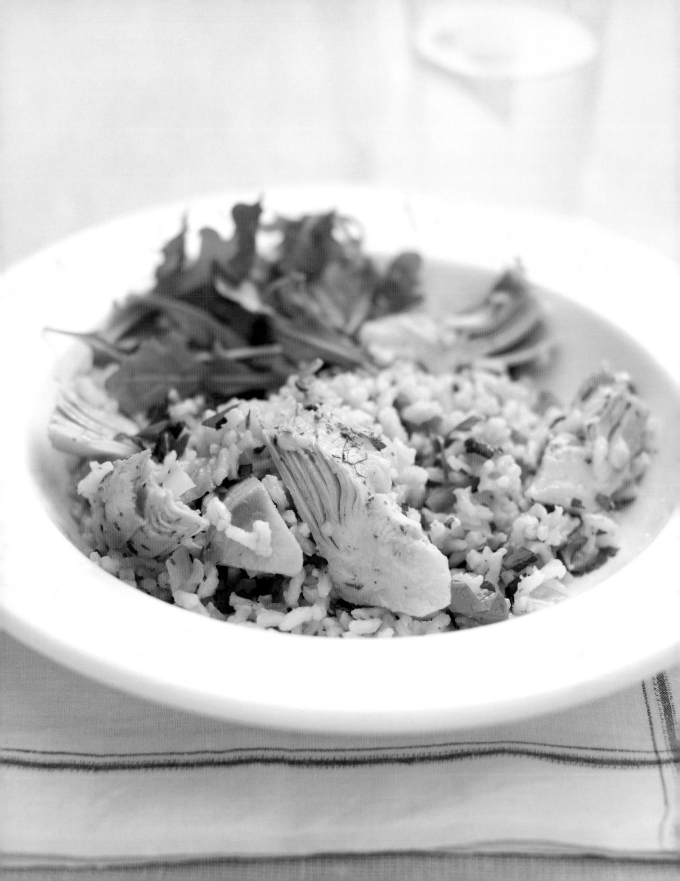

BROWN RICE, RED PEPPER AND ARTICHOKE RISOTTO

GUIDELINES PER SERVING:

● ● ○ GI
● ● ○ CALORIES
● ○ ○ SATURATED FAT
● ● ○ SALT

SERVES 4   **PREP** 10 MINS   **COOK** 50 MINS–1 HOUR

Not a risotto in the true sense, but a great mix of flavours and textures.

1 tbsp olive oil
1 onion, finely chopped
salt and freshly ground black pepper
2 sweet pointed red peppers, halved,
　deseeded and chopped
pinch of chilli flakes

280g (10oz) brown rice
1 litre (1¾ pints) vegetable stock
280g jar of artichoke hearts,
　drained and roughly chopped
handful of flat-leaf parsley,
　finely chopped

1 Heat the oil in a large frying pan then add the onion and cook on a low heat until soft and transparent. Season with a pinch of sea salt and some freshly ground black pepper. Add the red peppers and cook for a few minutes until they soften.

2 Add the chilli flakes, then stir in the rice. Raise the heat a little, pour in a ladleful of the stock, and bring to the boil. Reduce to a simmer and cook gently for 40–50 minutes, adding a little more stock each time the liquid is absorbed, until the rice is cooked.

3 Stir through the artichokes and cook for a couple of minutes to heat through, then taste and season as required. Cover with a lid, remove from the heat and leave for 10 minutes, then stir through the chopped parsley and transfer to plates or bowls. You could serve this with a rocket salad on the side.

COOK'S TIP
Artichokes bought in a jar will taste far better than the canned ones. Do save the oil as you can use it for a dressing. If you can't find the pointed peppers, just use regular peppers - they're just as tasty but not quite as sweet.

STATISTICS PER SERVING:

Energy 406kcals/1,713kJ

Carbohydrate 67g

Sugar 9g

Fibre 4g

Fat 13.5g

Saturated fat 1g

Salt 1.2g

PEA AND LEMON RISOTTO

SERVES 4   **PREP** 5 MINS   **COOK** 30-40 MINS

Frozen peas contain just as much vitamin C as fresh peas, so it's a good idea to keep a bag in the freezer for a convenient way to boost the nutritional content of meals.

2 tbsp olive oil
1 large onion, finely chopped
2 garlic cloves, crushed
  or finely chopped
300g (10oz) arborio (risotto) rice
150ml (5fl oz) white wine
600-750ml (1-1¼ pints) hot
  vegetable stock

400g (14oz) frozen peas
zest and juice of 1 lemon
salt and freshly ground black pepper
60g (2oz) freshly grated Parmesan
  cheese, plus some shavings
  to garnish

1 Heat the oil in large saucepan, add the onion and cook over a medium heat for about 2 minutes or until beginning to soften. Stir in the garlic and rice and continue to cook, stirring, for 1–2 minutes. Add the wine and cook until the liquid has evaporated.

2 Pour in just enough stock to cover the rice and continue to cook, stirring frequently, until most of the liquid has been absorbed. Continue adding the stock in this way until the rice is tender.

3 Stir in the peas, lemon juice and zest, and seasoning to taste. Cook, stirring, for 2–3 minutes.

4 Remove from the heat and stir in the Parmesan cheese. Garnish with shavings of fresh Parmesan and serve immediately.

STATISTICS PER SERVING:

Energy 537kcals/2,337kJ

Carbohydrate 76g

Sugar 5.5g

Fibre 6g

Fat 13g

Saturated fat 4.5g

Salt 1g

MUSHROOM AND CORIANDER RICE

SERVES 4   **PREP** 5 MINS   **COOK** 30 MINS

This fragrant rice dish combines earthy-tasting mushrooms with plenty of spice.

GUIDELINES PER SERVING:

● ● ○ GI

● ● ○ CALORIES

● ● ● SATURATED FAT

● ○ ○ SALT

1 tbsp olive oil
2 tsp mustard seeds
250g (9oz) basmati rice
75g (2½oz) creamed coconut, grated
2 tbsp fresh coriander

1 green chilli, deseeded
1 tsp turmeric
250g (9oz) chestnut mushrooms
salt and freshly ground black pepper

1 Heat the oil in a large frying pan, add the mustard seeds and cook for a few minutes until they pop. Set aside.

2 Pour the rice into a large saucepan, cover with water and cook for 10–15 minutes until tender, or according to the instructions on the packet. Put the lid on the pan and set aside.

3 Put the coconut, coriander, chilli, and turmeric into a food processor or blender and whiz until ground together. Add the mixture to the mustard seeds and return the pan to a low heat. Cook, stirring, for about 5 minutes.

4 Pulse the mushrooms in the food processor a few times until they are just broken up, then stir them into the coconut and coriander mixture. Cook for 5–10 minutes or until the mushrooms begin to release their juices. Tip in the cooked rice and stir well, then taste and season as required.

COOK'S TIP
Wrap the remaining coconut cream in cling film and keep in the refrigerator for using to make a curry.

STATISTICS PER SERVING:

Energy 383kcals/1,623kJ

Carbohydrate 52g

Sugar 2g

Fibre 1g

Fat 17g

Saturated fat 12g

Salt 0.5g

MUSHROOM AND CHILLI PILAF

SERVES 4   **PREP** 10 MINS   **COOK** 50 MINS

Nutty-flavoured rice with an added zing of chilli.

1 tbsp olive oil
1 red onion, finely chopped
salt and freshly ground black pepper
2 green chillies, deseeded and
 finely chopped

450g (1lb) mushrooms, chopped
225g (8oz) brown basmati rice
600ml (1 pint) vegetable
 or chicken stock

1 Heat the olive oil in a large, heavy pan, add the onion and cook for 7–8 minutes over a low heat until soft. Season with a pinch of salt and some black pepper. Add the chillies and cook for a few minutes more. Tip in the mushrooms and cook, stirring, until they release their juices (about 5 minutes). Add a little more oil if necessary.

2 Pour in the rice and stir until it is coated with the juices in the pan, then add the stock, increase the heat and bring to the boil. Reduce to a simmer, cover, and cook gently for 30 minutes or until the rice is just tender but retains some bite. Stir occasionally and add extra water, a little at a time, if needed.

3 Remove from the heat and set aside, still covered with the lid, for a further 10 minutes. Taste, season as needed, and serve.

COOK'S TIP
Brown rice takes longer to cook than white, so be patient; it will continue cooking as it steams while set aside with the lid on.

STATISTICS PER SERVING:

Energy 294kcals/1,243kJ

Carbohydrate 50g

Sugar 3g

Fibre 3g

Fat 7g

Saturated fat 1g

Salt 1.1g

LEEK AND TOMATO PILAF

SERVES 2   **PREP** 5 MINS   **COOK** 30 MINS

This version of a pilaf uses pearl barley instead of rice.

GUIDELINES PER SERVING:

GI

CALORIES

SATURATED FAT

SALT

2 tbsp olive oil
1 large leek, trimmed and roughly
  chopped
85g (3oz) pearl barley, rinsed
400g can chopped tomatoes
1 tbsp tomato purée
pinch of smoked paprika

500ml (16fl oz) vegetable stock
150g (5½oz) frozen soya beans
pinch of chilli flakes
salt and freshly ground black pepper
15g (½oz) Parmesan cheese shavings,
  to serve

1 Heat the oil in a large, deep frying pan, put the leek in and fry it for 2–3 minutes. Stir in the pearl barley and cook for a further minute.

2 Add the tomatoes, tomato purée, paprika, and 400ml (14fl oz) of the stock. Cover and simmer for 20 minutes, stirring occasionally and adding more stock as it is absorbed.

3 Stir in the soya beans and chilli flakes, and season to taste with salt and pepper. Cook for a further 5 minutes or until the barley is soft and the soya beans are heated through. Serve immediately, sprinkled with Parmesan shavings.

STATISTICS PER SERVING:

Energy 490kcals/2,048kJ

Carbohydrate 55g

Sugar 8g

Fibre 6g

Fat 20g
Saturated fat 4.4g

Salt 1.4g

KASHA PILAF

SERVES 6   **PREP** 5 MINS   **COOK** 25 MINS

Kasha is a healthy and delicious wholegrain cereal that is prepared similarly to risotto.

2 tbsp polyunsaturated margarine
1 large onion, chopped
2 celery sticks, sliced
1 large egg
200g (7oz) coarse kasha
  (buckwheat groats) or whole kasha

1 tsp ground sage
1 tsp ground thyme
115g (4oz) raisins
115g (4oz) walnut pieces,
  coarsely chopped
salt

1 In a large frying pan, melt the margarine and gently fry the onion and celery for 3 minutes, or until the vegetables begin to soften.

2 In a small bowl, mix the egg with the kasha, then add the mixture to the pan. Cook, stirring constantly, for 1 minute, or until the grains are dry and separated. Add 500ml (16fl oz) water, the sage, and the thyme to the kasha. Bring to the boil, then reduce the heat, cover, and simmer for 10–12 minutes.

3 Stir the raisins and walnuts into the kasha. Cook for a further 4–5 minutes, or until the kasha is tender and all the liquid has been absorbed. Season to taste with salt.

STATISTICS PER SERVING:

Energy 370kcals/1,537kJ

Carbohydrate 45g

Sugar 15g

Fibre 2g

Fat 19g

Saturated fat 2.5g

Salt 0.2g

KASHA WITH VEGETABLES

GUIDELINES PER SERVING:

⬤◯◯ GI

⬤◯◯ CALORIES

⬤◯◯ SATURATED FAT

⬤◯◯ SALT

SERVES 4   **PREP** 10 MINS   **COOK** 40 MINS

Added vegetables and goat's cheese make this kasha dish a hearty vegetarian main course.

2 tbsp olive oil
1 onion, finely chopped
1 carrot, finely chopped
1 garlic clove, finely chopped
2 flat mushrooms, sliced
1 celery stick, finely chopped
550g (1¼lb) kasha

120ml (4fl oz) dry white wine
1.2 litres (2 pints) hot vegetable
  stock or water
1 beetroot, steamed or roasted
  until tender, chopped
2 tbsp chopped parsley
60g (2oz) goat's cheese, crumbled

1 Heat the oil in a large saucepan. Add the onion, carrot, garlic, mushrooms, and celery and sauté for 8–10 minutes, stirring frequently, until brown. Add the kasha and cook, stirring for another 2–3 minutes. Add the wine and continue stirring until all the liquid has been absorbed.

2 Gradually add the hot vegetable stock, 120ml (4fl oz) at a time, and stirring until it has been absorbed before adding more. Cook for a further 20 minutes, or until the kasha is soft and chewy.

3 Toss in the chopped cooked beetroot and remove from the heat. Sprinkle over the parsley and goat's cheese, and serve.

STATISTICS PER SERVING:

Energy 362kcals/1,521kJ

Carbohydrate 55g

Sugar 8g

Fibre 4.5g

Fat 11.5g

Saturated fat 4g

Salt 0.7g

● ● ○ GI

● ● ○ CALORIES

● ○ ○ SATURATED FAT

● ○ ○ SALT

TURKISH-STYLE STUFFED PEPPERS

SERVES 2   **PREP** 15 MINS   **COOK** 1 HOUR

A good dish to make use of leftover rice.

125g (4½oz) basmati rice
1 tbsp olive oil, plus extra
  for drizzling
1 red onion, peeled and finely
  chopped
salt and freshly ground black pepper
small handful of flat-leaf parsley,
  finely chopped
small handful of fresh thyme
  leaves, chopped

pinch of dried oregano
1 tomato, diced
½ tsp paprika
2 tsp pine nuts, toasted (see
  Cook's Tip, below)
1 tbsp pitted and chopped
  black olives
2 red peppers, tops removed
  and retained, seeds removed

1 First cook the rice according to pack instructions, drain and put to one side. Preheat the oven to 200°C (400°F/Gas 6).

2 Heat the olive oil in a frying pan, add the onion and season with salt and black pepper. Cook over a low heat for 3–4 minutes until soft, add the garlic and cook for a few seconds more, then remove from the heat and allow to cool. Stir in the herbs, tomato, paprika, pine nuts, and olives, then add the cooked rice and stir again. Taste and season if needed.

3 Spoon the mixture into the peppers, packing them tightly so they hold together while cooking. Place them upright in a roasting tin, topped with the lids, drizzle with olive oil, and cook for 30–45 minutes until the peppers begin to soften and char slightly. Cover with foil towards the end of cooking if the rice is beginning to dry out too much. Serve hot.

STATISTICS PER SERVING:

Energy 535kcals/1,475kJ

Carbohydrate 67g

Sugar 14.5g

Fibre 4g

Fat 6g

Saturated fat 0.5g

Salt 0.2g

COOK'S TIP

Toast the pine nuts on a baking sheet in a hot oven or in a small dry frying pan over a moderate heat. Cook for a few minutes, keeping a close eye on them to make sure they don't burn.

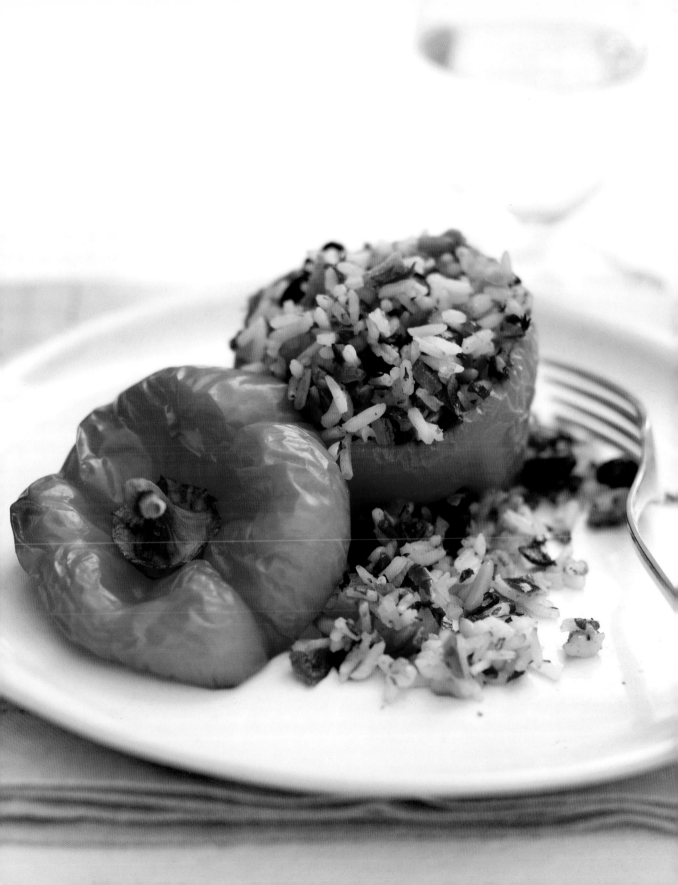

TANDOORI PANEER KEBABS

SERVES 4   **PREP** 20 MINS   **COOK** 10 MINS
PLUS MARINATING

Paneer is a firm Indian cheese that takes up the flavour of other ingredients.

150g (5½oz) thick natural yogurt
1 tbsp tandoori curry paste
1 tbsp lemon juice
250g (9oz) paneer, cut into
  2.5cm (1in) cubes
1 red pepper, deseeded and cut
  into 2.5cm (1in) chunks

12 button mushrooms
1 large courgette, cut into
  1cm (½in) slices
2 tbsp vegetable oil

1 In a bowl, mix the yogurt, curry paste, and lemon juice. Add the paneer, and stir well. Cover, chill, and marinate for up to 24 hours.

2 Thread the paneer cubes on to skewers, alternating with the pepper, mushrooms, and courgette. Brush with oil and grill or barbecue for 10 minutes, or until the vegetables are cooked.

COOK'S TIP
If using wooden skewers, soak them in cold water for 30 mins before using to prevent them burning.

STATISTICS PER SERVING:

Energy 172kcals/715kJ

Carbohydrate 8g

Sugar 8g

Fibre 1g

Fat 10g

Saturated fat 3g

Salt 0.7g

VEGETABLE CURRY

SERVES 4 **PREP** 20 MINS **COOK** 35-45 MINS **FREEZE** 3 MONTHS

In Indian cooking, cardamom, cloves, coriander, and cumin seeds are all considered "warming spices" that heat the body from within, making this an excellent winter dish.

GUIDELINES PER SERVING:

● ○ ○ GI

● ○ ○ CALORIES

● ○ ○ SATURATED FAT

● ○ ○ SALT

4 tbsp sunflower oil
300g (10oz) waxy potatoes, diced
5 green cardamom pods, cracked
3 cloves
1 cinnamon stick, broken in half
2 tsp cumin seeds
1 onion, finely chopped
2 tsp fresh root ginger, peeled
  and grated
2 large garlic cloves, crushed
1½ tsp turmeric
1 tsp ground coriander

salt and freshly ground black pepper
400g can chopped tomatoes
2 carrots, peeled and diced
2 green chillies, deseeded (optional)
  and sliced
150g (5½oz) Savoy cabbage or green
  cabbage, sliced
150g (5½oz) cauliflower florets
150g (5½oz) peas
2 tbsp chopped coriander leaves
almond flakes, toasted, to garnish

1 Heat the oil in a large deep-sided frying pan over a high heat. Add the potatoes and stir-fry for 5 minutes, or until golden brown. Remove from the pan with a slotted spoon and set aside to drain on kitchen paper.

2 Reduce the heat to medium, add the cardamom pods, cloves, cinnamon, and cumin seeds and cook, stirring, just until the seeds begin to crackle. Add the onion and continue stir-frying for 5–8 minutes, or until softened. Add the ginger, garlic, turmeric, and ground coriander, then season to taste with salt and pepper and stir for 1 minute.

3 Stir in the tomatoes. Return the potatoes to the pan, add the carrots, chillies, and 250ml (8fl oz) water, and bring to the boil, stirring often. Reduce the heat to low and simmer for 15 minutes, or until the carrots are just tender, stirring occasionally. Add a little water, if needed.

4 Stir in the cabbage, cauliflower, and peas, and increase the heat to medium. Let the liquid gently bubble for a further 5–10 minutes, or until all the vegetables are tender. Discard the cardamom pods and cloves and stir in the coriander. Transfer to a serving bowl and sprinkle with almond flakes.

STATISTICS PER SERVING:

Energy 275kcals/1,145kJ

Carbohydrate 30g

Sugar 11g

Fibre 7g

Fat 15g
Saturated fat 2g

Salt 0.2g

VEGETABLE MOUSSAKA

SERVES 4   **PREP** 20 MINS   **COOK** 1 HOUR 30 MINS   **FREEZE** 1 MONTH

Lentils replace the lamb, and yogurt is a light alternative to béchamel sauce, in this vegetarian version.

2 aubergines, about 600g (1lb 5oz) in total, cut into 1cm (½in) slices
2 courgettes, thickly sliced
2 onions, thickly sliced
2 red peppers, cored, deseeded, and thickly sliced
4 tbsp olive oil
salt and freshly ground black pepper
2 garlic cloves, coarsely chopped
1 tbsp chopped thyme leaves

400g can chopped tomatoes
300g can green lentils, drained and rinsed
2 tbsp chopped flat-leaf parsley
2 eggs, lightly beaten
300g (10oz) Greek-style yogurt
pinch of paprika
85g (3oz) feta cheese, crumbled
2 tbsp white sesame seeds

1 Preheat the oven to 220°C (425°F/Gas 7). Place the aubergines, courgettes, onions, and red peppers into a roasting tin. Drizzle over the olive oil,
toss together to coat the vegetables evenly, then season to taste with salt and pepper.

2 Roast for 10 minutes, toss, add the garlic and thyme, and roast for a further 30–35 minutes, or until the vegetables are tender. Reduce the temperature to 180°C (350°F/Gas 4).

3 Stir the tomatoes with their juices, the lentils, and the parsley into the roast vegetables. Taste and adjust the seasoning, if necessary. Transfer the vegetables to a 23cm (9in) square ovenproof serving dish.

4 Beat the eggs and yogurt with the paprika, and season to taste with salt and pepper. Spread the mixture over the vegetables, and sprinkle the feta cheese on top. Put the dish on a baking tray and bake for 40 minutes. Sprinkle with the sesame seeds and bake for 10 minutes, or until the top is golden. Leave to stand for at least 2 minutes, then serve while still warm.

STATISTICS PER SERVING:

Energy 505kcals/2,103kJ

Carbohydrate 33g

Sugar 17g

Fibre 8g

Fat 32g

Saturated fat 11.5g

Salt 1.1g

TUSCAN BEAN STEW

SERVES 4   **PREP** 15 MINS   **COOK** 1 HOUR 20 MINS   **FREEZE** 3 MONTHS

This classic dish, *Ribollita*, is named after the traditional method of reboiling soup from the day before.

GUIDELINES PER SERVING:

● ○ ○ GI

● ● ○ CALORIES

● ○ ○ SATURATED FAT

● ● ○ SALT

4 tbsp extra virgin olive oil,
  plus extra for drizzling
1 onion, chopped
2 carrots, sliced
1 leek, sliced
2 garlic cloves, chopped
400g can chopped tomatoes
1 tbsp tomato purée
900ml (1½ pints) chicken stock

salt and freshly ground black pepper
400g can borlotti beans, flageolet
  beans, or cannellini beans,
  drained and rinsed
250g (9oz) baby spinach leaves
  or spring greens, shredded
grated Parmesan cheese,
  for sprinkling

1 Heat the oil in a large saucepan and fry the onion, carrot, and leek over a low heat for 10 minutes, or until softened but not coloured. Add the garlic and fry for 1 minute. Add the tomatoes, tomato purée, and stock. Season to taste with salt and pepper.

2 Mash half the beans with a fork and add to the pan. Bring to the boil, then lower the heat and simmer for 30 minutes.

3 Add the remaining beans and spinach to the pan. Simmer for a further 30 minutes.

4 To serve, spoon the soup into the bowls, top with a sprinkling of Parmesan, and drizzle with a little more olive oil.

COOK'S TIP

This stew improves with reheating, so it benefits from being made 1 day in advance. Reheat gently over a low heat.

STATISTICS PER SERVING:

Energy 313kcals/1,304kJ

Carbohydrate 27g

Sugar 11g

Fibre 9g

Fat 15g
Saturated fat 3g

Salt 1.5g

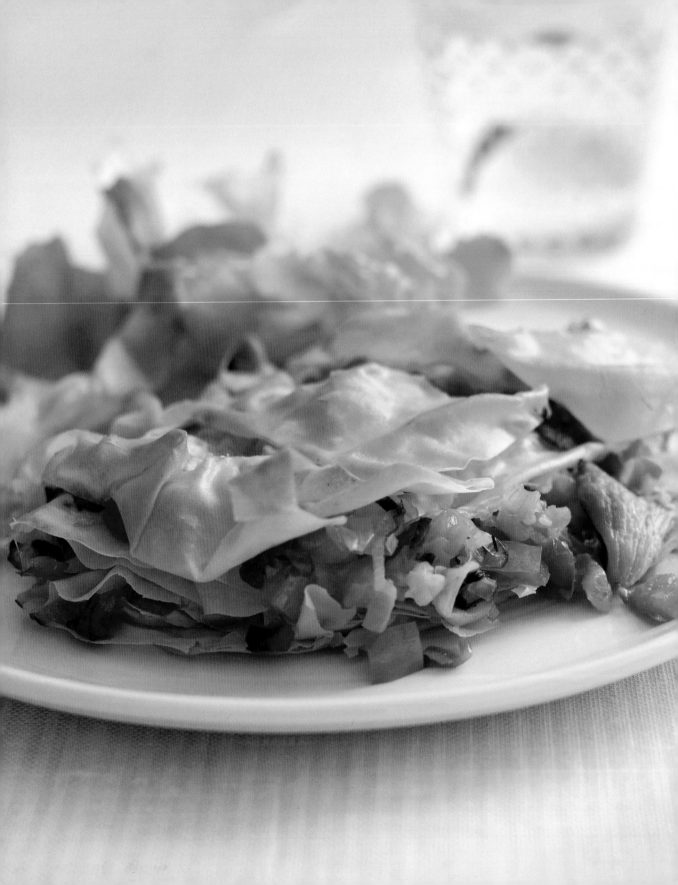

MUSHROOM, LEEK, AND RED PEPPER FILO PIE

SERVES 4   **PREP** 15 MINS   **COOK** 40 MINS

A layered pie to be eaten hot or cold.

GUIDELINES PER SERVING:

●●○ GI

●○○ CALORIES

●○○ SATURATED FAT

●○○ SALT

1 tbsp oil, plus extra for brushing
1 onion, finely chopped
salt and freshly ground black pepper
small handful fresh thyme,
  finely chopped
1 leek, finely sliced
2 red peppers, finely chopped

250g (9oz) mushrooms (chestnut
  and oyster varieties; keep them
  separate), chopped
150ml (5fl oz) vegetable stock
about 18 sheets filo pastry
butter, melted, for brushing

1 Preheat the oven to 190ºC (375ºF/Gas 5). Heat the oil in a large frying pan then add the onion, season with salt and black pepper, and add the thyme. Cook over a low heat for 2–3 minutes until the onion begins to soften, then stir in the leek and red peppers and cook for 5–8 minutes more.

2 Add the chestnut mushrooms and cook for 5 minutes or until they begin to release their juices, then add the oyster mushrooms and cook for 2 minutes more. Pour in a little stock, increase the heat and allow to bubble, then gradually add the rest and cook until the liquid is almost soaked up.

3 Lay a double layer of filo pastry sheets in a small–medium oblong pie dish or roasting tin to cover the base (about 6 sheets), and brush with oil. Spoon over half the mixture, then arrange another double layer of pastry sheets on top and brush with oil. Repeat with the remaining mixture and a third double layer of pastry, tucking the edges down the sides of the dish. Brush liberally with melted butter and transfer to the oven to cook for 20–25 minutes until golden and crispy. Cut into 4 portions and serve. You might try it with a dressed mixed salad on the side.

COOK'S TIP
This brittle pastry requires oiling so it doesn't break up. If you prefer not to oil, work quickly between layering and keep the filo wrapped in cling film.

STATISTICS PER SERVING:

Energy 259kcals/1,078kJ

Carbohydrate 35g

Sugar 10g

Fibre 3g

Fat 10g
Saturated fat 2.5g

Salt 0.7g

VEGETARIAN SAUSAGES

SERVES 4   **PREP** 20 MINS   **COOK** 25 MINS

These vegetarian sausages are rich in flavour and provide a less fatty alternative to meat sausages.

2 tbsp olive oil, plus extra for greasing
1 onion, finely diced
1 leek, trimmed and finely sliced
1 courgette, finely diced
salt and freshly ground black pepper
1 egg

150g (5½oz) lightly toasted
  breadcrumbs
80g (2½oz) Parmesan cheese,
  finely grated
pinch of paprika

1 Preheat the oven to 180°C (350°F/Gas 4). Heat the oil in a large frying pan and pop in the onion, leek, and courgette. Season with salt and black pepper and then cook over a low heat for about 10 minutes until soft.

2 Allow to cool, then put in a mixing bowl and add the egg, half the breadcrumbs, the Parmesan cheese, and the paprika. Stir until the mixture is evenly combined (you don't need more seasoning as the Parmesan is salty-tasting).

3 Using your hands, form the mixture into 8 sausages and roll each one in the remaining breadcrumbs. Place the sausages on an oiled baking sheet and cook in the oven for 15–20 minutes until just beginning to turn golden.

STATISTICS PER SERVING:

Energy 306kcals/1,285kJ

Carbohydrate 32g

Sugar 3g

Fibre 2g

Fat 14g

Saturated fat 5g

Salt 1.1g

MUSHROOM STRUDEL

SERVES 4   **PREP** 15 MINS   **COOK** 35 MINS

Reduced-fat cream cheese gives this dish a creamy taste
without adding too many calories or a lot of fat.

GUIDELINES PER SERVING:

● ○ ○ GI

● ○ ○ CALORIES

● ● ○ SATURATED FAT

● ○ ○ SALT

2 tbsp olive oil
450g (1lb) mixed mushrooms,
  roughly chopped
2 sticks celery, finely chopped
1 bunch of spring onions, trimmed
  and roughly chopped
225g (8oz) reduced-fat soft cheese
  with garlic and herbs

4 tbsp chopped fresh chives
salt and freshly ground black pepper
8 large sheets of filo pastry
  (about 200g/7oz)
30g (1oz) polyunsaturated margarine,
  melted

1 Preheat the oven to 180°C (350°F/Gas 4). Heat the oil in a large frying pan
and add the mushrooms, celery, and spring onions. Cook over a medium
heat, stirring occasionally, for 5 minutes or until the mushrooms are soft
and all the liquid has evaporated.

2 Allow the mushroom mixture to cool thoroughly, then stir in the soft
cheese and chives. Season the filling to taste.

3 Lay 4 pieces of filo pastry side by side on a clean tea towel, overlapping
the long edges by about 5cm (2in). Brush with a little melted margarine.
Place the 4 remaining sheets of pastry on top and brush with a little more
margarine. Cover the pastry with a clean, damp tea towel to help prevent it
from drying out; uncover when you are ready to add the filling.

4 Carefully spread the mushroom mixture over the pastry, leaving a border
of 2.5cm (1in) around the edges, then roll it up from a short edge, just as
you would a Swiss roll. Carefully transfer to a baking sheet, making sure
that the seam is underneath. Using a sharp knife, make light diagonal
slashes across the top of the pastry.

5 Brush the strudel with the remaining margarine and bake in the oven for
20 minutes or until the pastry is crisp and golden. Leave to stand for
5 minutes and then cut into slices. Serve warm.

STATISTICS PER SERVING:

Energy 274kcals/1,139kJ

Carbohydrate 15g

Sugar 4g

Fibre 2g

Fat 20g
Saturated fat 6g

Salt 0.7g

● ○ ○ GI

● ○ ○ CALORIES

● ○ ○ SATURATED FAT

● ○ ○ SALT

BUTTERNUT SQUASH AND SPINACH CURRY

SERVES 6   **PREP** 15 MINS   **COOK** 30-35 MINS   **FREEZE** 3 MONTHS

A mildly spiced, low-fat curry, rich in B vitamins and betacarotene, which the body can convert to Vitamin A.

2 tbsp vegetable oil
1 large onion, peeled and chopped
1 medium butternut squash, about
  1.25kg (2¾lb), peeled and cut into
  2cm (¾in) cubes
2 cloves garlic, peeled and crushed
2–3 tbsp curry paste

400g can chopped tomatoes
360ml (12fl oz) vegetable stock
  or chicken stock
225g (8oz) bag fresh washed
  baby spinach
salt and freshly ground black pepper

1 Heat the oil in a large, deep pan, add the onion and cook gently for 2–3 minutes. Add the butternut squash, garlic, and curry paste and cook for a further 2–3 minutes.

2 Add the tomatoes and stock. Bring the boil, then reduce the heat, cover, and simmer for 15 minutes, stirring occasionally. Remove the lid and simmer for a further 10 minutes. Add a little extra stock or water if it becomes too dry.

3 Stir in the spinach, cover and cook for 1–2 minutes until just wilted. Season to taste with salt and pepper and spoon into serving bowls. If desired, you could add a spoonful of yogurt to serve.

STATISTICS PER SERVING:

Energy 194kcals/817kJ

Carbohydrate 26g

Sugar 16g

Fibre 6g

Fat 8g

Saturated fat 0.8g

Salt 0.6g

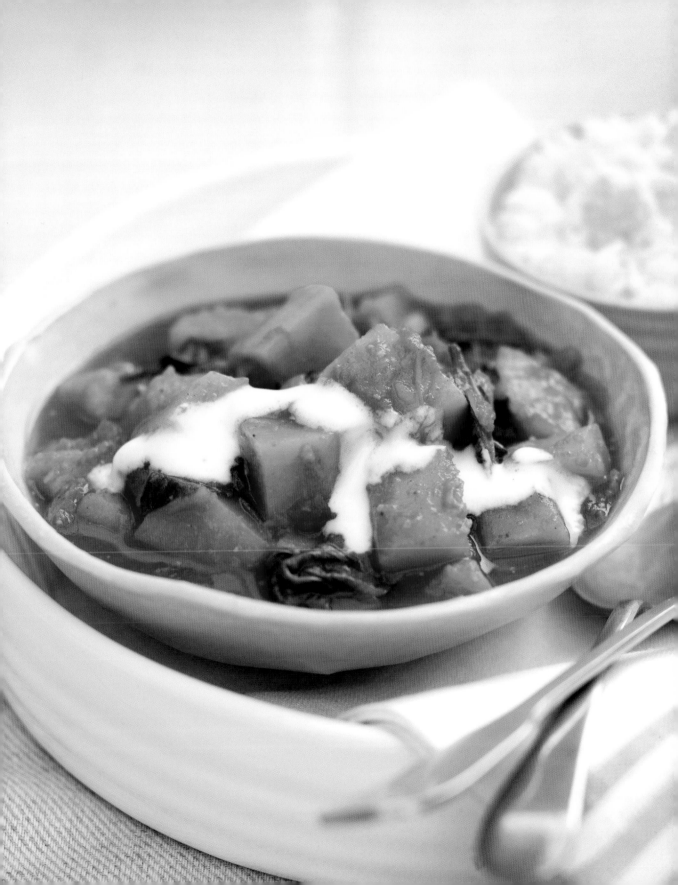

CAULIFLOWER MORNAY

SERVES 4   **PREP** 20 MINS   **COOK** 25 MINS   **FREEZE** 1 MONTH

A satisfying dish that's a favourite with everyone.

2 slices of wholemeal bread
1 large cauliflower, cut into florets
  (retain a few green leaves)
25g (scant 1oz) polyunsaturated
  margarine
1 tbsp flour

450ml (15fl oz) semi-skimmed milk
2 tsp grainy mustard
125g (4½oz) reduced-fat mature
  Cheddar cheese
salt and freshly ground black pepper

1 Preheat the oven to 180°C (350°F/Gas 4). Put the bread into a food processor or blender and whiz until it forms breadcrumbs. Tip out onto a baking sheet and toast in the oven for a few minutes until golden. Set aside.

2 Chop the cauliflower leaves roughly. Put the cauliflower and the leaves into a large pan of salted boiling water and cook for about 8 minutes or until starting to soften. Drain and allow to dry.

3 Melt the margarine in a pan, then stir in the flour and blend well. Remove from the heat, stir in a little milk, then put back on the heat and add the remaining milk slowly, stirring continually, to make a smooth sauce. Remove from the heat, stir in the mustard and a third of the cheese, and season with salt and black pepper.

4 Lay the cauliflower and leaves in the base of an ovenproof dish, pour the cheese sauce over it and then sprinkle with the breadcrumbs and the remaining cheese. Cook in the oven for 10–15 minutes until golden and bubbling, then serve.

COOK'S TIP
Don't be tempted to set the oven at a higher temperature, or the sauce may split and curdle.

STATISTICS PER SERVING:

Energy 276kcals/1,150kJ

Carbohydrate 19g

Sugar 8g

Fibre 3g

Fat 14g

Saturated fat 6g

Salt 1g

VEGETABLE CHOP SUEY

GUIDELINES PER SERVING:

⬤◯◯ GI

⬤◯◯ CALORIES

⬤◯◯ SATURATED FAT

⬤⬤◯ SALT

SERVES 4   **PREP** 15 MINS   **COOK** 5 MINS

A super-quick dish that makes a perfect midweek supper.

2 tbsp vegetable oil
1 onion, finely chopped
2 carrots, finely sliced
200g (7oz) baby corn
200g (7oz) mangetout
3 garlic cloves, finely chopped
200g can bamboo shoots, drained
200g (7oz) oyster mushrooms, large
  ones halved

400g (14oz) beansprouts
bunch of spring onions, trimmed
  and sliced
1 tbsp dark soy sauce
splash of sesame oil
freshly ground black pepper
15g (½oz) dry-roasted peanuts,
  chopped

1 Heat the oil in a wok and when just starting to smoke, add the onion and carrots and stir-fry for a few minutes. Then add the baby corn and mangetout and stir-fry for 1 minute.

2 Add the garlic, bamboo shoots, mushrooms, beansprouts, and spring onions, and stir-fry for another minute or two. Keep everything moving all the time.

3 Add the soy sauce and sesame oil and season with black pepper. Stir-fry for 1 minute and then tip out the vegetables onto a serving dish and top with the peanuts.

COOK'S TIP
Prepare all the vegetables before you start frying, so you can work fast. The fried vegetables should still have a crunch to them – don't overcook or they will become lifeless and soggy.

STATISTICS PER SERVING:

Energy 188kcals/786kJ

Carbohydrate 16g

Sugar 11g

Fibre 6.5g

Fat 10g
Saturated fat 1.5g

Salt 0.9g

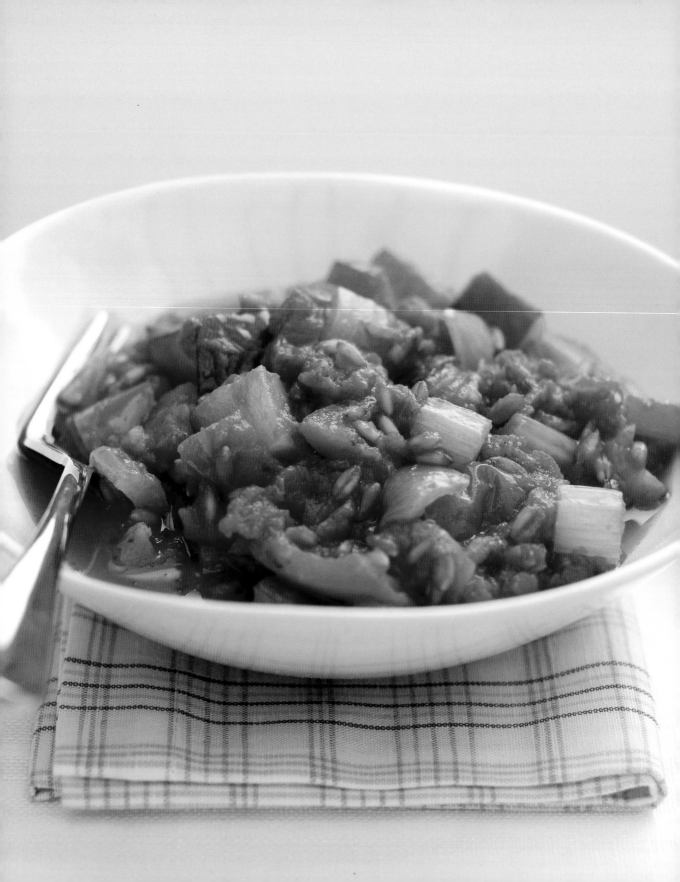

MEDITERRANEAN VEGETABLES WITH FARRO

GUIDELINES PER SERVING:

● ○ ○ GI

● ○ ○ CALORIES

● ○ ○ SATURATED FAT

● ○ ○ SALT

SERVES 4   **PREP** 15 MINS   **COOK** 40 MINS   **FREEZE** 1 MONTH

A hearty mix of chunky vegetables thickened with grains.

1 tbsp olive oil
1 onion, chopped
salt and freshly ground black pepper
3 celery stalks, chopped
pinch of dried oregano
1 red pepper, chopped

2 courgettes, chopped
squeeze of tomato purée
2 x 400g cans of tomatoes
900ml (1½ pints) vegetable stock
50g (1¾oz) farro

1 Heat the oil in a large pan then add the onion and cook over a low heat for 5 minutes or until soft and transparent. Season with salt and black pepper and add the celery and oregano and cook for 5 minutes or until the celery is soft.

2 Add the red pepper and courgettes and cook for 5 more minutes. Stir in the tomato purée, add the canned tomatoes and stock, and bring to the boil. Reduce the heat to a simmer, add the farro, and cook for 30–40 minutes, stirring occasionally and topping up with hot water or more stock if needed. Taste, season as required, and serve hot.

COOK'S TIP

Farro is a delicious healthy grain with a chewy texture. Used a lot in Italian cooking, you will find it in health food stores or in the special selection of some supermarkets.

STATISTICS PER SERVING:

Energy 237kcals/1,000kJ

Carbohydrate 25g

Sugar 11g

Fibre 3g

Fat 3g
Saturated fat 1.5g

Salt 0.3g

● ○ ○   GI

● ● ○   CALORIES

● ○ ○   SATURATED FAT

● ● ○   SALT

BEANS, SWISS CHARD, AND ARTICHOKES

SERVES 4   **PREP** 15 MINS   **COOK** 30 MINS   **FREEZE** 1 MONTH

A simple and hearty one-pot dish. Swiss chard contains vitamin K, which is good for bone health.

1 tbsp olive oil
1 onion, finely chopped
3 garlic cloves, finely chopped
2 red peppers, deseeded and
  finely chopped
pinch of ground cumin
pinch of paprika
1 bay leaf
salt and freshly ground black pepper
½ tbsp white wine vinegar

900ml (1½ pints) vegetable
  or chicken stock
400g can each of butter beans,
  cannellini beans, and red kidney
  beans, drained and rinsed
250g (9oz) Swiss chard, stems and
  leaves separated and roughly
  chopped
200g jar artichoke hearts in oil,
  drained, rinsed, and halved

1 Heat the olive oil in a large, heavy pan, add the onion and cook for about 5 minutes or until soft. Stir in the garlic and red peppers along with the cumin, paprika, and bay leaf. Season well with salt and black pepper.

2 Add the vinegar and increase the heat a little, stirring the contents of the pan, then pour in a little stock and bring to the boil. Reduce to a simmer, tip in the beans, stir, pour in the rest of the stock, and simmer gently for about 15 minutes with the pan partially covered.

3 Add the stems of the chard and cook for 5 more minutes. Add the leaves and the artichokes, and cook for a couple of minutes or until the leaves have wilted. Taste and, if needed, add more seasoning and a little more stock. Remove the bay leaf, then ladle into bowls.

COOK'S TIP
Swiss chard is grown in varieties that have green, red, or multicoloured stems. Choose a colourful variety to add drama to the dish.

STATISTICS PER SERVING:

Energy 421kcals/1,776kJ

Carbohydrate 12g

Sugar 10g

Fibre 15g

Fat 12g

Saturated fat 1g

Salt 1.5g

AUBERGINE AND COURGETTE TAGINE WITH COUSCOUS

SERVES 4   **PREP** 10 MINS   **COOK** 35–40 MINS   **FREEZE** 3 MONTHS
(TAGINE ONLY)

A colourful dish that is packed with aromatic Middle Eastern spices.

1 tbsp olive oil, plus 2–3 tbsp
  extra for frying
1 red onion, sliced
1 tsp coriander seeds, ground
2 tsp dried mint
1 heaped tsp paprika
salt and freshly ground black pepper
1 aubergine, chopped into bite-sized
  pieces
2–3 small courgettes, chopped into
  bite-sized pieces

600ml (1 pint) vegetable stock,
  plus extra for the couscous
4 preserved lemons, halved, pith and
  skin removed and discarded,
  chopped
225g (8oz) couscous
50g (2oz) pine nuts, toasted
1 tbsp chopped coriander leaves, to
  garnish

1 Heat 1 tablespoon of olive oil in a large, wide, heavy pan and add the onion, ground coriander, dried mint, paprika, and salt and black pepper. Cook over a low heat for about 5 minutes or until the onion starts to soften. Tip in the aubergine and, adding more oil as needed, cook until golden. Add the courgettes and continue cooking until they begin to colour.

2 Add a little of the stock and bring to the boil, then reduce to a simmer and add the remaining stock. Cook gently, partially covered, for about 20 minutes or until the liquid has reduced, adding a little more hot water if needed. Stir in the preserved lemons for the last 10 minutes of cooking.

3 Put a lid on the pan of tagine and set it aside while you prepare the couscous. Tip the couscous into a bowl and pour in just enough stock to cover it, leave for 5 minutes, then fluff up with a fork to separate the grains. Season well and then pile onto individual plates and spoon the vegetable mixture over it. Sprinkle with the pine nuts and coriander leaves.

STATISTICS PER SERVING:

Energy 370kcals/1,537kJ

Carbohydrate 37g

Sugar 5g

Fibre 3g

Fat 20g
Saturated fat 2.5g

Salt 1.2g

● ● ○ GI

● ● ○ CALORIES

● ○ ○ SATURATED FAT

● ○ ○ SALT

ROAST ROOT VEGETABLES WITH ROMESCO SAUCE

SERVES 4   **PREP** 20 MINS   **COOK** 45–50 MINS   **FREEZE** 3 MONTHS

The delicious smoky flavour of the romesco sauce complements the roasted vegetables perfectly.

2 sweet potatoes, cut into
  1cm (½in) cubes
2 large carrots, cut into 1cm (½in)
  cubes
2 parsnips, cut into 1cm (½in)
  cubes
1 small celeriac, cut into 1cm (½in)
  cubes
4 garlic cloves
4 tbsp olive oil
salt and freshly ground black pepper

For the romesco sauce
2 red peppers, deseeded and roughly
  chopped into 2cm (¾in) chunks
3 large tomatoes, deseeded and cut
  into quarters
3 tbsp olive oil
25g (scant 1oz) blanched almonds
2 garlic cloves, crushed or finely
  chopped
½ tsp smoked paprika
½ tsp cayenne pepper, or to taste
1–2 tbsp red wine vinegar

1 Preheat the oven to 220°C (425°F/Gas 7). Toss all the root vegetables and the 4 garlic cloves in 3 tablespoons of the olive oil, season to taste with salt and black pepper, and transfer to a large roasting tin. Roast in the oven for 40–50 minutes, or until tender.

2 To make the romesco sauce, place the peppers and tomatoes in a separate roasting tin. Drizzle with 1 tablespoon of the oil and cook in the oven for 20 minutes, then add the almonds and cook for a further 5 minutes. Remove from the oven and set aside to cool.

3 Place the cooled peppers and tomatoes in a food processor or a blender with the garlic, paprika, cayenne pepper, and vinegar. Process until smooth. Transfer to a small bowl and adjust the seasoning.

4 Arrange the roasted vegetables on a serving plate and drizzle the romesco sauce over them.

STATISTICS PER SERVING:

Energy 390kcals/1,622kJ

Carbohydrate 37g

Sugar 20g

Fibre 13g

Fat 25g

Saturated fat 3g

Salt 0.4g

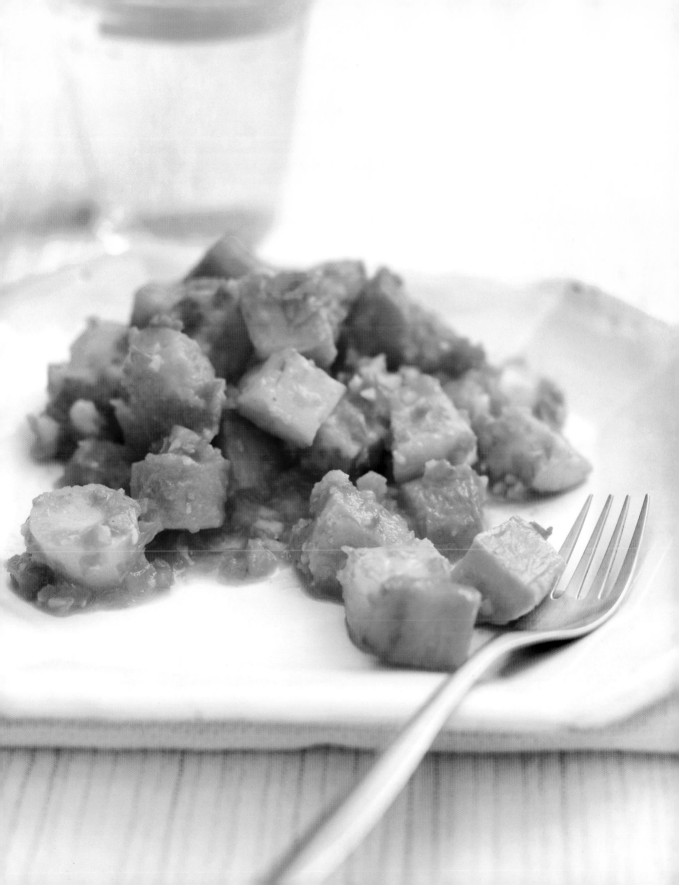

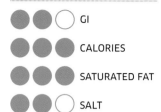

BLACK-EYED BEAN AND COCONUT CASSEROLE

SERVES 4   **PREP** 15 MINS   **COOK** 45 MINS   **FREEZE** 1 MONTH
WITHOUT THE RICE

A rich and satisfying dish that incorporates American and Asian influences.

1 tbsp olive oil
1 onion, finely chopped
2 garlic cloves, finely chopped
5cm (2in) piece of fresh root ginger, peeled and finely chopped
1 bay leaf
1 tsp coriander seeds, crushed
2 x 400g cans black-eyed beans, drained and rinsed

400g can coconut milk
600ml (1 pint) vegetable stock
3 potatoes, peeled and cut into bite-sized pieces
salt and freshly ground black pepper
200g (7oz) basmati rice

1 Heat the oil in a large pan, add the onion and cook until soft. Stir in the garlic, ginger, bay leaf, and coriander seeds and cook for a couple of minutes, being careful not to burn the garlic.

2 Stir in the beans, then add the coconut milk and stock and bring to the boil. Reduce the heat and simmer, partially covered, for about 15 minutes. Add the potatoes and cook for a further 10 minutes or until they are done. If the casserole needs more liquid, top up with stock but don't let it become runny. Taste and season as needed and remove the bay leaf.

3 Meanwhile, put the rice in a large pan, cover with water and cook for 10–15 minutes or according to the instructions on the packet. Once the rice is cooked, remove it from the heat, cover the pan, and leave it to steam for a few more minutes. Either add the rice to the casserole, or serve it separately.

STATISTICS PER SERVING:

Energy 726kcals/3,048kJ

Carbohydrate 100g

Sugar 5g

Fibre 12g

Fat 22g

Saturated fat 16g

Salt 0.8g

PUY LENTIL AND VEGETABLE HOTPOT

SERVES 4   **PREP** 20 MINS   **COOK** 1 HOUR   **FREEZE** 3 MONTHS

Sweet potatoes and cinnamon add a delicious sweetness to this tasty hotpot.

1 tbsp olive oil
2 onions, roughly chopped
1 cinnamon stick
1 bay leaf
3 celery sticks, finely diced
salt and freshly ground black pepper
2 garlic cloves, finely chopped
3 carrots, roughly chopped

400g (14oz) puy lentils, well rinsed
 and any grit removed
1.2 litres (2 pints) vegetable stock
handful of curly kale or dark green
 cabbage, roughly chopped
2 sweet potatoes, diced
handful of flat-leaf parsley, finely
 chopped

1 Heat the oil over a low heat in a large, heavy saucepan, add the onions and cook for a few minutes or until the onions soften a little. Add the cinnamon stick, bay leaf and celery and cook for a further 5 minutes to sweat the celery. Season with salt and some black pepper.

2 Stir in the garlic and carrots, cook for a couple of minutes, then add the lentils and stir until coated. Pour in the stock, bring it to the boil then reduce the heat to a simmer and cook, partially covered, for about 40 minutes or until the lentils are done. Stir occasionally and top up with more hot water if the mixture begins to dry out.

3 Add the cabbage and sweet potatoes to the pan, cover, and cook for a final 10 minutes or until the potato is soft and the cabbage is cooked. Remove the cinnamon stick and bay leaf, then stir through the parsley. Taste and season as needed, ladle into bowls, and serve.

COOK'S TIP
Curly kale is a member of the cabbage family and is full of nutrients. Trim away any tough bits of stalk before using and rinse the leaves well to remove dirt. Kale requires a slightly longer cooking time than cabbage, so do check that it is cooked before serving.

STATISTICS PER SERVING:

Energy 523kcals/2,214kJ

Carbohydrate 84g

Sugar 17g

Fibre 15g

Fat 8g
Saturated fat 1g

Salt 1.6g

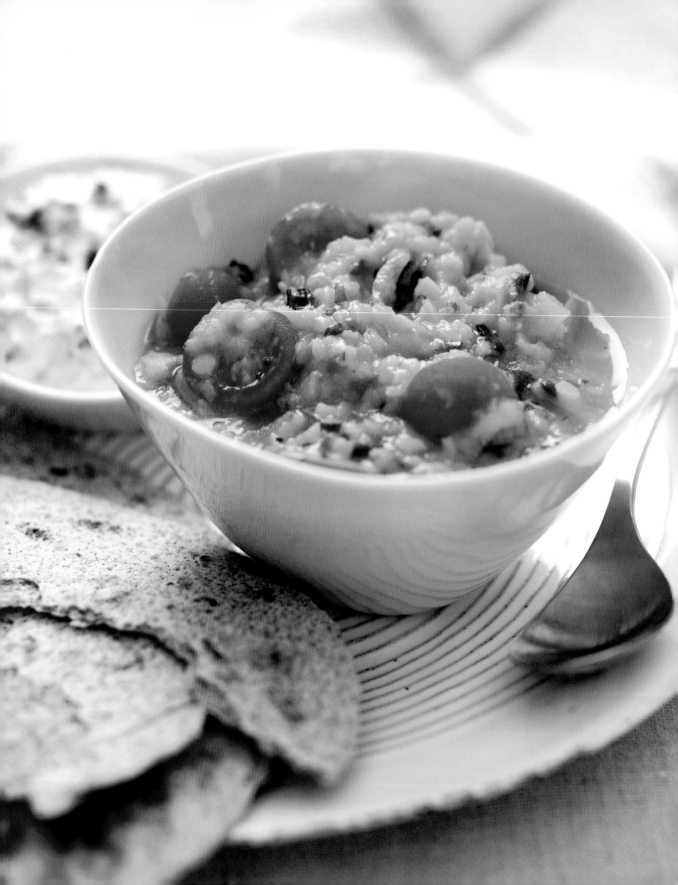

RED LENTIL DHAL WITH CHERRY TOMATOES

SERVES 4   **PREP** 10 MINS   **COOK** 40 MINS

A quick and tasty lunch or supper. Unlike other pulses, lentils don't need to be soaked before cooking.

2 tbsp vegetable oil
1 large onion, peeled and
 finely chopped
3 cloves of garlic, peeled and
 crushed or finely chopped
5mm (1/4in) piece of fresh ginger,
 peeled and finely chopped
200g (7oz) red lentils, rinsed

1 red chilli, deseeded and
 finely chopped
1/2 tsp salt
freshly ground black pepper
200g (7oz) cherry tomatoes, halved
1 tsp black mustard seeds (optional)
3 tbsp chopped fresh coriander

1 Heat the oil in a large saucepan, add the onion and cook over a low heat, stirring occasionally, for 5 minutes. Add the garlic and ginger and continue to cook for 1–2 minutes.

2 Add the lentils, chilli, salt, and 750ml (1 1/4 pints) water. Bring to the boil, reduce the heat, and simmer for 30 minutes or until the lentils are soft. Season to taste with freshly ground black pepper.

3 Stir in the tomatoes, mustard seeds if using, and coriander. Serve with chapattis (see page 338) and riata.

STATISTICS PER SERVING:

Energy 231kcals/965kJ

Carbohydrate 33g

Sugar 4.5g

Fibre 3.5g

Fat 7g

Saturated fat 1g

Salt 0.1g

● ○ ○ GI

● ● ○ CALORIES

● ● ○ SATURATED FAT

● ● ○ SALT

LENTIL LOAF

SERVES 6   **PREP** 15 MINS   **COOK** 1 HOUR 20 MINS

Lentils are a good source of protein and iron, and this substantial loaf can be eaten hot or cold.

175g (6oz) red lentils
450ml (15fl oz) vegetable stock
1 tbsp olive oil
1 onion, sliced
2 sticks celery, finely chopped
1 red pepper, deseeded and diced
1 clove garlic, crushed
1 small red chilli, deseeded and
  finely chopped

125g (4½oz) shiitake mushrooms,
  finely chopped
150g (5½oz) half-fat Cheddar cheese,
  grated
225g (8oz) wholemeal breadcrumbs
3 tbsp chopped fresh coriander
1 egg, beaten
salt and freshly ground black pepper

1 Put the lentils in a saucepan and add the stock. Bring to the boil, then reduce the heat, cover and simmer over a low heat for 15–20 minutes or until the lentils are very soft.

2 Preheat the oven to 180°C (350°F/Gas 4). Grease and line the bottom of a 1.2 litre (2 pint) loaf tin. Heat the oil in a frying pan, add the onion and cook for 2–3 minutes or until softened. Add the celery, red pepper, garlic, chilli, and mushrooms. Cook, stirring, for 10 minutes.

3 Tip the vegetables into the lentil mixture, then stir in the cheese, breadcrumbs, coriander, and egg. Mix well and season to taste with salt and pepper.

4 Spoon the mixture into the prepared loaf tin and bake for 1 hour or until firm to the touch.

5 Cool in the tin for 10 minutes before turning out. Cut into thick slices and serve hot or cold.

STATISTICS PER SERVING:

Energy 300kcals/1,265kJ

Carbohydrate 35g

Sugar 3.5g

Fibre 4g

Fat 9g

Saturated fat 3.5g

Salt 1.3g

LENTILS WITH TURNIPS AND CHESTNUTS

GUIDELINES PER SERVING:

● ○ ○ GI

● ● ○ CALORIES

● ○ ○ SATURATED FAT

● ● ○ SALT

SERVES 4   **PREP** 10 MINS   **COOK** 50 MINS   **FREEZE** 3 MONTHS

A chunky vegetable dish with versatility: serve it as a soup or a casserole.

1 tbsp olive oil
1 onion, finely chopped
salt and freshly ground black pepper
2 garlic cloves, finely chopped
2 turnips, cut into chunks
200g vacuum pack of chestnuts

3 sage leaves, roughly chopped
1 tbsp fresh parsley,
  roughly chopped
350g (12oz) Puy lentils, rinsed
  and any grit removed
1.2 litres (2 pints) vegetable stock

1 Heat the oil in a large, heavy pan, put in the onion and cook until soft. Season with salt and black pepper, then stir in the garlic, turnips, chestnuts, sage, and parsley.

2 Stir in the lentils so they are coated with the vegetable mixture, then pour in the stock and bring to the boil. Reduce to a simmer, partially cover the pan and cook gently for about 40 minutes or until the lentils are soft, topping up with more stock if needed.

3 Season to taste, then ladle into bowls and serve.

STATISTICS PER SERVING:

Energy 442kcals/1,872kJ

Carbohydrate 67g

Sugar 8g

Fibre 11g

Fat 8g
Saturated fat 1.5g

Salt 1.4g

SPICED LEMONY LENTILS WITH ROAST POTATOES

SERVES 4   **PREP** 15 MINS   **COOK** 40-50 MINS   **FREEZE** 3 MONTHS

A tasty vegetarian dish, made extra substantial by the inclusion of chickpeas and roast potatoes.

175g (6oz) Puy lentils, rinsed and any grit removed
900ml (1½ pints) vegetable stock
salt and freshly ground black pepper
3 potatoes, peeled and cut into 2.5cm (1in) cubes
2 tbsp olive oil
2 red chillies, deseeded and finely chopped
2 tsp cumin seeds

2 garlic cloves, finely chopped
zest of 1 lemon
1 onion, finely chopped
1 red pepper, deseeded and finely chopped
400g can chickpeas, drained and rinsed
juice of 2 lemons
1 tbsp flat-leaf parsley, finely chopped

1 Preheat the oven to 200°C (400°F/Gas 6). Put the lentils in a large pan and cover with the stock. Season well and bring to the boil, remove any scum on the surface of the liquid, and then simmer gently for 30–40 minutes or until the lentils are soft. (If the lentils look as if they are drying out, top up with a little more stock.) Drain and set aside.

2 While the lentils are cooking, toss the potatoes in 1 tablespoon of the olive oil and put them in a large roasting tin along with the chillies and cumin seeds. Season well with salt and black pepper. Roast in the oven for 30–35 minutes, giving them a shake or a stir halfway through, and add the garlic and lemon zest at the same time.

3 Heat 1 tablespoon of the oil in a large, heavy, deep frying pan. Add the onion and red pepper, and cook for about 5 minutes or until the pepper softens. Tip in the chickpeas and the cooked lentils, stir well, and then stir in the lemon juice and parsley. If you prefer a wetter mixture, add a little hot stock and let it cook for a few minutes. Serve topped with a spoonful of the crispy roast potatoes.

STATISTICS PER SERVING:

Energy 456kcals/1,925kJ

Carbohydrate 67g

Sugar 7g

Fibre 7g

Fat 9g

Saturated fat 1.5g

Salt 1.1g

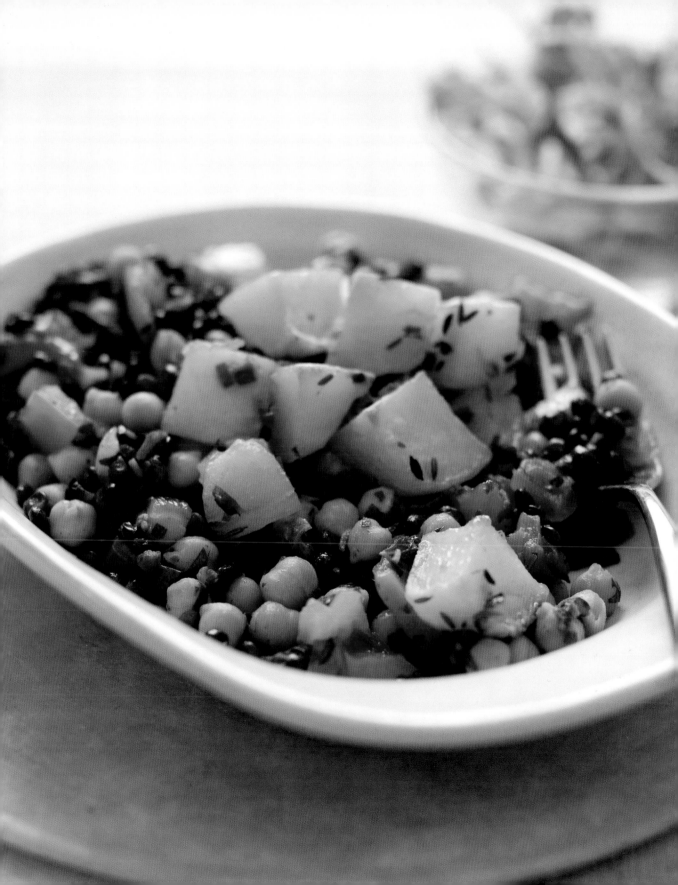

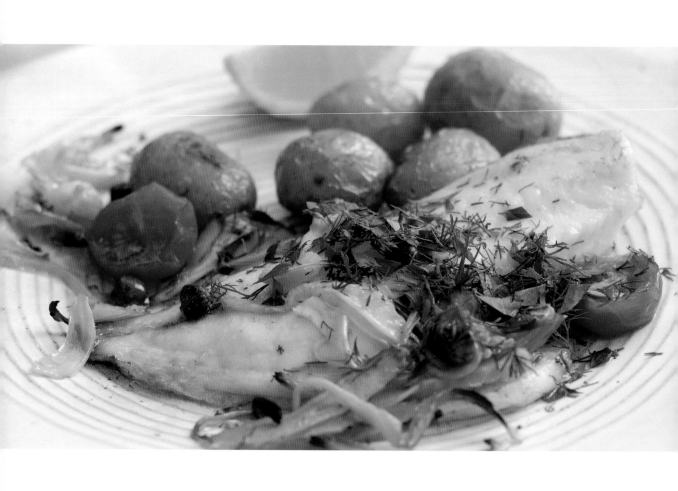

SIMPLE SUPPERS
– FISH

◑◯◯ GI

●●◯ CALORIES

●●◯ SATURATED FAT

●◯◯ SALT

TUNA WITH BLACK-EYED BEAN AND AVOCADO SALSA

SERVES 4   **PREP** 10 MINS   **COOK** 15 MINS

Serving fish or meat with a spicy salsa like this one is a great way to add to your intake of fruit and vegetables.

400g can black-eyed beans, rinsed and drained
2 ripe avocados, peeled, stoned, and diced
200g (7oz) plum tomatoes, cut into quarters, deseeded and diced
1 small red onion, finely chopped

4 tbsp chopped fresh coriander
zest and juice of 2 limes
salt and freshly ground black pepper
4 fresh tuna steaks (about 150g/5½oz each)
1 tbsp olive oil

1 To make the salsa, mix together the beans, avocados, tomatoes, and onion in a large bowl. Stir in the coriander, lime zest and juice, and season to taste.

2 Brush the tuna steaks with oil. Place on a hot griddle pan and sear for 4–5 minutes each side.

3 Transfer the tuna to a warm serving plate and serve with the salsa.

STATISTICS PER SERVING:

Energy 480kcals/2,014kJ

Carbohydrate 20g

Sugar 5g

Fibre 9g

Fat 25g

Saturated fat 6g

Salt 0.2g

STEAMED SEA BASS WITH SOY, GINGER, AND LEMONGRASS

GUIDELINES PER SERVING:

● ○ ○ GI

● ○ ○ CALORIES

● ○ ○ SATURATED FAT

● ● ● SALT

SERVES 4   **PREP** 5 MINS   **COOK** 15 MINS

Sea bass is a delicate-tasting fish; here it is enhanced with aromatic spices and cooked in foil to seal in all the juices.

4 sea bass fillets, skin on
4 tbsp soy sauce
5cm (2in) piece of fresh root ginger, finely sliced
2 stalks lemongrass, trimmed and finely sliced

1 bunch of spring onions, trimmed and sliced on the diagonal
1 tbsp fresh coriander, leaves only

1 Preheat the oven to 180°C (350°F/Gas 4). Rinse the fish and pat dry. Lay a large piece of foil in a roasting tin and place the fish on it. Pour the soy sauce over it and sprinkle with the ginger and lemongrass.

2 Bring the edges of the foil together and squeeze so they are secure, but leave plenty of room around the fish. Put in the oven and cook for 8–10 minutes until the fish flakes when poked with a sharp knife.

3 Remove the fish to a serving dish and top with the spring onions and coriander, then pour the soy sauce from the foil over it.

STATISTICS PER SERVING:

Energy 165kcals/697kJ

Carbohydrate 3.5g

Sugar 3g

Fibre 0.4g

Fat 4g

Saturated fat 0.6g

Salt 2.9g

ROASTED MONKFISH WITH ROMESCO SAUCE

GUIDELINES PER SERVING:

● ○ ○ GI
● ● ○ CALORIES
● ○ ○ SATURATED FAT
● ○ ○ SALT

SERVES 4   **PREP** 15 MINS   **COOK** 20-25 MINS

A meaty fish such as monkfish works so well with this piquant red pepper sauce.

2 red peppers
1 bulb of garlic
1.1kg (2½lb) monkfish tails, washed and thin membrane removed, patted dry
4 tbsp olive oil
salt and freshly ground black pepper

2 tomatoes, quartered
2 tbsp breadcrumbs
25g (scant 1oz) blanched almonds or hazelnuts
2 tbsp red wine vinegar
pinch of chilli flakes

1 Preheat the oven to 200°C (400°F/Gas 6). Put the peppers and garlic in a roasting tin and place in the oven for about 20 minutes or until the peppers begin to soften and char very lightly. Remove the peppers, put them in a plastic bag and leave to cool. Set the garlic aside to cool. Leave the oven on.

2 While the vegetables are cooling, lightly rub the fish with a little olive oil and season with salt and black pepper. Put in a roasting tin and cook in the oven for 20–25 minutes or until the fish is cooked through.

3 Remove the skin from the red peppers and discard it along with the stem and seeds. Heat a little of the olive oil in a frying pan, add the tomatoes and cook for a couple of minutes until they soften. Tip into a food processor or blender and whiz until blended. Add the breadcrumbs and whiz again. Squeeze the garlic cloves from their skins and put them in the mixture along with the peeled red peppers, then whiz again. Add the nuts, vinegar, remaining oil, and chilli flakes. Season well with salt and black pepper. Blend to a smooth paste. Taste and adjust the seasoning if needed, and serve with the roasted fish.

COOK'S TIP
For ease, you could use ready-roasted peppers from a 340g jar, drained and blended as per the recipe.

STATISTICS PER SERVING:

Energy 345kcals/1,450kJ

Carbohydrate 13g

Sugar 6g

Fibre 2g

Fat 16g

Saturated fat 2g

Salt 0.3g

SWORDFISH WITH A SPICY COATING

SERVES 4　　**PREP** 5 MINS　　**COOK** 10 MINS

This firm, rich-textured fish is perfect for griddling and here's a quick and zesty way to enjoy it at its freshest.

1 tsp cayenne pepper
1 tbsp olive oil
1 tbsp fresh flat-leaf parsley, finely
　chopped

juice and zest of 1 lime
salt and freshly ground black pepper
4 x 200g (7oz) swordfish steaks
4 lime segments, to serve

1 In a small bowl, mix together the cayenne pepper, olive oil, parsley, lime juice and zest. Season with salt and black pepper.

2 Lay the swordfish steaks on a plate, pour the spicy mixture over them and rub to coat. Heat a griddle pan over a high heat, then pop in the steaks, two at a time if there is not enough room for all of them, and cook for 3–5 minutes each side until cooked through. Remove and serve with a squeeze of lime.

GUIDELINES PER SERVING:

● ○ ○　GI
● ○ ○　CALORIES
● ○ ○　SATURATED FAT
● ○ ○　SALT

STATISTICS PER SERVING:

Energy	243kcals/1,018kJ
Carbohydrate	0g
Sugar	0g
Fibre	0g
Fat	11g
Saturated fat	2g
Salt	0.6g

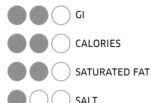

SPICY MACKEREL AND BEETROOT ROAST

SERVES 4   **PREP** 15 MINS   **COOK** 10 MINS

Mackerel, an oily fish that is rich in essential fatty acids, marries well with sweet beetroot and Indian spices.

4 whole fresh mackerel, cleaned, gutted, and slashed
300g (10oz) cooked beetroot
1 tbsp olive oil
1 tbsp fresh coriander, to garnish

For the spice rub
1 tsp cumin seeds
1 tsp coriander seeds

2 garlic cloves, roughly chopped
1 red chilli, deseeded and chopped
½ tbsp sherry vinegar or red wine vinegar
1 tbsp olive oil
salt and freshly ground black pepper

1 Preheat the oven to 200°C (400°F/Gas 6). First, make the spice rub. Put all the ingredients in a food processor or blender and whiz until ground. Alternatively, grind in a pestle and mortar.

2 Rub the paste all over the fish and into the slashes. Put the beetroot in a roasting tin and toss in 1 tablespoon of oil. Add the fish and place in the oven for 8–10 minutes or until cooked and crispy. Sprinkle with the coriander to serve. You could accompany this with a little brown or basmati rice.

COOK'S TIP
Mackerel needs to be cooked and eaten as soon as possible after purchase.

STATISTICS PER SERVING:

Energy 414kcals/1,730kJ

Carbohydrate 7g

Sugar 6g

Fibre 1.5g

Fat 29g

Saturated fat 6g

Salt 0.5g

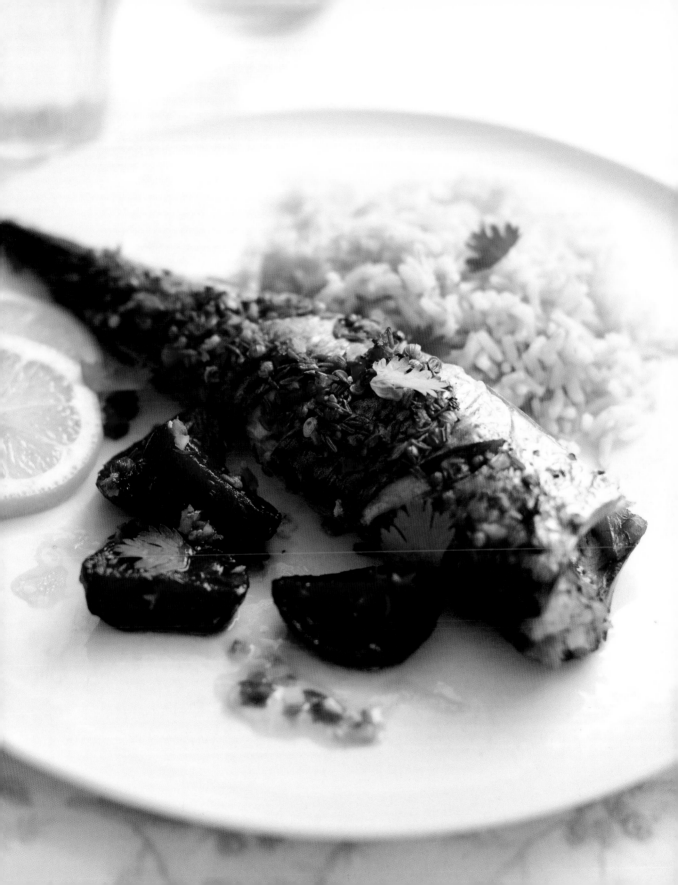

- ●○○ GI
- ●○○ CALORIES
- ●○○ SATURATED FAT
- ●○○ SALT

MONKFISH WITH SALSA VERDE

SERVES 4   **PREP** 15 MINS   **COOK** 15 MINS

Salsa verde, or green sauce, is a piquant Italian recipe that can work magic with roasted or grilled fish and meat.

2 x 350g (12oz) pieces of chunky
  prepared monkfish, outer film
  removed
1 tbsp olive oil

For the salsa verde
1 tbsp fresh flat-leaf parsley
1 tbsp fresh basil

1 tbsp fresh mint leaves
2 tbsp capers, rinsed
2 anchovy fillets
2 garlic cloves
1 tbsp red wine vinegar
100ml (3½fl oz) good-quality, fruity
  olive oil

1 Preheat the oven to 200°C (400°F/Gas 6). First, make the salsa verde. Put all the ingredients for the sauce in a food processor or blender and pulse until the mixture is well combined but still fairly coarse.

2 Slash the monkfish a few times, then spoon a little of the salsa verde into the slashes, making sure that it includes some of the oil.

3 Heat the olive oil in a large frying pan over a gentle heat, add the monkfish, and cook for about 4 minutes each side. Carefully remove the fish from the pan and transfer to a roasting tin. Cook in the oven for 6–8 minutes, depending on the thickness of the pieces, until done.

4 Spoon a little of the salsa verde over the monkfish and put the remainder in a small bowl to serve alongside.

COOK'S TIP
Monkfish is covered with a thin film that the fishmonger may remove for you; if you do it yourself, simply use a small, sharp knife to peel it away.

STATISTICS PER SERVING:

Energy 303kcals/1,263kJ

Carbohydrate 0.5g

Sugar 0g

Fibre 0g

Fat 22g

Saturated fat 3g

Salt 0.8g

COD IN A RICH TOMATO SAUCE

SERVES 4   **PREP** 10 MINS   **COOK** 40-45 MINS   **FREEZE** 3 MONTHS
(SAUCE ONLY)

GUIDELINES PER SERVING:

● ○ ○ GI

● ○ ○ CALORIES

● ○ ○ SATURATED FAT

● ● ○ SALT

Like all white fish, cod is low in fat, making it an excellent choice for anyone watching their weight.

2 tbsp olive oil
1 large red onion, finely chopped
2 sticks celery, finely chopped
2 cloves garlic, crushed
large pinch of chilli flakes
1 tsp ground coriander
1 tsp ground cumin

2 x 400g cans chopped tomatoes
2 tbsp tomato purée
150ml (5fl oz) red wine
salt and freshly ground black pepper
4 skinless cod fillets
50g (1¾oz) pitted black olives

1 Heat half the oil in large saucepan, tip in the onion and cook for 2–3 minutes. Add the rest of the oil, the celery, garlic, chilli, coriander, and cumin. Cook for 5 minutes or until the onion is beginning to soften.

2 Empty in the tomatoes, tomato purée, and red wine. Season to taste, bring to the boil and then simmer for about 30 minutes or until the sauce is reduced by about half.

3 Bury the fish in the tomato sauce and scatter with the olives. Cover and cook gently for 10 minutes or until the fish is done. Check the seasoning and serve immediately.

STATISTICS PER SERVING:

Energy 269kcals/1,130kJ

Carbohydrate 11g

Sugar 9g

Fibre 3g

Fat 9g
Saturated fat 1g

Salt 0.8g

SALMON EN PAPILLOTE

SERVES 4   **PREP** 25 MINS   **COOK** 15 MINS

Cooking in a tightly sealed parchment packet or *papillote* ensures that the cooking juices are retained and keeps the fish moist.

olive oil, for greasing
4 tomatoes, sliced
4 salmon steaks or fillets,
  175g (6oz) each

2 lemons, sliced
8 sprigs of tarragon
freshly ground black pepper

1 Cut 8 circles of greaseproof paper large enough for the salmon steaks to fit on half of a circle. Place 2 circles on top of each other to create a double thickness of paper. Lightly grease the top circle's surface with olive oil. Repeat with the other circles.

2 Preheat the oven to 160°C (325°F/Gas 3). Divide the tomato slices among the circles, placing them on one half. Place the salmon on the tomatoes, then top with the lemon slices and tarragon and season to taste with pepper. Fold up the paper to enclose the fish. Crimp the edges to create a tight seal. Place the parcels on a baking tray and bake for 15 minutes.

3 Place the salmon on warm plates, and serve immediately.

COOK'S TIP
The salmon parcels can be prepared several hours in advance and chilled until needed.

STATISTICS PER SERVING:

Energy 345kcals/1,441kJ

Carbohydrate 3g

Sugar 3g

Fibre 1g

Fat 21g
Saturated fat 3.5g

Salt 0.2g

MEDITERRANEAN-STYLE GRILLED SARDINES

SERVES 4   **PREP** 15 MINS   **COOK** 5 MINS
PLUS MARINATING

Popular in coastal regions all over southern Europe, this is the way to enjoy these oily fish at their very best.

8 large whole sardines, cleaned
8 sprigs of thyme or lemon thyme,
 plus extra to garnish
4 lemons

3 tbsp olive oil
2 garlic cloves, crushed
1 tsp ground cumin

1 Rinse the sardines inside and out, and pat dry. Put a sprig of thyme or lemon thyme inside each fish, and place them in a shallow non-metallic dish. Grate the zest and squeeze the juice from 3 of the lemons and place in a small bowl. Add the oil, garlic, and cumin, and whisk together. Pour this mixture over the sardines, cover, and leave to marinate in the refrigerator for at least 2 hours.

2 Preheat the grill on its highest setting. Transfer the sardines to a grill pan and grill for 2–3 minutes on each side, basting with the marinade.

3 Cut the remaining lemon into 8 wedges. Transfer the sardines to a heated serving plate and serve immediately, garnished with lemon wedges and sprigs of thyme.

GUIDELINES PER SERVING:

GI

CALORIES

SATURATED FAT

SALT

STATISTICS PER SERVING:

Energy 322kcals/1,341kJ

Carbohydrate 0g

Sugar 0g

Fibre 0g

Fat 22g
Saturated fat 3g

Salt 0.4g

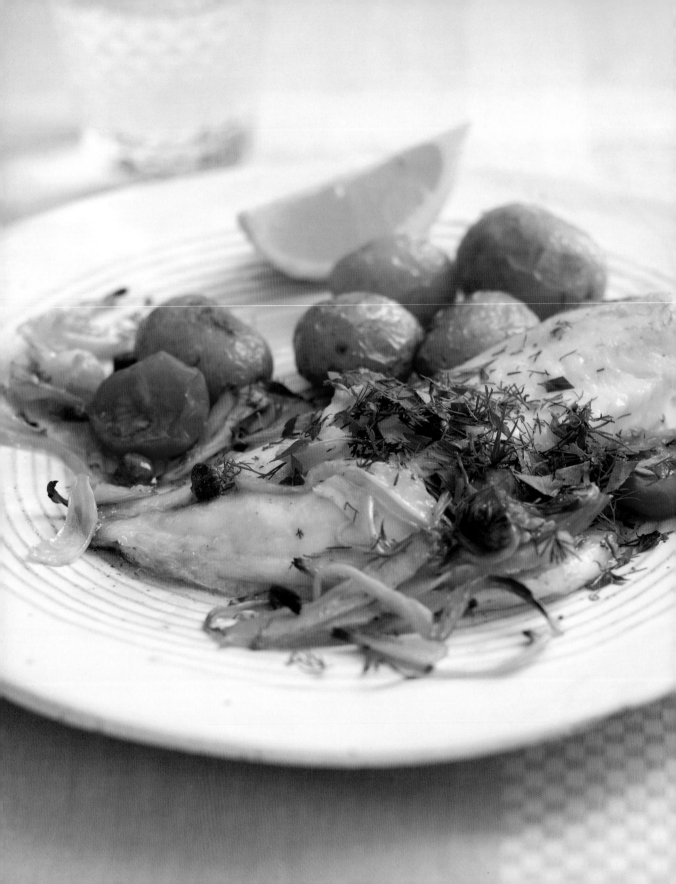

ROASTED SNAPPER WITH NEW POTATOES AND FENNEL

SERVES 4   **PREP** 15 MINS   **COOK** 30 MINS

An easy and healthy all-in-one roast.

GUIDELINES PER SERVING:

● ● ○ GI

● ○ ○ CALORIES

● ○ ○ SATURATED FAT

● ○ ○ SALT

300g (10oz) baby new potatoes
2 tbsp olive oil
salt and freshly ground black pepper
8 cherry tomatoes, finely chopped
1 fennel bulb, finely chopped
2 tsp capers, rinsed

4 fillets of snapper (about 140g/5oz each), skin on
1 tbsp fresh flat-leaf parsley, finely chopped
1 tbsp fresh dill, finely chopped

1 Preheat the oven to 200°C (400°F/Gas 6). Put the potatoes in a roasting tin and drizzle with 1 tablespoon of the olive oil. Mix to coat, using your hands, and arrange so that they have plenty of room around them. Season well with salt and black pepper, then roast for about 15 minutes.

2 While the potatoes are cooking, combine the tomatoes, fennel, and capers with the remaining olive oil. Season to taste. Smother the fish fillets with the tomato mixture. Remove the tin of potatoes from the oven, sit the coated fish on top, and return the tin to the oven to cook for a further 15 minutes, or until the potatoes and fish are done.

3 Sprinkle with the parsley and dill and serve immediately.

STATISTICS PER SERVING:

Energy 244kcals/1,028kJ

Carbohydrate 13g

Sugar 2g

Fibre 1.5g

Fat 8g

Saturated fat 1.5g

Salt 0.6g

MONKFISH WITH WILTED GREENS AND CHILLI

SERVES 4   **PREP** 15 MINS   **COOK** 25 MINS

Earthy greens livened up with chilli and sherry are an excellent accompaniment to white fish.

2 tbsp olive oil
1.1kg (2½lb) monkfish tails, washed,
  thin membrane removed and
  patted dry
salt and freshly ground black pepper

500g (1lb 2oz) young spinach leaves
3 garlic cloves, finely chopped
1 tsp chilli flakes
1 tbsp dry sherry
lemon wedges, to serve

1 Preheat the oven to 200°C (400°F/Gas 6). Heat 1 tablespoon of the oil in a large frying pan. Season the fish with salt and black pepper, add to the pan, and cook for 5 minutes on each side or until it is sealed. Transfer the fish to a roasting tin and bake in the oven for 15 minutes or until cooked through.

2 While the fish is cooking, wipe out the pan with a piece of kitchen paper and heat the remaining olive oil. Add the spinach and cook for a minute then add the garlic and chilli and cook for a further 2–3 minutes or until the spinach begins to wilt. Increase the heat, add the sherry and a little salt and pepper, and cook for 2–3 minutes more or until the sherry has evaporated.

3 Divide up the spinach onto plates, then slice the monkfish and arrange on top. Serve with lemon wedges for squeezing over.

STATISTICS PER SERVING:

Energy 267kcals/1,126kJ

Carbohydrate 2g

Sugar 1.5g

Fibre 2.5g

Fat 7.5g
Saturated fat 1g

Salt 0.6g

TUNA KEBABS WITH SALSA VERDE

SERVES 4   **PREP** 15 MINS   **COOK** 10 MINS

Tuna's firm, meaty texture makes it good for kebabs.

450g (1lb) tuna, cut into
   12 bite-sized pieces
75g (2½oz) Parma ham,
   cut into 12 strips
12 small cherry tomatoes
olive oil, for brushing

For the salsa verde
1 tsp Dijon mustard
8 tbsp olive oil

2 anchovy fillets
handful of flat-leaf parsley
handful of mint
handful of basil
1 tbsp capers, rinsed
2 garlic cloves, peeled
juice of 1 lemon

1 First make the salsa verde: place all the ingredients in a food processor and whiz for 30 seconds or until smooth.

2 Preheat the grill to high. Wrap each piece of tuna in a strip of Parma ham and thread onto 4 skewers, alternating with cherry tomatoes. Brush the kebabs with a little oil and place under the grill for 3–4 minutes, then turn and cook for a further 3 minutes or until cooked to your liking. Serve with the salsa verde.

GUIDELINES PER SERVING:

● ○ ○ GI
● ● ○ CALORIES
● ● ○ SATURATED FAT
● ○ ○ SALT

STATISTICS PER SERVING:

Energy 345kcals/1,432kJ

Carbohydrate 1g

Sugar 1g

Fibre 0.5g

Fat 27g

Saturated fat 4g

Salt 0.6g

SEAFOOD CEVICHE

SERVES 4   **PREP** 20 MINS
PLUS MARINATING

"Ceviche" describes a brief, light pickling of raw fish in citrus juice, which brings out its true flavour.

450g (1lb) very fresh, firm-fleshed
  fish such as salmon, turbot, halibut,
  or monkfish
1 red onion, thinly sliced
juice of 2 lemons or limes

1 tbsp olive oil
½ tsp pimentón picante
1 chilli, deseeded and finely chopped
salt and freshly ground black pepper
2 tbsp finely chopped parsley

1 With a sharp knife, slice the fish into very thin slivers.

2 Spread the onion slices evenly in the bottom of a shallow, nonmetallic dish. Pour the lemon juice over the onion, then sprinkle the pimentón picante and chilli on top.

3 Place the fish slivers on the layer of onion slices, gently turning them so that they are all fully coated with the marinade.

4 Leave to marinate in the refrigerator for at least 20 minutes, preferably for over 1 hour. Season to taste with salt and pepper, then sprinkle with parsley and serve.

COOK'S TIP
Pimentón picante is a medium-hot paprika pepper.

STATISTICS PER SERVING:

Energy 238kcals/988kJ

Carbohydrate 2g

Sugar 1.5g

Fibre 0.3g

Fat 15g

Saturated fat 2.5g

Salt 0.2g

HADDOCK AND GREEN BEAN PIE

SERVES 4   **PREP** 10 MINS   **COOK** 30 MINS   **FREEZE** 1 MONTH

Flakes of fish in a creamy tarragon sauce, topped with crispy breadcrumbs.

2 slices of wholemeal bread
1 tbsp olive oil
1 onion, finely chopped
salt and freshly ground black pepper
200g (7oz) green beans, trimmed
  and halved
3 garlic cloves, finely chopped

1 tbsp white wine vinegar
1 tbsp plain flour
300ml (10fl oz) milk
few tarragon leaves, finely chopped
500g (1lb 2oz) haddock fillets,
  skinned

1 Preheat the oven to 200°C (400°F/Gas 6). Put the bread in a food processor or blender and whizz until it forms breadcrumbs, then set aside.

2 Heat the olive oil in a large frying pan, add the onion and cook for about 3 minutes until soft and translucent. Season with some salt and black pepper, then add the beans and garlic and cook for a further minute. Add the vinegar, increase the heat and cook for 1 minute.

3 Remove the pan from the heat, stir in the flour to combine, add a little milk and stir again until all the flour is mixed in. Reduce the heat, return the pan to the hob and slowly pour in the rest of the milk, stirring continuously to make a smooth sauce (you can use a balloon whisk to prevent lumps forming).

4 Remove the pan from the heat and stir in the tarragon. Season to taste. Lay the fish in an ovenproof baking dish, pour the sauce over it and stir to combine. Sprinkle with the breadcrumbs and cook in the oven for about 20 minutes or until the fish is done and the breadcrumbs are golden.

STATISTICS PER SERVING:

Energy   246kcals/1,037kJ

Carbohydrate   17g

Sugar   6g

Fibre   2g

Fat   7g

Saturated fat   2.5g

Salt   0.5g

SALMON AND SWEET POTATO PIE

SERVES 4   **PREP** 25 MINS   **COOK** 40-45 MINS   **FREEZE** 1 MONTH

Salmon topped with a golden, sweet mash makes a flavoursome mix that is rich in nutrients.

4 salmon fillets, skinned (about 450g/1lb in total)
750g (1lb 10oz) sweet potatoes, sliced
25g (scant 1oz) polyunsaturated margarine

1 tbsp flour
500ml (16fl oz) semi-skimmed milk
salt and freshly ground black pepper
75g (2½oz) frozen or fresh peas
1 bunch of chives, snipped

1 Preheat the oven to 200°C (400°F/Gas 6). Put the salmon in a roasting dish and cook for 10–15 minutes or until it flakes when you poke it. Don't let it dry out too much. Meanwhile, boil the sweet potatoes in a pan of lightly salted water for 10–15 minutes, until soft when pierced with a knife. Drain and mash using a potato masher.

2 Next, make the sauce. Melt the margarine in a pan, remove from the heat and stir in the flour. Add a little of the milk and stir with a wooden spoon until smooth. Put the pan back on the heat, and gradually add the remaining milk, stirring all the time. Cook, stirring, until it thickens into a smooth sauce. Season well with salt and black pepper. Stir the peas and chives into the sauce.

3 Put the cooked fish in an ovenproof dish and flake it slightly. Pour or spoon the sauce over it, then mix gently to combine. Top with the sweet potato mash, patterning the surface with the back of a fork. Put the pie in the oven to cook for about 30 minutes or until golden brown.

STATISTICS PER SERVING:

Energy 500kcals/2,096kJ

Carbohydrate 50g

Sugar 16g

Fibre 6g

Fat 21g

Saturated fat 5g

Salt 0.5g

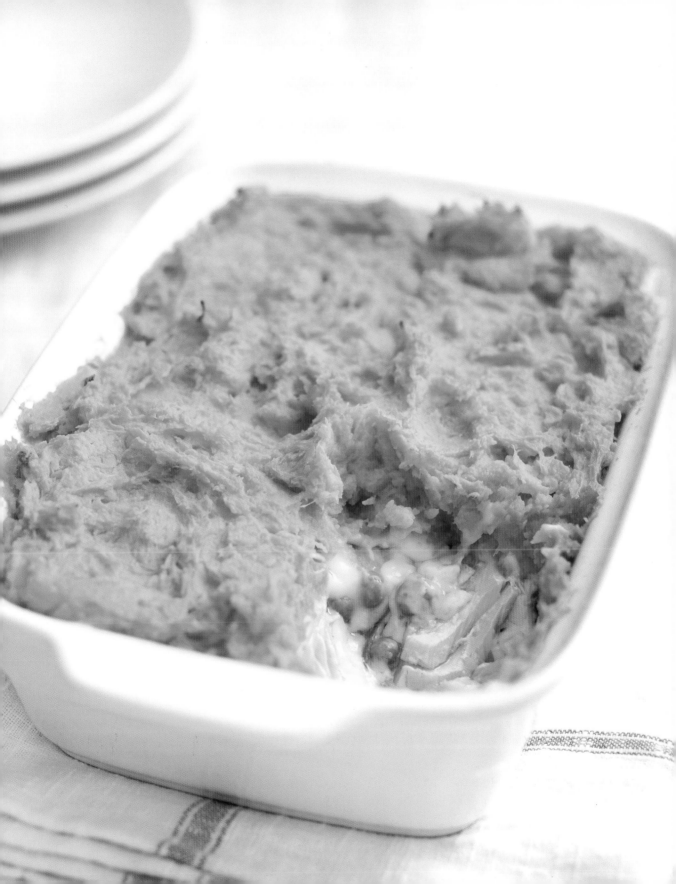

⬤◯◯ GI

⬤⬤◯ CALORIES

⬤◯◯ SATURATED FAT

⬤◯◯ SALT

CURRIED SALMON KEBABS

SERVES 4 **PREP** 5 MINS **COOK** 10 MINS
PLUS CHILLING

These kebabs are perfect for an easy supper. You could also make miniature versions and serve as canapés with a tzatziki dip (see opposite).

3 tbsp tandoori curry paste
150g (5½oz) plain yogurt
4 skinless salmon fillets, sliced
 into bite-sized cubes
1 lemon, cut into 4 wedges, to serve

1 Stir the curry paste into the yogurt and mix well. Add the salmon to the yogurt mix and cover the dish. Set aside in the refrigerator for 15 minutes.

2 Thread the salmon cubes onto metal kebab skewers.

3 Preheat the grill to a medium-high temperature. Line a grill pan with foil and put the kebabs under the grill for 7–10 minutes, or until cooked through. Serve with the lemon wedges.

STATISTICS PER SERVING:

Energy 318kcals/1,331kJ

Carbohydrate 3.5g

Sugar 3g

Fibre 0g

Fat 19g

Saturated fat 3g

Salt 0.7g

SALMON AND SWEET POTATO FISHCAKES

SERVES 4   **PREP** 15 MINS   **COOK** 30 MINS
PLUS CHILLING

Salmon is a great source of omega-3 fats, which help to keep your heart healthy.

500g (1lb 2oz) sweet potatoes, cut into even-sized chunks
2 tbsp reduced-fat mayonnaise
400g can red salmon, drained
85g (3oz) smoked salmon, roughly chopped
plain flour, for dusting
1 large egg, beaten
115g (4oz) fresh wholemeal breadcrumbs

3 tbsp sunflower oil
4 lemon wedges, to serve

For the tzatziki
1 small cucumber
200ml (7fl oz) reduced-fat Greek yogurt
2 tbsp chopped fresh mint
salt and freshly ground black pepper

1 Put the sweet potatoes in a pan of salted water, bring to the boil and cook for 20 minutes, or until tender. Drain well, add the mayonnaise and mash.

2 To make the tzatziki, slice the cucumber in half lengthways and, using a teaspoon, remove the seeds. Dice the flesh and mix with the yogurt and mint. Season with salt and black pepper to taste, cover and set aside.

3 Place the canned salmon in a large bowl and mash it. Add the mashed sweet potato and smoked salmon, and season to taste. Mix well, then cover and place in the refrigerator for 1 hour.

4 Preheat the oven to its lowest setting. Turn out the mixture onto a lightly floured surface and shape it into 8 fishcakes. Dip each one into the beaten egg, then into the breadcrumbs, making sure that they are evenly coated.

5 Heat half the oil in a large frying pan over a high heat and cook half the fishcakes for 4 minutes each side, or until golden brown. Drain the fishcakes on kitchen paper, then transfer to a plate and keep warm in the oven while you cook the rest. Serve with the tzatziki and lemon wedges.

STATISTICS PER SERVING:

Energy 580kcals/2,456kJ

Carbohydrate 54g

Sugar 10g

Fibre 4g

Fat 25g

Saturated fat 4.5g

Salt 2.5g

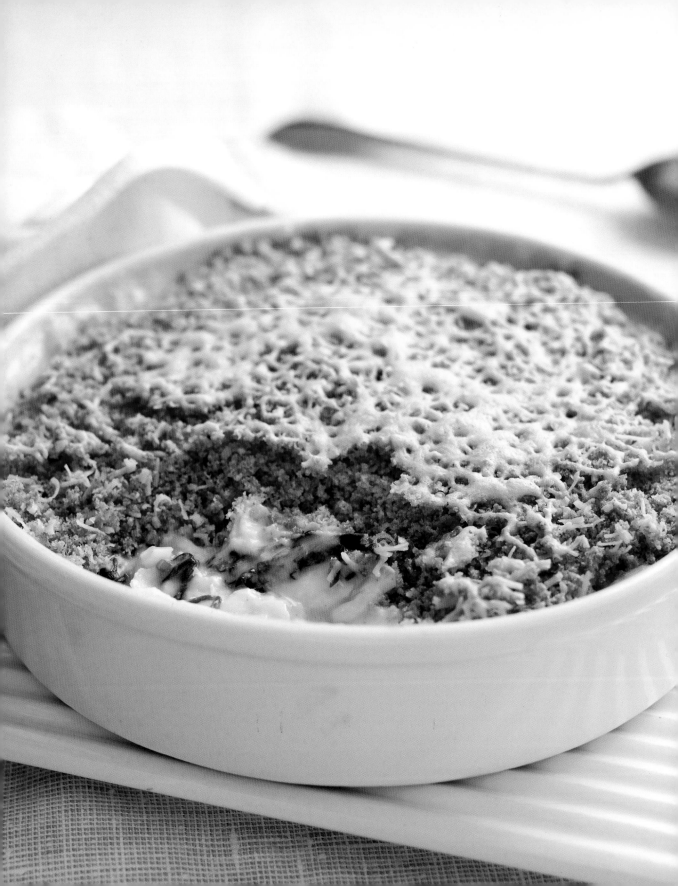

HADDOCK AND SPINACH GRATIN

GUIDELINES PER SERVING:

● ● ○ GI

● ● ○ CALORIES

● ● ○ SATURATED FAT

● ● ○ SALT

SERVES 4   **PREP** 15-20 MINS   **COOK** 20 MINS   **FREEZE** 1 MONTH

A hearty and healthy fish pie topped with golden wholemeal breadcrumbs.

3 slices wholemeal bread, torn
350g (12oz) skinless and
  boneless haddock
600ml (1 pint) semi-skimmed milk
salt and freshly ground black pepper
25g (scant 1oz) polyunsaturated
  margarine
1 tbsp flour

pinch of paprika
150g (5½oz) young spinach leaves,
  roughly torn
3 spring onion stalks, finely chopped
25g (scant 1oz) Parmesan cheese,
  grated
pinch of chilli flakes

1 Preheat the oven to 200°C (400°F/Gas 6). Put the bread in a food processor or blender and whiz to make breadcrumbs. Tip these into a shallow tin and cook in the oven for 5–8 minutes until beginning to turn golden. Remove from the oven and tip back into the food processor .

2 Put the fish in a pan and cover with the milk. Season well. Simmer gently over a low heat for 5 minutes, or until the fish breaks up when poked. Remove with a slotted spoon and put on a plate. Pour the milk into a jug.

3 Melt the margarine in the pan, remove it from the heat and stir in the flour and a little of the reserved cooking milk. Return the pan to the heat and gradually add the remainder of the milk, stirring continually. Cook, stirring, until it thickens into a smooth sauce. Stir in the paprika and season really well with lots of black pepper.

4 Stir the spinach into the sauce (you could precook the spinach for a couple of minutes if you wish) along with the spring onions. Mix the sauce with the fish, taking care not to break up the fish. Spoon the mixture into an ovenproof dish or individual dishes.

5 Add the Parmesan cheese and chilli flakes to the breadcrumbs in the food processor. Whiz again until a fine blend, then scatter evenly over the fish mixture. Cook in the oven for 10–15 minutes until bubbling around the edges; the top should be golden.

STATISTICS PER SERVING:

Energy 335kcals/1,411kJ

Carbohydrate 25g

Sugar 8g

Fibre 3g

Fat 13.5g

Saturated fat 5g

Salt 1.2g

TUNA AND CHICKPEA PATTIES

SERVES 4 **PREP** 15 MINS **COOK** 10 MINS
PLUS CHILLING

An easy dish that can be whipped up from ingredients that are usually lurking in the storecupboard.

2 x 400g cans chickpeas, drained
  and rinsed
2 x 180g cans tuna in spring water,
  drained

1 tbsp mild curry paste
2 tbsp plain flour
2 tbsp vegetable oil
salt and freshly ground black pepper

1 Place the chickpeas, tuna, and curry paste in a food processor or blender and process until just blended. Season to taste.

2 On a lightly floured surface, shape the mixture into 8 patties and then place them in the refrigerator for at least 1 hour.

3 Heat 1 tablespoon of oil in a large, non-stick frying pan, add half the patties, and cook for 4–5 minutes on either side. Put on a plate and transfer to the oven to keep warm. Add 1 more tablespoon of oil to the pan and cook the remaining patties in the same way. You could serve the fishcakes with Coleslaw (see page 299).

COOK'S TIP
Although fresh tuna contains good amounts of omega-3 fats, not all canned tuna does. For optimum health benefit, make the effort to find a variety that is rich in omega-3.

STATISTICS PER SERVING:

Energy 365kcals/1,535kJ

Carbohydrate 32g

Sugar 2g

Fibre 7g

Fat 10g

Saturated fat 1g

Salt 0.4g

CARIBBEAN-FLAVOURED FISH AND RICE

SERVES 4   **PREP** 10 MINS   **COOK** 20 MINS

A sweet-marinated fish dish with a bit of fire to it, to bring some Caribbean sunshine to your table.

GUIDELINES PER SERVING:

●●○ GI

●●○ CALORIES

●○○ SATURATED FAT

●○○ SALT

juice of 4 oranges
50g (1¾oz) black olives, pitted and sliced
1 tbsp thyme stalks, leaves only
1-2 red chillies, deseeded and finely chopped

salt and freshly ground black pepper
700g (1½lb) firm white fish fillets (such as haddock or hake)
225g (8oz) long-grain rice
1 tbsp coriander leaves, to garnish

1 Preheat the oven to 180°C (350°F/Gas 4). Mix together the orange juice, olives, thyme, and chillies. Season with salt and lots of black pepper.

2 Place the pieces of fish in an ovenproof dish and pour the orange juice mixture over them. Cover the dish tightly with foil, so the fish will steam in the oven. Cook in the oven for 15–20 minutes or until the fish flakes when poked with a fork. Remove from the oven and set aside for 5 minutes before serving.

3 While the fish is in the oven, cook the rice. Tip the rice into a large saucepan, cover with water and add a pinch of salt. Cook for 10–15 minutes until the rice is tender, or according to the instructions on the packet. Serve the fish with the rice, sprinkled with the coriander.

STATISTICS PER SERVING:

Energy 396kcals/1,655kJ

Carbohydrate 54g

Sugar 8.5g

Fibre 0.3g

Fat 3.5g
Saturated fat 0.5g

Salt 0.6g

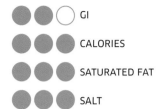

KEDGEREE

SERVES 4   **PREP** 20 MINS   **COOK** 20 MINS

This Anglo-Indian brunch dish is traditionally made with just smoked haddock, but this version also includes salmon for added colour, texture, and flavour.

300g (10oz) undyed smoked haddock
300g (10oz) salmon fillets
200g (7oz) basmati rice
pinch of saffron threads
60g (2oz) butter

4 eggs, hard boiled
2 tbsp chopped parsley, plus extra
  to garnish
salt and freshly ground black pepper
1 lemon, cut into wedges, to serve

1 Place the haddock and salmon in a single layer in a large frying pan. Pour over enough water to cover and heat gently to simmering point. Simmer for 5 minutes, then drain.

2 Meanwhile, cook the rice in boiling, salted water with the saffron threads for 10–12 minutes, or according to packet instructions. When the rice is cooked, drain and stir in the butter.

3 Flake the fish into large chunks and add them to the rice. Discard the skin and bones.

4 Remove the yolks from the hard boiled eggs and reserve. Chop the egg whites and stir into the rice. Add the chopped parsley, and season to taste with salt and pepper.

5 Divide the mixture between heated plates and crumble the reserved egg yolks across the top with more chopped parsley. Serve garnished with lemon wedges.

STATISTICS PER SERVING:

Energy 574kcals/2,395kJ

Carbohydrate 40g

Sugar 3g

Fibre 2g

Fat 28g

Saturated fat 11g

Salt 1.9g

PAELLA

SERVES 4   **PREP** 10 MINS   **COOK** 30 MINS

This Spanish rice dish has many regional variations. This
version contains a delicious mix of seafood.

GUIDELINES PER SERVING:

● ● ○ GI

● ● ○ CALORIES

● ○ ○ SATURATED FAT

● ○ ○ SALT

1.2 litres (2 pints) hot fish stock
large pinch of saffron threads
2 tbsp olive oil
1 onion, finely chopped
2 garlic cloves, crushed
2 large tomatoes, skinned and diced
12 king prawns, peeled

225g (8oz) squid, sliced into rings
400g (14oz) paella rice
85g (3oz) fresh or frozen peas
4 langoustines or Dublin Bay prawns
12-16 mussels, scrubbed and
  debearded
1 tbsp chopped parsley, to garnish

1 Pour a little of the hot fish stock into a cup or jug, add the saffron threads,
and set aside to infuse. Heat the oil in a paella pan or large frying pan, and
fry the onion and garlic until softened. Add the tomatoes and cook for
2 minutes, then add the prawns and squid and fry for 1–2 minutes, or until
the prawns turn pink.

2 Stir in the rice, then add the saffron liquid, peas, and 900ml (1½ pints)
of the stock. Simmer, uncovered, without stirring, over a low heat for
12–14 minutes, or until the stock has evaporated and the rice is just tender
(add a little extra stock if necessary).

3 Meanwhile, cook the langoustines in 150ml (5fl oz) simmering stock for
3–4 minutes, or until cooked through. Transfer to a warm plate with a slotted
spoon. Add the mussels to the stock, cover, and cook over a high heat for
2–3 minutes, or until open. Remove from the pan with a slotted spoon,
discarding any that have not opened.

4 Reserve 8 mussels for garnish. Remove the rest from their shells and stir
into the paella. Arrange the reserved mussels and langoustines on top, and
garnish with parsley.

COOK'S TIP
Tap the mussels prior to cooking and discard any that do not close.

STATISTICS PER SERVING:

Energy 552kcals/2,312kJ

Carbohydrate 88g

Sugar 5g

Fibre 3.5g

Fat 8g

Saturated fat 1g

Salt 0.9g

● ● ○ GI

● ● ○ CALORIES

● ○ ○ SATURATED FAT

● ● ○ SALT

WILD RICE, COURGETTE, FENNEL, AND PRAWN PAN-FRY

SERVES 4   **PREP** 15 MINS   **COOK** 35 MINS

Wild rice adds a delicate, nutty flavour to this pan-fry.

2 tbsp olive oil
1 red onion, finely chopped
3 courgettes, diced
salt and freshly ground black pepper
1 fennel bulb, trimmed and finely
  chopped
225g (8oz) mixed long-grain and
  wild rice.

900ml (1½ pints) vegetable stock
200g (7oz) peeled prawns, raw
2 garlic cloves, chopped
1 tbsp flat-leaf parsley,
  finely chopped
4 lemon wedges, to serve

1 Heat half the oil in a large frying pan and add the onion. Cook over a low heat for 5 minutes, or until it softens. Stir in the courgettes and cook for 5 minutes, or until they begin to colour slightly. Season well with salt and black pepper.

2 Add the fennel and continue cooking over a low heat for 5 minutes, or until it softens. Stir in the mixed rice. Pour in a little of the stock and bring to the boil. Reduce the heat to a simmer, then add most of the remaining stock and cook for 20–25 minutes or until the wild rice starts to split. Add more hot stock if needed.

3 Meanwhile, heat the remaining oil in a frying pan, add the prawns, and cook for a few minutes until they turn pink. Throw in the garlic and toss with the prawns. Remove from the heat and stir in the parsley. Spoon the rice mixture into a large serving dish, and tip the prawns over it. Serve with the lemon wedges.

COOK'S TIP

Alternatively, you could use cooked prawns for ease; once the rice is cooked, just stir them in and warm through.

STATISTICS PER SERVING:

Energy 366kcals/1,528kJ

Carbohydrate 52g

Sugar 4g

Fibre 2g

Fat 8g

Saturated fat 1.5g

Salt 1.4g

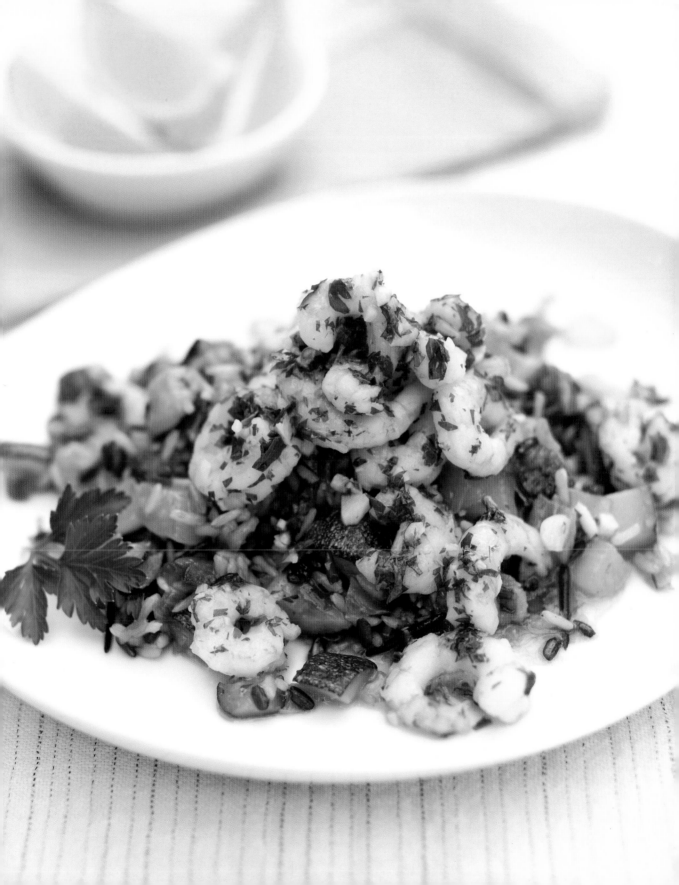

● ○ ○ GI

● ● ○ CALORIES

● ○ ○ SATURATED FAT

● ○ ○ SALT

MOROCCAN FISH TAGINE

SERVES 4   **PREP** 10 MINS   **COOK** 25 MINS

This dish is just the thing to warm you up on a cold winter's night. It is healthy, low in fat, and can be put together in a matter of minutes.

4 cloves garlic, crushed
½ tsp ground cumin
½ tsp ground turmeric
¼ tsp paprika
¼ tsp hot chilli powder
zest and juice of 1 lemon
3 tbsp olive oil
4 skinless cod fillets or any
 firm white fish
1 large red onion, thinly sliced
2 tsp harissa paste
85g (3oz) dried apricots,
 roughly chopped

2 large carrots, thickly sliced
1 red pepper, deseeded
 and roughly chopped
salt and freshly ground black pepper
400ml (14fl oz) hot fish
 stock or vegetable stock
400g can chickpeas, drained
 and rinsed
225g (8oz) cherry tomatoes,
 sliced in half
2 tbsp roughly chopped fresh
 coriander

1 Combine half the garlic with the cumin, turmeric, paprika, chilli powder, lemon zest and juice, and 1 tablespoon of olive oil. Rub the mixture over the fish fillets.

2 Heat the remaining oil in a large saucepan, add the onion and cook for 2–3 minutes or until beginning to soften. Add the remaining garlic and harissa paste, and cook for a further minute.

3 Add the apricots and all the vegetables to the pan and stir. Pour in the stock and bring to the boil. Season to taste, cover and simmer for 15 minutes.

4 Add the chickpeas and cherry tomatoes, and stir to combine. Place the fish on top of the vegetables, cover the pan and cook for a further 10 minutes or until the fish is done. Scatter with the coriander to serve.

STATISTICS PER SERVING:

Energy 389kcals/1,631kJ

Carbohydrate 36g

Sugar 19g

Fibre 8g

Fat 12g

Saturated fat 1.5g

Salt 0.5g

SWEET POTATO AND MUSSEL STEW

GUIDELINES PER SERVING:

● ● ○ GI

● ○ ○ CALORIES

● ○ ○ SATURATED FAT

● ● ○ SALT

SERVES 4   **PREP** 20 MINS   **COOK** 30 MINS

The chilli cuts through the richness with a subtle underlying heat. Portion sizes are on the small side – you might consider serving this as an impressive starter.

2 tbsp olive oil
1 onion, finely chopped
2 celery sticks, finely chopped
salt and freshly ground black pepper
2 leeks, trimmed and chopped
1 tsp paprika
½ tsp chilli flakes

3 garlic cloves, finely chopped
few fresh thyme stalks
500ml (16fl oz) vegetable stock
2 sweet potatoes, cut into
  bite-sized pieces
1.1kg (2½lb) fresh mussels,
  scrubbed and debearded

1 Heat the olive oil in a large, deep pan. Put in the onion and celery, and cook over a low heat for a couple of minutes until they soften. Season with salt and black pepper, then add the leeks and cook for about 3 minutes.

2 Add the paprika, chilli flakes, garlic, and thyme. Cook for 1 minute. Pour in a little of the vegetable stock and let it boil, then add the remaining stock and simmer gently for 8–10 minutes, partially covered. Taste, and add a little more seasoning if needed.

3 Tip the sweet potatoes into the pan and cook for about 10 minutes until they are just beginning to soften. Add the mussels, put the lid on and cook for 5–8 minutes until the mussels start to open. Remove the thyme stalks before serving.

COOK'S TIP
Do not cook mussels if the shells are already open – throw them away. After cooking mussels, don't eat any that haven't opened.

STATISTICS PER SERVING:

Energy 242kcals/1,013kJ

Carbohydrate 27g

Sugar 8g

Fibre 4g

Fat 9g

Saturated fat 1g

Salt 1.5g

⬤⬤◯ GI

⬤⬤⬤ CALORIES

⬤◯◯ SATURATED FAT

⬤◯◯ SALT

FISHERMAN'S TUNA STEW

SERVES 4   **PREP** 10 MINS   **COOK** 35 MINS

This fish stew, which Basque fisherman call *marmitako de bonito*, was originally made at sea to provide for a hungry crew.

900g (2lb) potatoes
750g (1lb 10oz) fresh tuna
350g (12oz) jar roasted red peppers, drained
3 tbsp olive oil
1 large onion, finely sliced

2 garlic cloves, crushed
1 bay leaf
salt and freshly ground pepper
400g (14oz) can chopped tomatoes
300g (10oz) frozen petits pois
2 tbsp chopped parsley

1 Peel the potatoes and cut into thick rounds. Cut the tuna into pieces roughly the same size as the potatoes, and slice the red peppers into strips.

2 Heat the oil in a flameproof casserole, stir in the onion, garlic, and bay leaf, and cook, stirring, until the onions are translucent. Add the potatoes, stir well, season to taste with salt and pepper, then cover with water. Boil for 10 minutes, or until the potatoes are almost cooked, then add the tomatoes, and continue to cook for a further 5 minutes.

3 Reduce the heat to low, add the tuna, and cook for a further 5 minutes, then add the petits pois and the red peppers, and cook very gently for 10 minutes. Sprinkle with the parsley and serve.

STATISTICS PER SERVING:

Energy 625kcals/2,630kJ

Carbohydrate 50g

Sugar 6g

Fibre 10g

Fat 24g

Saturated fat 3.5g

Salt 0.5g

FISH SOUP WITH SAFFRON AND FENNEL

SERVES 6   **PREP** 10 MINS   **COOK** 1 HOUR

This rustic, Mediterranean-style fish soup is simple to prepare and sure to please.

GUIDELINES PER SERVING:

●●○ GI

●○○ CALORIES

●○○ SATURATED FAT

●○○ SALT

5 tbsp olive oil
1 large fennel bulb, finely chopped
2 garlic cloves, crushed
1 small leek, sliced
4 ripe plum tomatoes, chopped
3 tbsp brandy
¼ tsp saffron threads, infused
 in a little hot water
zest of ½ orange
1 bay leaf
1.7 litres (3 pints) fish stock

300g (10oz) potatoes, diced and
 parboiled for 5 minutes
4 tbsp dry white wine
500g (1lb 2oz) fresh black mussels,
 scrubbed and debearded
salt and freshly ground black pepper
500g (1lb 2oz) monkfish or firm white
 fish, cut into bite-sized pieces
6 raw whole tiger prawns
parsley, chopped, to garnish

1 Heat 4 tbsp of the oil in a large, deep pan. Stir in the fennel, garlic, and leek, and fry over a moderate heat, stirring occasionally, for 5 minutes, or until softened and lightly browned.

2 Stir in the tomatoes, add the brandy, and boil rapidly for 2 minutes, or until the juices are reduced slightly. Stir in the saffron, orange zest, bay leaf, fish stock, and potatoes. Bring to the boil, then reduce the heat and skim off any scum from the surface. Cover and simmer for 20 minutes, or until the potatoes are tender. Remove the bay leaf.

3 Meanwhile, heat the remaining oil with the wine in a large deep pan until boiling. Add the mussels, cover, and continue on high heat for 2–3 minutes, shaking the pan often. Discard any mussels that do not open. Strain, reserving the liquid, and set the mussels aside. Add the liquid to the soup and season to taste. Bring to the boil, add the monkfish and prawns, then reduce the heat, cover, and simmer gently for 5 minutes, or until the fish is just cooked and the prawns are pink. Add the mussels to the pan and bring almost to the boil. Serve the soup sprinkled with chopped parsley.

STATISTICS PER SERVING:

Energy 265kcals/1,112kJ

Carbohydrate 15g

Sugar 5g

Fibre 4g

Fat 11g
Saturated fat 1.5g

Salt 0.7g

● ● ○ GI

● ● ○ CALORIES

● ○ ○ SATURATED FAT

● ○ ○ SALT

LINGUINE WITH SARDINES

SERVES 4   **PREP** 5 MINS   **COOK** 10 MINS

A classic combination that can be made with storecupboard ingredients.

300g (10oz) linguine
1 tbsp olive oil
1 red onion, finely chopped
salt and freshly ground black pepper
2 garlic cloves, finely chopped

120g can sardines in oil, drained
3 tsp capers (rinsed, if salty)
juice of 1 lemon
1 tbsp flat-leaf parsley,
  finely chopped

1 Put the linguine in a pan of salted boiling water and cook for 8–10 minutes, or according to the instructions on the packet.

2 Meanwhile, heat the olive oil in a large frying pan, add the onion and cook for about 5 minutes over a low heat until it begins to soften. Season with a little salt and black pepper. Stir in the garlic and cook for a few seconds, then add the sardines and stir gently to break them up. Add the capers and lemon juice, and cook for about 5 minutes.

3 Drain the linguine, reserving some of the cooking water, then return it to the pan with a little of the water. Add the sardine sauce and the parsley and toss to combine.

COOK'S TIP
You can, of course, use fresh sardines if you wish: grill until cooked, then flake them and serve with the pasta.

STATISTICS PER SERVING:

Energy 362kcals/1,530kJ

Carbohydrate 60g

Sugar 3g

Fibre 3g

Fat 8.5g

Saturated fat 1.5g

Salt 0.6g

PASTA WITH CLAMS

SERVES 4 **PREP** 10 MINS **COOK** 15 MINS

Salty, meaty clams tossed with delicate linguine pasta and aromatic fresh parsley.

GUIDELINES PER SERVING:

● ● ○ GI

● ● ○ CALORIES

● ○ ○ SATURATED FAT

● ○ ○ SALT

1.1kg (2½lb) clams
1 tbsp olive oil
1 onion, finely chopped
2 garlic cloves, finely chopped
1 red chilli, deseeded and
   finely chopped

350g (12oz) linguine
1 tbsp flat-leaf parsley,
   finely chopped
freshly ground black pepper

1 First, wash the clams, throwing away any that are already open. Set aside.

2 Pour the olive oil into a large frying pan, add the onion and cook for 5 minutes until soft. Put a pan of salted water on to boil for the pasta.

3 Stir the garlic and chilli into the onion and cook for a minute or two, being careful not to burn the garlic. Add 2 tablespoons of water, tip in the clams, cover the pan and cook for 3–5 minutes.

4 Put the linguine in the pan of boiling water and cook for 8–10 minutes, or according to the instructions on the packet. Drain, reserving some of the cooking water, then return the linguine to the pan with a little of the water. Add the clams and the parsley, and toss to coat. Season with black pepper if needed.

COOK'S TIP
Do not cook clams that are already open: throw them away.
After cooking clams, discard any that haven't opened.

STATISTICS PER SERVING:

Energy 415kcals/1,764kJ

Carbohydrate 71g

Sugar 3g

Fibre 3g

Fat 6g
Saturated fat 1g

Salt 0.7g

●●○ GI

●●○ CALORIES

●○○ SATURATED FAT

●●○ SALT

VERMICELLI NOODLES WITH PRAWNS AND CRAB

SERVES 4   **PREP** 10 MINS   **COOK** 20 MINS

A light, quick, Asian-style dish full of aromatic flavours, prepared in a wok.

5cm (2in) piece of fresh root ginger, roughly chopped
2 tsp Sichuan pepper
3 garlic cloves
1 stalk lemongrass, trimmed and woody outer leaf removed
salt and freshly ground black pepper
2 tbsp sunflower oil
250g (9oz) peeled prawns, raw

¼ small pumpkin or butternut squash (about 140g/5oz), grated
200g (7oz) fresh white crabmeat
1 tbsp rice vinegar
400ml (14fl oz) vegetable or chicken stock
225g (8oz) vermicelli noodles
1 bunch of spring onions, finely chopped, to garnish

1 Put the ginger, Sichuan pepper, garlic, and lemongrass in a food processor or blender and whiz until chopped. Season with salt and black pepper and whiz again. Heat 1 tablespoon of oil in a wok, swirling it around to coat. When the oil is hot, add the prawns and cook until pink (2–4 minutes). Remove and set aside.

2 Pour the remaining oil into the wok, add the ginger mixture to the pan and stir for a couple of minutes. Add the grated pumpkin and cook for a further 5 minutes, until the pumpkin has softened. Stir in the crabmeat.

3 Add the rice vinegar and the stock, and bring to the boil. Toss in the vermicelli noodles and stir for 5–8 minutes until the clump breaks down and the noodles begin to soften. Stir the cooked prawns into the mixture. Taste, season if needed, and then sprinkle with the spring onions to serve.

COOK'S TIP
Use ready-cooked prawns if you prefer: simply stir them in at the end of cooking.

STATISTICS PER SERVING:

Energy 392kcals/1,640kJ

Carbohydrate 51g

Sugar 4g

Fibre 1g

Fat 9g

Saturated fat 1g

Salt 1g

PRAWN AND
NEW POTATO BALTI

SERVES 4   **PREP** 10 MINS   **COOK** 20-25 MINS

In common with other shellfish, prawns are low in fat, making them a good option for a healthy curry.

2 tbsp oil
1 large red onion, sliced
2 cloves garlic, crushed
400g (14oz) baby new potatoes, unpeeled, sliced in half

2 tbsp balti curry paste
400g can cherry tomatoes
200ml (7fl oz) vegetable stock
225g (8oz) peeled prawns, raw
200g (7oz) baby spinach leaves

1 Heat the oil in a deep frying pan and cook the onion for 2–3 minutes. Add the garlic, potatoes, and curry paste. Cook, stirring, for 2 minutes.

2 Add the tomatoes and stock, bring to a simmer and cook for 15 minutes, stirring occasionally, until the potatoes are tender. Add a little more stock if necessary.

3 Gently stir in the prawns and spinach, and simmer gently for 3 minutes until the prawns are cooked through.

STATISTICS PER SERVING:

Energy 255kcals/1,068kJ

Carbohydrate 25g

Sugar 8g

Fibre 3.5g

Fat 9g

Saturated fat 1g

Salt 0.9g

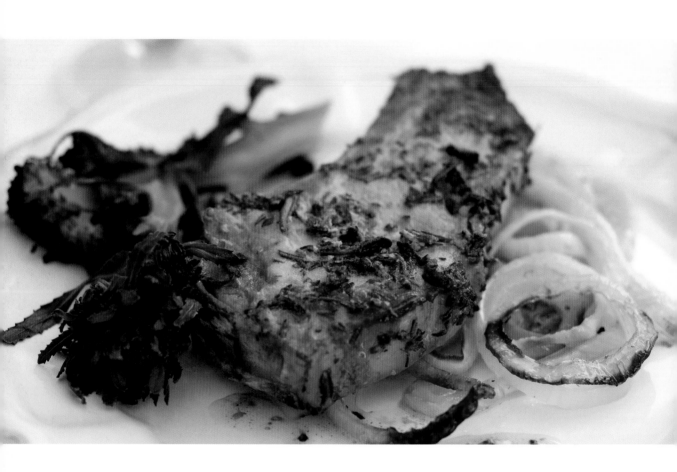

SIMPLE SUPPERS
– MEAT

GRIDDLED STEAK CHUNKS WITH HERBY RICE

SERVES 4   **PREP** 10 MINS   **COOK** 30 MINS

A tasty and filling dish for red meat lovers.

2 tbsp olive oil
1 red onion, finely chopped
salt and freshly ground black pepper
2 cloves garlic, finely chopped
225g (8oz) basmati rice
900ml (1½ pints) vegetable stock
125g (4½oz) frozen peas

handful of flat-leaf parsley,
   finely chopped
handful of fresh mint,
   finely chopped
handful of fresh coriander,
   finely chopped
500g (1lb 2oz) lean steak

1 Heat 1 tablespoon of the oil in a large frying pan and add half the onion. Cook over a low heat for 5 minutes or until soft. Season with salt and pepper, then stir in the garlic. Add the rice and stir to coat with the oil.

2 Pour in a little of the stock and let it bubble, add a little more, and stir again. Gradually add the rest of the stock as it is absorbed and cook for 15 minutes until the rice is soft and tender, then stir in the peas. Heat through for 1–2 minutes, then remove from the heat and stir in the herbs. Cover with a lid and set aside.

3 Coat the steak with the remaining olive oil and season. Heat a griddle pan until hot, then add the steak and grill for 3–5 minutes each side or until cooked to your liking. Remove and let rest for a few minutes, then slice and arrange over the rice. Sprinkle over the remaining onion and serve.

STATISTICS PER SERVING:

Energy 488kcals/2,039kJ

Carbohydrate 52g

Sugar 2.5g

Fibre 2g

Fat 13g

Saturated fat 3.5g

Salt 1.3g

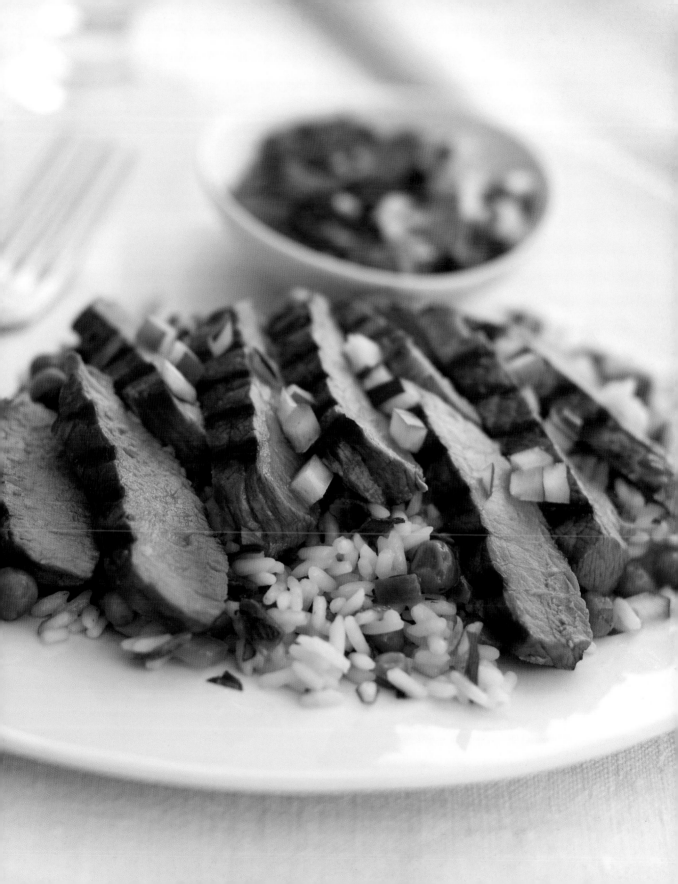

BEEF AND GREEN BEAN STIR-FRY

SERVES 4   **PREP** 10 MINS   **COOK** 15 MINS
PLUS MARINATING

An instant meal full of punchy flavour and nutrients. Beef is a good source of protein, iron, B-vitamins, and zinc.

½ tbsp soy sauce
½ tbsp Worcestershire sauce
juice of 1 orange
2 garlic cloves, finely chopped
1 green chilli, deseeded and
   finely chopped

salt and freshly ground black pepper
400g (14oz) beef steak, cut into strips
1 tbsp sesame oil
300g (10oz) fine green beans,
   topped and tailed
250g (9oz) baby spinach leaves

1 Combine the soy sauce, Worcestershire sauce, orange juice, garlic, and chilli. Season with salt and black pepper. Put the beef in a shallow bowl and pour the marinade over it. Leave to marinate for 15–30 minutes.

2 Meanwhile, put the beans in a pan of salted boiling water and cook for 3 minutes. Drain and refresh with cold water, then set aside. Heat the oil in a wok over a high heat, then add the strips of beef, shaking them a little first to remove excess marinade.

3 Stir-fry the beef for about 5 minutes, moving it around the pan until it is no longer pink. Add the beans and stir-fry for a few more minutes. With the heat on high, tip in the marinade and let it bubble and cook for a few minutes. Finally, add the spinach and stir until it wilts.

COOK'S TIP
The key to this stir-fry is to use good-quality, tender beef, as this will require only a little cooking, and to keep everything moving over a high heat.

STATISTICS PER SERVING:

Energy 185kcals/773kJ

Carbohydrate 4g

Sugar 3g

Fibre 3g

Fat 8g
Saturated fat 2g

Salt 0.7g

SPICY COTTAGE PIE
WITH LENTILS

SERVES 4   **PREP** 20 MINS   **COOK** 1 HOUR   **FREEZE** 3 MONTHS

In this recipe, some of the meat has been replaced with lentils to reduce the fat content of the dish and boost fibre.

GUIDELINES PER SERVING:

●○○ GI
●●● CALORIES
●●○ SATURATED FAT
●●○ SALT

2 tbsp olive oil
400g (14oz) extra-lean minced beef
1 large onion, finely chopped
3 sticks celery, finely chopped
2 garlic cloves, crushed
1 red pepper, deseeded and diced
2 tbsp plain flour
½ tsp ground cinnamon
2 tbsp tomato purée
150ml (5fl oz) red wine
1 tsp dried thyme
300–400ml (10–14fl oz) beef stock
1 tsp Worcestershire sauce

pinch of dried chilli flakes
400g can lentils, rinsed and drained

For the mash
450g (1lb) white potatoes, peeled and
  cut into even-sized chunks
600g (1lb 5oz) sweet potatoes, peeled
  and cut into even-sized chunks
150ml (5fl oz) hot semi-skimmed milk
25g (scant 1oz) polyunsaturated
  margarine
salt and freshly ground black pepper
1 tbsp sunflower or pumpkin seeds

1 Preheat the oven to 200°C (400°F/Gas 6). Heat 1 tablespoon of oil in a non-stick frying pan. Brown the mince over a high heat for 1–2 minutes; set it aside. Using the remaining oil, cook the onion over a medium heat for 2 minutes. Add the celery, garlic, and red pepper. Cook for 2 minutes.

2 Return the meat to the pan. Add the flour, cinnamon, tomato purée, and wine. Cook, stirring, for 1 minute. Add the thyme, 300ml (10fl oz) stock, the Worcestershire sauce, and chilli flakes. Season to taste. Bring to the boil and reduce the heat. Cover and simmer for 30 minutes, adding more stock if necessary. Remove from the heat and stir in the lentils.

3 Boil the potatoes and sweet potatoes for 15–20 minutes, or until tender. Drain well, then return to the pan and dry off over a low heat for 1 minute. Add the milk and margarine, and mash well. Season to taste. Spoon the meat mixture into an ovenproof dish, spread the mash on top, and sprinkle with the seeds. Place the cottage pie on a baking tray and cook in the oven for 20–25 minutes, or until the top begins to brown.

STATISTICS PER SERVING:

Energy 683kcals/2,878kJ

Carbohydrate 75g

Sugar 17g

Fibre 10g

Fat 26g
Saturated fat 7g

Salt 1g

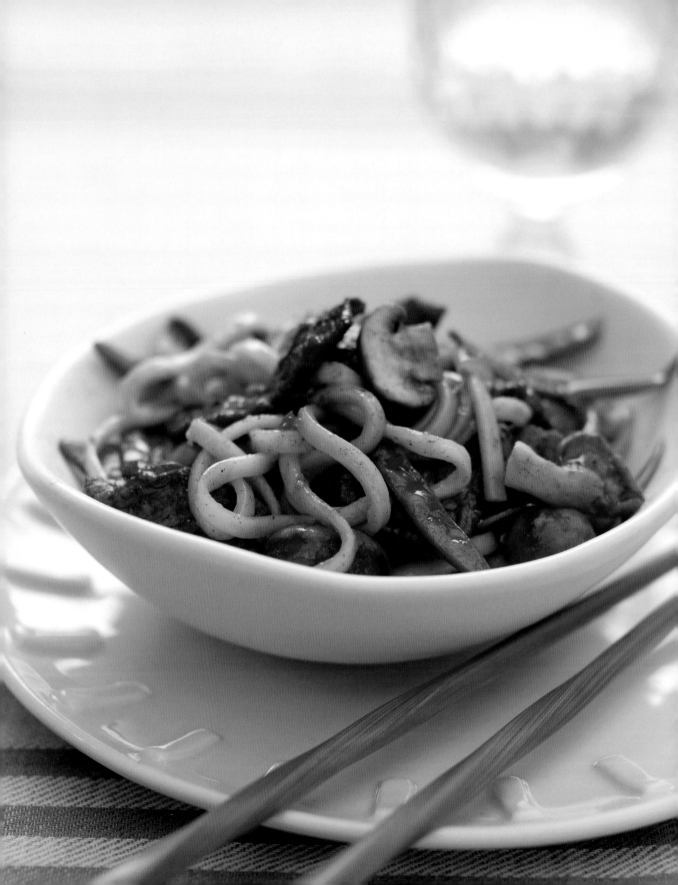

CINNAMON AND GINGER BEEF WITH NOODLES

SERVES 4   PREP 10 MINS   COOK 15 MINS

A quick dish with punchy flavours.

- ●●○ GI
- ●●○ CALORIES
- ●○○ SATURATED FAT
- ●●○ SALT

500g (1lb 2oz) lean steak, thinly sliced
2 tsp ground cinnamon
1 tbsp sunflower oil
1 onion, sliced
5cm (2in) piece of fresh ginger,
  peeled and shredded
1 red chilli, deseeded and
  finely chopped
2 garlic cloves, finely chopped

1 tbsp fish sauce
1 tbsp sesame oil
200g (7oz) mixed exotic mushrooms,
  such as oyster, shiitake and hon
  shimeji, trimmed or chopped
200g mange tout
400g (14oz) medium or thick
  straight-to-wok udon noodles

1 Put the steak in a bowl, sprinkle over the cinnamon and stir to coat. Heat the sunflower oil in a wok, add the onion, and stir-fry over a high heat for 1 minute. Add the ginger and chilli and stir-fry for a further minute.

2 Now add the steak, garlic, fish sauce, and sesame oil and continue to cook, stirring, until the meat is no longer pink. Add the mushrooms and mange tout and continue to stir-fry for a further 1–2 minutes.

3 Add the noodles and stir-fry for about 3 minutes until the noodles become sticky. Serve immediately.

COOK'S TIP
Always cook quickly over a high heat when using a wok, and have all your ingredients to hand.

STATISTICS PER SERVING:

Energy 378kcals/1,584kJ

Carbohydrate 33g

Sugar 2.5g

Fibre 2.2g

Fat 12g

Saturated fat 3g

Salt 1.2g

SIMPLE SUPPERS – MEAT   247

LEBANESE SPICED BEEF AND OKRA

SERVES 4   **PREP** 10 MINS   **COOK** 35 MINS

A spiced and flavourful one-pot dish.

1 tbsp olive oil
1 onion, sliced
200g (7oz) okra, topped and
  halved horizontally
500g (1lb 2oz) lean steak, cut
  into 1cm (½in) pieces
1 tsp paprika

4 cloves garlic, finely chopped
juice of ½ lemon
400g can of chopped tomatoes
handful of fresh coriander,
  roughly chopped
salt and freshly ground black pepper

1 Heat the oil in a large frying pan, add the onion, and cook over a medium heat for 2 minutes until it begins to soften, then add the okra and cook for a further minute.

2 Add the beef, paprika, and garlic and cook, stirring, until the beef is no longer pink. Add the lemon juice, tomatoes, and coriander and season with salt and pepper. Bring to the boil then reduce to a simmer and cook, uncovered, for 20–30 minutes, stirring occasionally, until the sauce has reduced and thickened. Spoon into warmed bowls and serve. You could accompany this with some brown rice.

COOK'S TIP
Frying the okra before the other ingredients are added will prevent it from becoming gluey.

STATISTICS PER SERVING:

Energy 226kcals/947kJ

Carbohydrate 7.5g

Sugar 6g

Fibre 3g

Fat 8.5g

Saturated fat 2.5g

Salt 0.4g

BEEF AND BEAN STEW

SERVES 4   **PREP** 10 MINS   **COOK** 35 MINS   **FREEZE** 3 MONTHS

A hearty meal-in-one of tender beef simmered with tomatoes and beans.

GUIDELINES PER SERVING:

● ○ ○ GI

● ● ○ CALORIES

● ○ ○ SATURATED FAT

● ○ ○ SALT

2 tbsp olive oil
2 onions, roughly chopped
salt and freshly ground black pepper
500g (1lb 2oz) lean beef, diced
1 tsp hot paprika or cayenne pepper
1 tbsp cider vinegar
4 garlic cloves, finely chopped
400g can of black-eyed beans,
  drained and rinsed

400g can of chickpeas, drained
  and rinsed
400g can of chopped tomatoes
300ml (10fl oz) vegetable stock
handful of fresh flat-leaf parsley,
  chopped
4 spring onions, finely chopped,
  to serve

1 Heat the oil in a large pan, add the onions and cook for about 5 minutes until soft. Season with salt and black pepper, then add the beef and paprika, stir to coat, and cook for 2–3 minutes until the beef is no longer pink. Add the vinegar and cook for a minute or two until the liquid evaporates.

2 Add the garlic and cook for 1 minute, then tip in the beans and chickpeas and stir to combine. Add the tomatoes and stock, bring to the boil, then reduce to a simmer and cook gently for 20–30 minutes until thickened. Top up with a little extra stock or water if it dries out too much. Stir in the parsley and adjust the seasoning if required. Scatter over the chopped spring onions and serve straight away.

STATISTICS PER SERVING:

Energy 453kcals/1,910kJ

Carbohydrate 40g

Sugar 8g

Fibre 8g

Fat 14g
Saturated fat 3g

Salt 0.6g

CHILLI CON CARNE

SERVES 4   **PREP** 5 MINS   **COOK** 50 MINS   **FREEZE** 1 MONTH

A hearty and warming Tex-Mex classic.

1 tbsp olive oil
1 onion, thinly sliced
2 tbsp chilli sauce
1 garlic clove, crushed
1 tsp ground cumin

600g (1lb 5oz) extra lean minced beef
400g can red kidney beans,
   drained and rinsed
400g can chopped tomatoes
salt and freshly ground black pepper

1 Heat the oil in a large saucepan over a medium heat. Add the onions and fry for 5 minutes, or until softened. Stir in the chilli sauce, garlic, cumin, and beef, and fry for 3 minutes, or until the meat browns, stirring occasionally.

2 Stir in the kidney beans and tomatoes and bring to the boil. Reduce the heat, cover, and leave to simmer for 40 minutes, stirring occasionally. Season to taste with salt and pepper. You might want to try serving this with a spoonful of soured cream.

STATISTICS PER SERVING:

Energy 397kcals/1,664kJ

Carbohydrate 20g

Sugar 8g

Fibre 6g

Fat 18g

Saturated fat 7g

Salt 1g

NAVARIN OF LAMB

GUIDELINES PER SERVING:

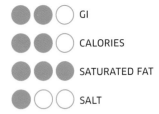

GI

CALORIES

SATURATED FAT

SALT

SERVES 4   **PREP** 30 MINS   **COOK** 1½ HOURS   **FREEZE** 3 MONTHS

This classic French stew is a complete one-pot meal, traditionally made with young spring vegetables.

2 tbsp olive oil
900g (2lb) middle neck of lamb,
  cut into pieces
2 small onions, quartered
1 tbsp plain flour
400ml (14fl oz) lamb stock
  or beef stock

2 tbsp tomato purée
1 bouquet garni
salt and freshly ground black pepper
300g (10oz) small new potatoes
300g (10oz) small whole carrots
300g (10oz) baby turnips
175g (6oz) French beans

1 Heat the oil in a large flameproof casserole, add the lamb chunks, and fry until brown on all sides. Add the onions and fry gently for 5 minutes, stirring frequently.

2 Sprinkle the flour over the meat and stir well for 2 minutes, or until the pieces are evenly coated. Stir in the stock, then add the tomato purée and bouquet garni, and season to taste with salt and pepper. Bring to the boil, then cover and simmer for 45 minutes.

3 Add the potatoes, carrots, and turnips. Cover and cook for a further 15 minutes, then stir in the beans, cover, and cook for a further 10–15 minutes, or until all the vegetables are tender.

STATISTICS PER SERVING:

Energy 543kcals/2,270kJ

Carbohydrate 32g

Sugar 15g

Fibre 7g

Fat 25g
Saturated fat 8.5g

Salt 0.7g

● ● ○ GI

● ● ○ CALORIES

● ● ○ SATURATED FAT

● ● ○ SALT

BULGUR WHEAT WITH LAMB AND CHICKPEAS

SERVES 6   **PREP** 10 MINS   **COOK** 45 MINS

The classic combination of chickpeas and lamb makes a filling supper dish.

plain flour, for dusting
salt and freshly ground black pepper
450g (1lb) lean lamb, cut into
  bite-sized pieces
2 tbsp oil
125g (4½oz) frozen peas
1 onion, finely chopped

1 tbsp fresh thyme, leaves only,
  chopped
2 x 400g cans chickpeas,
  drained and rinsed
1.2 litres (2 pints) vegetable stock
275g (9½oz) bulgur wheat
1 tbsp fresh dill, finely chopped

1 Season the flour with a pinch of salt and black pepper, and dust the meat with it until coated. Cook the meat in batches: heat 1 teaspoon of the oil in large frying pan, add some of the meat and cook until golden. Repeat for the rest of the meat. Remove the meat with a slotted spoon and set aside.

2 Tip the peas into a bowl of boiling water, leave for few minutes, then drain and refresh with cold water and set aside.

3 Heat 1 tablespoon of oil in the pan, add the onion and cook for 5 minutes, or until soft and transparent. Season well and stir in the thyme. Return the meat to the pan along with the chickpeas. Increase the heat, add a little of the stock and bring to the boil. Reduce to a simmer and then add most of the remaining stock, reserving 300ml (10fl oz). Cook over a low heat for about 20 minutes or until it thickens. Add more water if it needs it.

4 Meanwhile, tip the bulgur wheat into a bowl, pour in the reserved stock, cover with cling film, and leave for 8–10 minutes. Fluff up with a fork, stir in the peas and dill, and season to taste. Serve with the lamb mixture.

COOK'S TIP
Choose lean lamb such as leg, and dice it yourself rather than buying it ready cut. It is usually cheaper to do this, and you can easily remove any fat.

STATISTICS PER SERVING:

Energy 528kcals/2,203kJ

Carbohydrate 51g

Sugar 31g

Fibre 1.5g

Fat 16.5g

Saturated fat 5.5g

Salt 1g

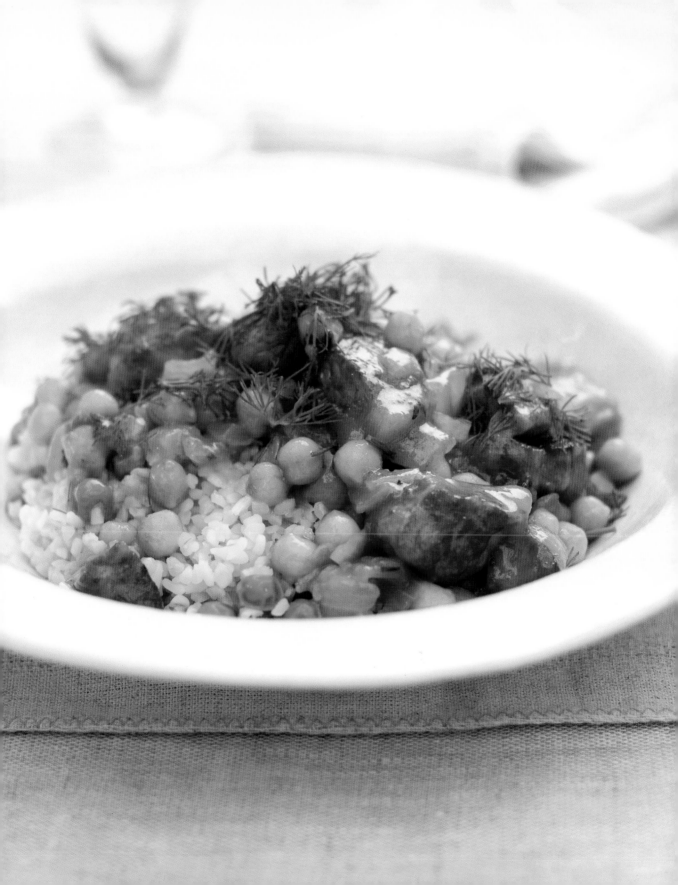

● ○ ○ GI

● ● ○ CALORIES

● ● ○ SATURATED FAT

● ○ ○ SALT

ROAST LAMB WITH FLAGEOLETS

SERVES 6   **PREP** 15 MINS   **COOK** 1 HOUR 40 MINS

A perfect Sunday lunch; the beans make a tasty change to the more traditional accompaniment of roast potatoes.

½ leg of lamb, about 1.35kg (3lb)
2–3 sprigs rosemary
1 tbsp olive oil
salt and freshly ground black pepper
4 garlic cloves, roughly chopped

250g (9oz) baby plum
  tomatoes, halved
410g can flageolet beans, drained
1 tbsp tomato purée
150ml (5fl oz) dry white wine

1 Preheat the oven to 180°C (350°F/Gas 4). With a small, sharp knife, make several deep cuts into the skin surface of the lamb. Push a few rosemary leaves into each cut. Place the lamb in a roasting tin, brush with oil, and season with salt and pepper. Roast for 1 hour.

2 Mix the remaining rosemary with the garlic, tomatoes, and flageolets. Remove the lamb from the oven and spoon the tomato and bean mixture around it. Mix the tomato purée with the wine and pour over the lamb.

3 Cover loosely with foil, then return to the oven for 30–40 minutes, or until the lamb is cooked but the juices are still slightly pink, stirring once. Allow the meat to rest for 10–15 minutes, loosely covered with foil, before carving.

COOK'S TIP
The lamb can be prepared and stuffed with the rosemary leaves, ready for roasting, a few hours in advance of cooking.

STATISTICS PER SERVING:

Energy 338kcals/1,414kJ

Carbohydrate 10g

Sugar 2.5g

Fibre 3.5g

Fat 16g

Saturated fat 6g

Salt 0.6g

LAMB CUTLETS WITH CHERMOULA

SERVES 6   **PREP** 15 MINS   **COOK** 10 MINS
PLUS MARINATING

GUIDELINES PER SERVING:

● ○ ○ GI
● ○ ○ CALORIES
● ● ● SATURATED FAT
● ○ ○ SALT

Chermoula is a classic Moroccan spice marinade, wonderful for grilled meats and fish.

12 lamb cutlets, trimmed
4 ripe plum tomatoes, chopped
salt and freshly ground
   black pepper
1 tbsp balsamic vinegar

For the marinade
1 red onion, finely chopped
2 garlic cloves, crushed

1 tsp ground cumin
¼ tsp smoked paprika
1 tsp ground coriander
grated zest and juice of 1 lemon
6 tbsp olive oil, plus extra
   for drizzling
handful of mint, roughly chopped
handful of coriander, chopped

1 Place the trimmed cutlets in a dish. In a mixing bowl, combine the red onion, garlic, cumin, paprika, ground coriander, lemon juice and zest, olive oil, and most of the chopped mint and coriander. Rub the marinade over the lamb and leave to marinate for at least 30 minutes.

2 Season the chopped tomatoes with salt and pepper, drizzle with a little olive oil, the balsamic vinegar, and the remaining coriander and mint. Set aside.

3 Preheat the grill on its highest setting. Remove the cutlets from the marinade and grill for 5 minutes each side, or until cooked and crisp. Serve the lamb with the tomato salad alongside.

COOK'S TIP
The meat can be left to marinate for up to 24 hours.

STATISTICS PER SERVING:

Energy 350kcals/1,451kJ

Carbohydrate 4g

Sugar 3.5g

Fibre 1g

Fat 23g
Saturated fat 7g

Salt 0.3g

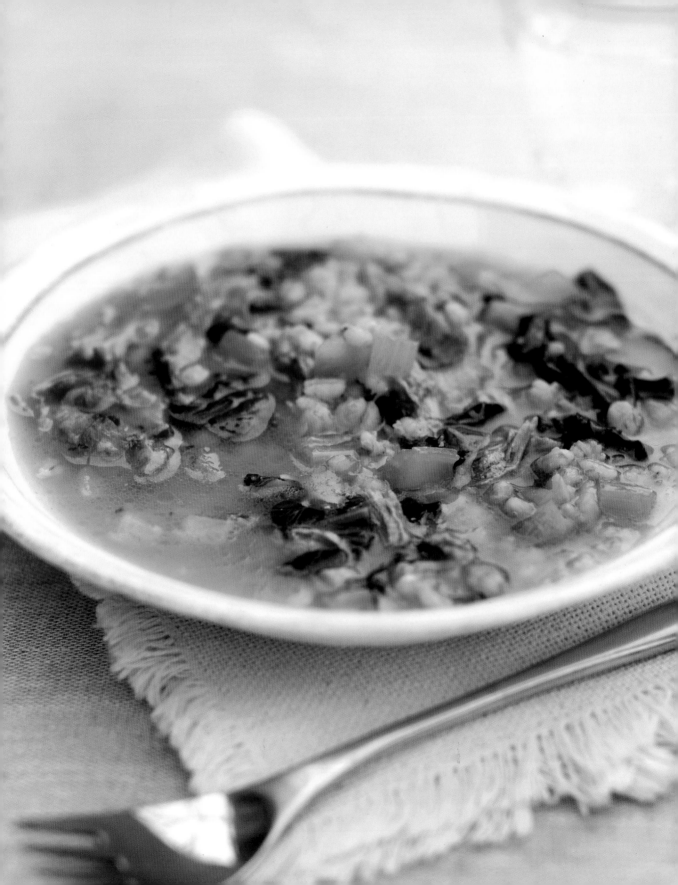

PEARL BARLEY, SPINACH, AND LAMB POT

SERVES 4   **PREP** 15 MINS   **COOK** 1 HOUR 25 MINS
PLUS SOAKING

GUIDELINES PER SERVING:

● ○ ○   GI

● ● ○   CALORIES

● ● ●   SATURATED FAT

● ○ ○   SALT

One-pot cooking at its best, this dish is easy to make and full of flavour and goodness.

1 tbsp olive oil
1 onion, finely chopped
2 cloves of garlic, finely chopped
3 carrots, diced
3 celery stalks, diced
few stalks of thyme
750g (1lb 10oz) neck of lamb
  on the bone, trimmed of fat

1.2 litres (2 pints) of vegetable stock
75g (2½oz) pearl barley,
  soaked overnight
450g (9oz) spinach leaves,
  roughly chopped
salt and freshly ground black pepper

1 Heat the oil in a large heavy-based pan, add the onion and cook over a low heat until it softens. Add the garlic, carrot, celery, and thyme and cook for a further 10 minutes. Add the lamb to the pan and cover with the stock. Bring to the boil and skim off any scum that comes to the surface. Reduce to a simmer, add the pearl barley, and cook gently for 1 hour until the lamb is tender and pearl barley is cooked. Top up with more stock or water if needed.

2 Remove the lamb from the pan, leave to cool slightly, and then shred the meat away from the bone. Meanwhile add the spinach to the pan and cook for 5 minutes or until it has wilted. Return the lamb to the pot and stir well then taste and season as required. Ladle into bowls and serve.

COOK'S TIP
This will taste even better the next day; put in the refrigerator once cooled and reheat when required.

STATISTICS PER SERVING:

Energy   570kcals/2,731kJ

Carbohydrate   28g

Sugar   9.5g

Fibre   5g

Fat   21g

Saturated fat   8g

Salt   0.8g

LAMB WITH AUBERGINE PURÉE

SERVES 6   **PREP** 15 MINS   **COOK** 40 MINS
PLUS MARINATING

Harissa makes a spicy crust for the lamb that goes well
with the creamy aubergine.

1 tbsp harissa
2 tbsp chopped mint,
  plus extra for garnish
5 tbsp lemon juice
3 tbsp olive oil
900g (2lb) lamb loin fillet
  or noisettes of lamb

2 aubergines
2 garlic cloves, crushed
2 tbsp tahini
120ml (4fl oz) Greek yogurt
salt and freshly ground black pepper

1 Preheat the oven to 220°C (425°F/Gas 7). Place the harissa, mint,
2 tablespoons of the lemon juice, and 1 tablespoon of the olive oil in a
bowl. Add the lamb and cover evenly in the marinade. Leave to marinate
for at least 30 minutes.

2 Place the aubergines on a baking tray, prick the skin with a fork several
times, and bake for 30 minutes, or until the skins have charred. Remove
from the oven and, when cool enough to handle, peel away the skins and
discard. Place the aubergine flesh in a colander, drain for 15 minutes, then
place in a food processor with the garlic, the remaining 3 tablespoons of
lemon juice, the tahini, and the Greek yogurt and process until smooth.
Season to taste with salt and pepper.

3 Remove the lamb from the marinade. Heat the remaining 2 tablespoons
of oil in a frying pan and brown the lamb on all sides. Roast in the oven for
10 minutes, or longer if desired. Remove, and let rest for 10 minutes.

4 Carve the lamb and serve on warmed plates with the purée. Pour the pan
juices over, and sprinkle with a little chopped mint.

COOK'S TIP
The aubergine purée can be made 1 day in advance and served at room
temperature. The lamb can marinate for up to 24 hours, chilled and covered.

STATISTICS PER SERVING:

Energy 348kcals/1,447kJ

Carbohydrate 2g

Sugar 2g

Fibre 1g

Fat 23g

Saturated fat 8g

Salt 0.4g

RAGOUT OF VENISON WITH WILD MUSHROOMS

SERVES 4   **PREP** 15 MINS   **COOK** 1¾–2¼ HOURS   **FREEZE** 3 MONTHS

This slowly simmered stew concentrates all the rich flavours of the venison and mushrooms.

1 tbsp olive oil
15g (½oz) butter
4 shallots, sliced
115g (4oz) smoked bacon, diced
600g (1lb 5oz) venison, diced
1 tbsp plain flour
3 tbsp brandy

250g (9oz) wild mushrooms, sliced
250ml (9fl oz) beef stock
1 tbsp tomato purée
1 tbsp Worcestershire sauce
1 tsp dried oregano
salt and freshly ground black pepper

1 Heat the oil and butter in the casserole and fry the shallots and bacon over a medium-high heat, stirring frequently, until beginning to brown.

2 Add the venison and fry for 3–4 minutes, or until browned on all sides, stirring frequently. Stir in the flour, then cook for 1–2 minutes, or until beginning to brown.

3 Add the brandy and stir for 30 seconds, then add the mushrooms and stock. Bring to the boil, stirring often.

4 Stir in the tomato purée, Worcestershire sauce, and oregano, and season to taste with salt and pepper. Reduce the heat to low, cover tightly with a lid, and simmer very gently for 1½–2 hours, or until the venison is tender (the cooking time will depend on the age of the meat). Serve hot, straight from the casserole.

COOK'S TIP
Leftovers can be reheated the next day. The flavour will improve with keeping.

STATISTICS PER SERVING:

Energy 362kcals/1,521kJ

Carbohydrate 10g

Sugar 7g

Fibre 2.5g

Fat 16g
Saturated fat 6g

Salt 2g

VENISON WITH ROAST CELERIAC AND REDCURRANT SAUCE

SERVES 2   **PREP** 10 MINS   **COOK** 50 MINS   **FREEZE** 3 MONTHS
(SAUCE ONLY)

Venison steaks contain just 1.5g of fat per 100g, which is considerably less than even the leanest cut of beef.

½ medium celeriac, cut into
  5cm (2in) chunks
4 tbsp olive oil
1 small red onion, finely chopped
1 clove garlic, finely chopped
200ml (7fl oz) chicken stock

200ml (7fl oz) fruity red wine
pinch of ground cinnamon
1 tbsp redcurrant jelly
salt and freshly ground black pepper
2 venison steaks, about 150g
  (5½oz) each

1 Preheat the oven to 180ºC (350ºF/Gas 4). Place the celeriac in a bowl, drizzle with 2 tablespoons of oil and stir to coat. Transfer to an ovenproof dish and put in the oven for 40 minutes or until cooked through

2 To make the sauce, heat 1 tablespoon of the oil in a non-stick pan. Put in the onion and garlic and cook, stirring occasionally, for about 2–3 minutes. Add the stock, red wine, and cinnamon. Bring to the boil and allow the sauce to bubble for about 10 minutes or until reduced by half. Strain the sauce and discard the onions. Season with salt and ground black pepper, and stir in the redcurrant jelly.

3 Brush the venison with the remaining oil and cook on a hot griddle pan for 2–3 minutes either side, or until done to your liking.

4 Place the venison and celeriac on a warm serving plate, then spoon a little of the sauce over the venison and serve.

COOK'S TIP
You can prepare the sauce up to two days in advance and keep it in the refrigerator. Simply reheat it in a small pan when needed.

STATISTICS PER SERVING:

Energy 484kcals/2,022kJ

Carbohydrate 9g

Sugar 7.5g

Fibre 5.6g

Fat 25g

Saturated fat 4.5g

Salt 1g

SLOW-ROAST PORK AND LENTILS

SERVES 4   **PREP** 10 MINS   **COOK** 1 HOUR 10 MINS

A comforting dish made from pork tenderloin, or fillet, which is a long, cylindrical cut of meat.

3 sage leaves
450g (1lb) pork tenderloin,
  slashed 3 times
½ tbsp olive oil
salt and freshly ground black pepper
350g (12oz) Puy lentils, rinsed and
  any grit removed

2 celery stalks, roughly chopped
3 carrots, roughly chopped
1 onion, roughly chopped
1 sweet potato, roughly chopped
900ml (1½ pints) vegetable stock

1 Preheat the oven to 200°C (400°F/Gas 6). Stuff the sage leaves into the cuts on the pork, drizzle with the oil and season well. Heat a large, cast-iron pot over a high heat, put the pork in and cook for about 5 minutes on each side to seal.

2 Add the lentils, celery, carrots, onion, and sweet potato. Season well. Pour in the stock, push the pork down to sit snugly in the lentils, put the lid on the pot and cook in the oven for about 1 hour. Check halfway through the cooking time to make sure the pork isn't drying out; if it is, top up with a little hot water.

COOK'S TIP
You could cook the lentils and pork separately. Cook the lentils up to one day ahead and keep in the refrigerator, then reheat when required. Roast the pork for about 30 minutes. Serve together.

GI

CALORIES

SATURATED FAT

SALT

STATISTICS PER SERVING:

Energy 520kcals/2,288kJ

Carbohydrate 63g

Sugar 11g

Fibre 11g

Fat 10g
Saturated fat 2.5g

Salt 1.4g

● ○ ○ GI

● ● ○ CALORIES

● ○ ○ SATURATED FAT

● ○ ○ SALT

PORK TENDERLOIN STUFFED WITH CHILLIES AND TOMATOES

SERVES 4   **PREP** 15 MINS   **COOK** 35 MINS

A fiery dish that looks impressive but is simple to make.

1–2 tbsp green jalapenos pickled
  in vinegar, drained
1 tbsp capers, rinsed if salty
8 large sun-dried tomatoes in
  oil, drained

450g (1lb) pork tenderloin
1 tbsp olive oil
salt and freshly ground black pepper

1 Preheat the oven to 200°C (400°F/Gas 6). Put the jalapenos, capers, and sun-dried tomatoes in a food processor or blender and process to form a paste.

2 Slice the pork along its length, making sure that you don't cut all the way through it. Smother with the oil and season with salt and black pepper.

3 Stuff the paste into the slit in the pork, spreading it evenly. Pull the edges of the pork up around the stuffing and transfer the meat to a roasting tin, cut-side down. Roast the pork for 30–35 minutes, or until it is cooked to your liking. Allow the meat to rest for 5 minutes before slicing, then serve. Try this with green vegetables and brown basmati rice.

STATISTICS PER SERVING:

Energy 177kcals/745kJ

Carbohydrate 3g

Sugar 0.5g

Fibre 0.5g

Fat 6.5g
Saturated fat 1.5g

Salt 0.5g

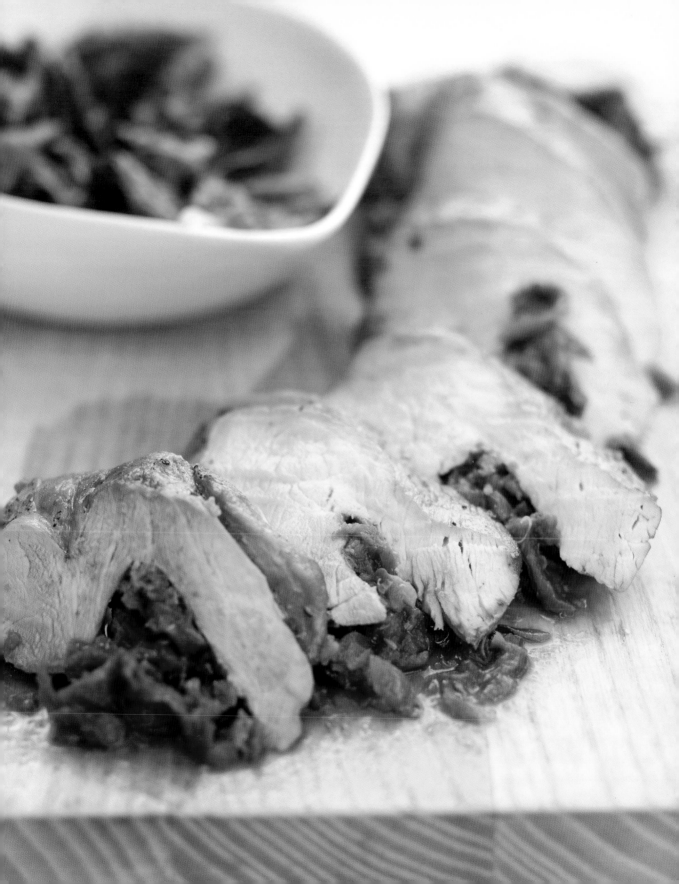

PORK CHOPS WITH SALSA VERDE

SERVES 4   **PREP** 10 MINS   **COOK** 10-12 MINS

A simple recipe for juicy pork.

large handful of flat-leaf parsley
handful of fresh basil leaves
handful of fresh mint leaves
2 tbsp red wine vinegar
2 garlic cloves, roughly chopped

2 anchovy fillets
2 tbsp capers, drained and rinsed
3-4 tbsp olive oil
4 lean pork chops, trimmed of fat
salt and freshly ground black pepper

1 Add the herbs, vinegar, garlic, anchovies, capers, and most of the olive oil to a food processor and whiz until chopped. Spoon out and transfer to a dish.

2 Rub the pork chops with a splash of the remaining oil and season well with salt and black pepper. Heat a griddle pan until hot, add the chops and leave undisturbed for 3–5 minutes, depending on their thickness, then turn them and cook the other side for the same length of time again or until they are no longer pink and are cooked through.

3 Serve the chops topped with the salsa verde and with a mixed salad.

STATISTICS PER SERVING:

Energy 266kcals/1,115kJ

Carbohydrate 0.5g

Sugar 0g

Fibre 0g

Fat 15g
Saturated fat 3g

Salt 1.1g

PORK STIR-FRY WITH CASHEW NUTS AND GREENS

GUIDELINES PER SERVING:

● ○ ○ GI

● ○ ○ CALORIES

● ○ ○ SATURATED FAT

● ● ● SALT

SERVES 4   **PREP** 15 MINS   **COOK** 10-15 MINS

A fast and flavoursome dish.

2 tbsp sunflower oil
1 onion, chopped
2.5cm (1in) piece of fresh root ginger,
  peeled and finely chopped
3 garlic cloves, finely chopped
1 red chilli, deseeded and finely
  sliced

400g (14oz) pork tenderloin,
  finely sliced
3 tbsp soy sauce
1 tbsp sesame oil
handful of cashew nuts
200g (7oz) bok choy, roughly
  sliced lengthways

1 Heat the oil in a wok, add the onion and stir-fry quickly for a minute then add the ginger, garlic, and chilli and cook, stirring continually to make sure the ingredients don't burn.

2 Throw in the pork, stir, and cook for 3–5 minutes until no longer pink, then add the remaining ingredients and cook for a further 3–5 minutes, stirring occasionally until the bok choy is tender and wilted. Serve immediately with noodles or rice.

STATISTICS PER SERVING:

Energy 265kcals/1,100kJ

Carbohydrate 6g

Sugar 4g

Fibre 2g

Fat 16g
Saturated fat 3g

Salt 2.3g

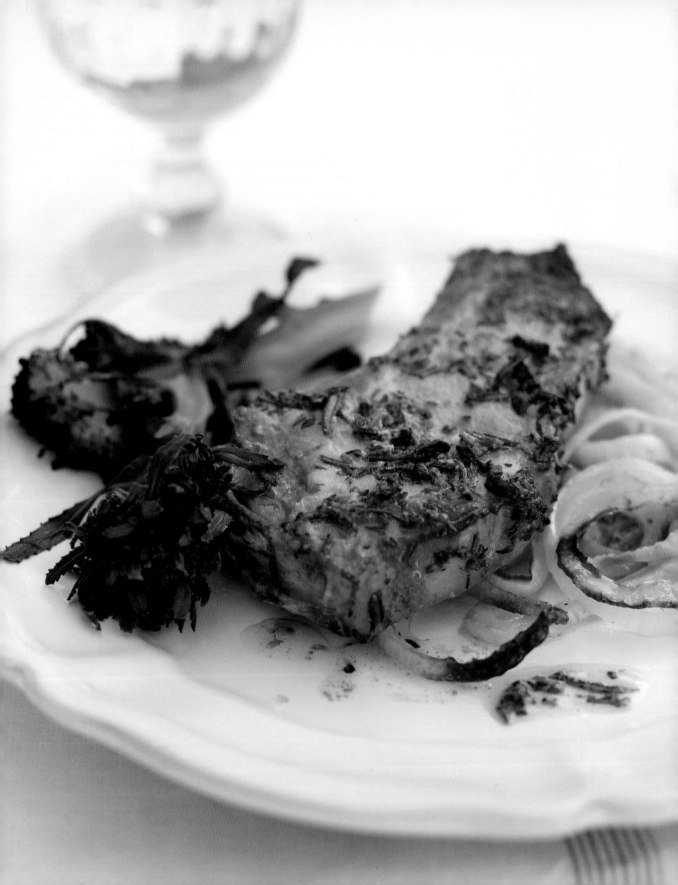

ROASTED PORK CHOPS WITH MUSTARD RUB

⬤◯◯ GI

⬤◯◯ CALORIES

⬤◯◯ SATURATED FAT

⬤◯◯ SALT

SERVES 4   **PREP** 10 MINS   **COOK** 40 MINS

Tasty pork chops paired with purple sprouting broccoli and roasted fennel.

4 tsp English mustard
few stalks thyme, leaves only,
  finely chopped
few stalks rosemary, leaves only,
  finely chopped
salt and freshly ground black pepper
4 chunky pork chops, trimmed of fat

2 onions, peeled and sliced
2 bulbs of fennel, trimmed and sliced
  horizontally
1 tbsp olive oil
handful of purple sprouting broccoli,
  stalks trimmed (prepared weight
  about 100g/3½oz)

1 Preheat the oven to 180°C (350°F/Gas 4). In a bowl, combine the mustard, thyme, and rosemary and season with salt and pepper. Rub this mixture all over the pork chops and put to one side.

2 Arrange the onions and fennel in a roasting tin, season, and drizzle over the olive oil. Add the pork chops, nestling them in amongst the vegetables. Transfer to the oven to cook for about 40 minutes or until the pork is cooked and the onions and fennel are starting to caramelize.

3 Meanwhile, add the purple sprouting broccoli to a pan of boiling salted water and cook for 8–10 minutes or until tender, then drain. Arrange the pork and roasted vegetables on plates with the broccoli on the side, and serve.

COOK'S TIP
Cover the tin with foil if the vegetables are beginning to brown too quickly.

STATISTICS PER SERVING:

Energy 244kcals/1,026kJ

Carbohydrate 5.5g

Sugar 4g

Fibre 2.5g

Fat 9g

Saturated fat 2.5g

Salt 0.4g

MINCED PORK WITH GREEN BEANS

SERVES 4   **PREP** 10 MINS   **COOK** 30 MINS

Choose this supper when you have had a long day at work – it's quick to make.

1 tbsp olive oil
1 large onion, finely diced
1 red chilli, deseeded and chopped
500g (1lb 2oz) lean pork mince
3 garlic cloves, finely chopped

1 tbsp fresh thyme stalks, leaves only
200g (7oz) fine green beans,
 trimmed and halved
300ml (10fl oz) vegetable stock
salt and freshly ground black pepper

1 Heat the oil in a large frying pan and add the onion. Cook for about 3 minutes until soft, then add the chilli and cook for 1 minute. Add the mince and cook for 3–5 minutes until no longer pink.

2 Stir in the garlic, thyme, and green beans. Cook for 1 minute, then add the stock. Season well with salt and black pepper, bring to the boil, then reduce to a simmer. Cook for about 15–20 minutes, partially covered, stirring occasionally. Top up with boiling water if it gets too dry.

STATISTICS PER SERVING:

Energy 223kcals/938kJ

Carbohydrate 6g

Sugar 4g

Fibre 2g

Fat 9g

Saturated fat 2g

Salt 0.6g

PORK MINCE WITH MUSHROOMS AND PASTA

GUIDELINES PER SERVING:

●●○ GI
●●○ CALORIES
●○○ SATURATED FAT
●○○ SALT

SERVES 4   **PREP** 10 MINS   **COOK** 30 MINS

An easy, everyday pasta dish: achieve tasty results with minimal effort.

1 tbsp olive oil
1 onion, finely chopped
salt and freshly ground black pepper
400g (14oz) lean pork mince
250g (9oz) chestnut mushrooms,
  roughly chopped

1 chilli, deseeded and finely chopped
2 garlic cloves, finely chopped
1 tsp dried oregano
400g can chopped tomatoes
350g (12oz) pappardelle pasta
1 tbsp fresh basil, chopped

1 Heat the oil in a large saucepan, add the onion and cook for about 5 minutes or until soft. Season with salt and black pepper, then add the pork mince and mash with the back of a fork. Cook for about 5 minutes or until no longer pink.

2 Add the mushrooms, chilli, garlic, and oregano. Cook for a further 5 minutes, then add the tomatoes, stir well and bring to the boil. Reduce to a simmer and cook for about 20 minutes, adding a little hot water if it starts to dry out too much.

3 Meanwhile, put the pasta in a pan of salted boiling water and cook for 10–12 minutes, or according to the instructions on the packet. Drain, reserving some of the cooking water, and return the pasta to the pan with a little of the water.

4 Add the basil to the mince, stir, and season if needed. Toss the mixture with the pasta.

COOK'S TIP
Use spaghetti, linguine, or fettucine as an alternative to pappardelle, if you wish.

STATISTICS PER SERVING:

Energy 485kcals/2,059kJ

Carbohydrate 70g

Sugar 6g

Fibre 4.5g

Fat 9g
Saturated fat 2g

Salt 0.3g

⬤◯◯ GI

⬤◯◯ CALORIES

⬤◯◯ SATURATED FAT

⬤◯◯ SALT

PORK AND APPLE PATTIES

SERVES 4   **PREP** 15 MINS   **COOK** 10 MINS   **FREEZE** 1 MONTH
(MAKES 8)   AFTER STEP 1

Miniature burgers made from a few simple ingredients.

450g minced pork
2 crisp eating apples, cored
  and finely diced
salt and freshly ground black pepper
1 egg

1 tsp paprika
4–5 stalks of fresh thyme, leaves only,
  finely chopped
oil for frying

1 Place the pork in a bowl with the apple, season well with salt and black pepper, and mix together. Add the egg, paprika, and thyme and mix until combined, then, using your hands, squeeze the mixture together until it is an even paste. Shape into 8 balls (2 per serving) and pat into patties.

2 Heat the oil in a large non-stick frying pan and add the patties, working in batches if necessary. Cook over a medium heat for 3–4 minutes each side, until a deep golden colour. Transfer to a plate lined with kitchen paper to drain, then serve.

COOK'S TIP
You could also oven bake these; sit them in a roasting tin and cook at 200ºC (400ºF/Gas 6) for 15–20 minutes.

STATISTICS PER SERVING:

Energy 126kcals/528kJ

Carbohydrate Carbohydrate 3g

Sugar 3g

Fibre 0.4g

Fat 7g

Saturated fat 1.5g

Salt 0.2g

BEEF BURGERS

SERVES 4   **PREP** 10 MINS
                PLUS CHILLING   **COOK** 15-20 MINS   **FREEZE** 3 MONTHS
                                                          AFTER STEP 2

Using lean mince, and oven baking rather than frying, stops these burgers being too fatty.

GUIDELINES PER BURGER:

● ○ ○ GI

● ○ ○ CALORIES

● ● ○ SATURATED FAT

● ● ○ SALT

500g (1lb 2oz) lean beef mince
2 tbsp capers, drained, rinsed,
   and very finely chopped

1 onion, very finely chopped
2 tsp grainy mustard

1 Add all the ingredients to a bowl and, using your hands, mix evenly until well combined.

2 Divide the mixture into four and roll each into a ball. Flatten into patties on a sheet of greaseproof paper set on a plate, and place in the fridge to firm up for 30 minutes.

3 Preheat the oven to 200°C (400°F/Gas 6). When hot, turn each patty onto a baking sheet and peel away the paper. Transfer the baking sheet to the oven for 15–20 minutes or until the burgers are cooked through. These are good served on wholemeal rolls with some fresh lettuce and tomato.

STATISTICS PER BURGER:

Energy 236kcals/988kJ

Carbohydrate 3.5g

Sugar 2g

Fibre 0.8g

Fat 12g
Saturated fat 5g

Salt 0.9g

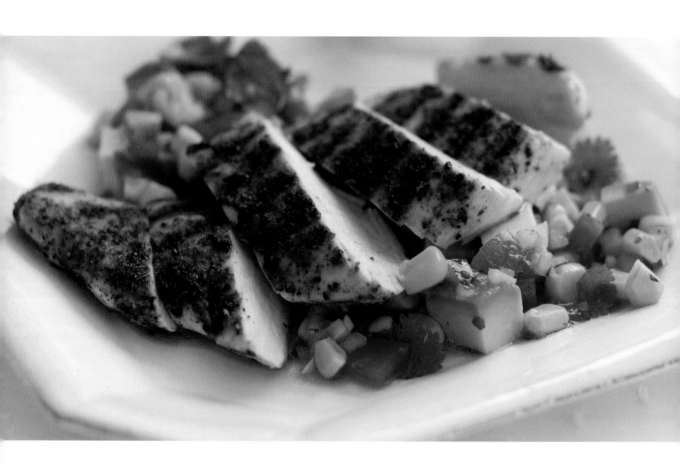

SIMPLE SUPPERS
– POULTRY

CHICKEN LIVERS WITH KALE AND BALSAMIC VINEGAR

SERVES 4   **PREP** 10 MINS   **COOK** 15-20 MINS

A robust and hearty dish that is full of flavour and packed with vitamins and minerals.

450g (1lb) chicken livers
200g (7oz) kale or spinach leaves
2 tbsp olive oil
2 red onions, thickly sliced
100g (3½oz) smoked lardons,
  or 4 rashers smoked back bacon,
  roughly chopped

2 garlic cloves, crushed or finely
  chopped
3 tbsp balsamic vinegar
150ml (5fl oz) dry sherry
salt and freshly ground black pepper
250g (9oz) baby cherry tomatoes

1 Rinse the chicken livers and chop roughly, discarding any fibrous bits.

2 Chop the kale or spinach leaves, removing the central stalk of the kale. Heat 1 tablespoon of oil in a large, nonstick frying pan. When the oil is hot, add the chicken livers and cook over a high heat for about 5 minutes or until just brown. Remove the livers from the pan and set aside.

3 Pour the remaining oil into the pan and reduce the heat. Add the onions, bacon, and garlic. Cook, stirring frequently, for about 5 minutes or until the onions are soft.

4 Add the balsamic vinegar and sherry and continue to cook for a further minute. Return the chicken livers to the pan and season with black pepper. Add the kale and tomatoes. Continue cooking over a low heat for 4–6 minutes or until the kale begins to wilt.

STATISTICS PER SERVING:

Energy 318kcals/1,326kJ

Carbohydrate 12g

Sugar 10g

Fibre 3g

Fat 13g

Saturated fat 3g

Salt 1.2g

POACHED CHICKEN WITH STAR ANISE, SOY, AND BROWN RICE

GUIDELINES PER SERVING:

●●○ GI

●●○ CALORIES

●○○ SATURATED FAT

●●● SALT

SERVES 4   **PREP** 5 MINS   **COOK** 50 MINS   **FREEZE** 1 MONTH
WITHOUT THE RICE

A light and aromatic chicken dish enjoyed with nutty brown rice.

225g (8oz) brown basmati rice
salt and freshly ground black pepper
2 tsp five-spice powder
4 chicken breasts, skinned
4 star anise
5cm (2in) piece of fresh root ginger,
  finely sliced

2 large red chillies, deseeded
  and finely sliced lengthways
3 tbsp dark soy sauce
100g (3½oz) sugarsnap peas,
  finely sliced lengthways

1 Put the rice in a large pan of salted water and cook for 30–35 minutes, or according to the instructions on the packet. Drain, return to the pan and set aside with the lid on.

2 Sprinkle the five-spice powder over the chicken and set it aside. Measure 1.7 litres (3 pints) water into a large pan and add the star anise, ginger, chillies, and soy sauce. Bring to the boil, then add the chicken. Reduce to a simmer and cook until the chicken is done – about 20 minutes (pierce it with a sharp knife: the juices should run clear). Remove the chicken from the pan and set aside.

3 Bring the liquid in the pan to the boil and reduce it by half. Taste, and season with black pepper if needed – it should be salty enough because of the soy sauce. Add the sugarsnap peas for the last couple of minutes of cooking. Slice or tear the chicken into bite-sized pieces (if you wish) and return it to the broth. Remove the star anise. Serve the rice in individual bowls, topped with the chicken, and with plenty of juice ladled over it.

COOK'S TIP
You could use the star anise for a garnish, but remember that it should not be eaten.

STATISTICS PER SERVING:

Energy 373kcals/1,584kJ

Carbohydrate 48g

Sugar 2.5g

Fibre 1.5g

Fat 3.5g

Saturated fat 1g

Salt 2.2g

BENGALI SPICE RUB CHICKEN

SERVES 4   **PREP** 15 MINS   **COOK** 40 MINS

An easy Indian-style dish you can make as hot as you wish.

1 tbsp turmeric
4 chicken breasts, skinned and cut
  into chunky pieces
1 onion, roughly chopped
5cm (2in) piece of fresh ginger, peeled
1–2 green chillies, deseeded
1 tsp mustard seeds
1 tsp cumin seeds
1 tsp onion seeds
1 tbsp sunflower oil
salt and freshly ground black pepper

6 tomatoes, roughly chopped
2 red peppers, roughly chopped
1 tbsp of tomato purée

For the yoghurt mixture
200g carton of thick natural yogurt
½ cucumber, halved lengthways,
  peeled, seeds removed, and diced
handful of fresh coriander leaves,
  finely chopped

1 First make the yoghurt mixture: mix all the ingredients together and season with a pinch of sea salt. Put to one side. Toss the chicken pieces in the turmeric to coat and put to one side. Put the onion, ginger and chillies in a food processor and whiz to a paste.

2 In a heavy-based deep frying pan, heat the mustard seeds over a medium heat for a minute or so until they begin to pop, then add the cumin and onion seeds and fry for 1–2 minutes more, being careful not to let the seeds burn. Add the oil to the pan, then add the chicken and cook for 5–10 minutes or until golden, then remove from the pan and set aside. Spoon in the onion mixture, season with salt and black pepper, and cook for 5 minutes.

3 Add the tomatoes, red peppers, and tomato purée and cook over a low heat for a further 5 minutes until softened. A little at a time, add 600ml (1 pint) water, stirring and allowing the mixture to bubble in between times. Return the chicken to the pan and cook on a low heat for 15 minutes. Serve with basmati rice, with the yoghurt on the side.

COOK'S TIP
If you prefer, you can skin the tomatoes before chopping, or use a 400g can of chopped tomatoes instead.

STATISTICS PER SERVING:

Energy 294kcals/1,240kJ

Carbohydrate 18g

Sugar 16g

Fibre 3.5g

Fat 8g

Saturated fat 2g

Salt 0.5g

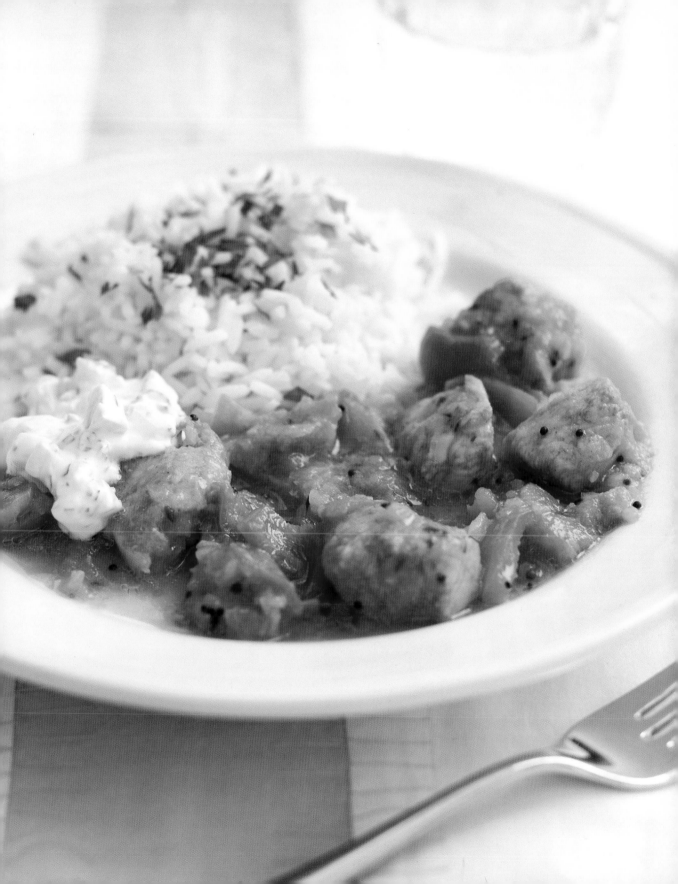

● ○ ○   GI

● ○ ○   CALORIES

● ○ ○   SATURATED FAT

● ● ○   SALT

CHICKEN, ONION, AND PEAS

SERVES 4   **PREP** 5 MINS   **COOK** 40 MINS

A simple, satisfying dish made with few ingredients.

4 chicken thighs or breasts
salt and freshly ground black pepper
2 tbsp oil
1 onion, finely chopped
2 garlic cloves
1 tbsp fresh thyme leaves

600ml (1 pint) mushroom
  or vegetable stock
225g (8oz) frozen garden peas
1 tbsp flat-leaf parsley,
  finely chopped
200g (7oz) brown rice

1 Season the chicken well with salt and black pepper. Pour 1 tablespoon of oil into a large, heavy pan and when hot, add the chicken pieces. Cook for about 5 minutes, or until golden, then turn and cook them on the other side for the same length of time. Remove with tongs and set aside.

2 Heat the remaining oil in the pan, add the onion and cook until soft. Season well, then throw in the garlic and thyme and cook for a few seconds. Return the chicken to the pan and add a small amount of stock. Let it bubble, then stir up any bits from the bottom of the pan before adding the remaining stock. Reduce to a simmer.

3 Tip in the peas and continue to cook, covered, over a low heat for 25–35 minutes or until the chicken is cooked (the juices should run clear when the chicken is pierced with a sharp knife). If the chicken begins to dry out, top up the pan with a little more hot stock or water.

4 Meanwhile, cook the rice according to the instructions on the packet. Drain, then serve with the chicken.

COOK'S TIP
Chicken breasts will not take as long to cook as thighs.
To prevent the chicken from drying out, don't have the heat too high.

STATISTICS PER SERVING:

Energy 468kcals/1,956kJ

Carbohydrate 50g

Sugar 3.5g

Fibre 4.1g

Fat 10.5g

Saturated fat 2.2g

Salt 0.8g

WILD RICE WITH CHICKEN, SAFFRON, AND PUMPKIN

SERVES 4   **PREP** 15 MINS   **COOK** 1 HOUR 15 MINS

A fruity and aromatic dish, full of colour. Bring a golden glow to a winter evening.

GUIDELINES PER SERVING:

●●○ GI

●●○ CALORIES

●○○ SATURATED FAT

●●● SALT

350g (12oz) chicken breast, cut into chunky, bite-sized pieces
1 tbsp olive oil
salt and freshly ground black pepper
1 onion, roughly chopped
2 carrots, roughly chopped
6 cloves garlic, unpeeled
900ml (1½ pints) vegetable stock
1 bay leaf

75g (2½ oz) bacon, chopped into bite-sized pieces
½ small pumpkin (about 300g/10oz), cut into bite-sized chunks
zest and juice of 1 orange
pinch of saffron threads, soaked in a little boiling water
350g (12oz) rice and wild rice, mixed

1 Preheat the oven to 200°C (400°F/Gas 6). Rub the chicken with the oil and season well with salt and black pepper. Heat a large, cast-iron casserole and add the chicken. Cook for about 6–8 minutes, turning, until brown on all sides.

2 Add the onion, carrots, garlic, and a little of the stock. Bring to the boil and stir, then pour in the remaining stock. Add the bay leaf, bacon, pumpkin, orange zest and juice, and saffron in its water. Season well and stir. Transfer the casserole to the oven and cook for 1 hour, topping it up with hot water if the mixture becomes too dry.

3 Meanwhile, cook the rice in salted boiling water for 20 minutes, or according to the instructions on the packet. Drain and keep warm. Remove the garlic cloves from the casserole with a slotted spoon, and then squeeze them out of their skins and back into the pot.

4 Divide the rice between 4 bowls or plates, and ladle in the chicken and pumpkin mixture.

STATISTICS PER SERVING:

Energy 558kcals/2,338kJ

Carbohydrate 79g

Sugar 6.5g

Fibre 2g

Fat 10g
Saturated fat 2.5g

Salt 2g

● ○ ○ GI

● ○ ○ CALORIES

● ○ ○ SATURATED FAT

● ○ ○ SALT

CHICKEN WITH HERBS AND CHILLIES

SERVES 4   **PREP** 5 MINS   **COOK** 35 MINS

A simple and healthy, but very tasty, way to serve chicken.

handful of curly parsley
handful of basil leaves
1–2 red chillies, deseeded
3 garlic cloves, peeled
juice of ½ lemon

1 tbsp olive oil, plus extra
  for oiling
salt and freshly ground
  black pepper
4 skinless chicken breasts

1 Preheat the oven to 200°C (400°F/Gas 6). Place the parsley, basil, chillies, garlic, lemon juice, and olive oil in a food processor and whiz until well combined. Season with salt and pepper and whiz again.

2 Slash the chicken breasts a few times horizontally then rub the herb mixture all over, making sure it goes into the slashes. Place the chicken in an oiled roasting tin and cook in the oven for 30–35 minutes or until the chicken is cooked through.

STATISTICS PER SERVING:

Energy 184kcals/775kJ

Carbohydrate 0g

Sugar 0g

Fibre 0g

Fat 4.5g

Saturated fat 0.8g

Salt 0.3g

CHICKEN NUGGETS

GUIDELINES PER SERVING:

● ○ ○ GI

● ○ ○ CALORIES

● ○ ○ SATURATED FAT

● ○ ○ SALT

SERVES 4   **PREP** 20 MINS   **COOK** 20 MINS   **FREEZE** 1 MONTH

Tender bites of moist chicken in a golden coating.

4 slices of white bread
1 tsp paprika
salt and freshly ground black pepper
1–2 eggs, lightly beaten

plain flour, for dusting
2 skinless chicken breasts,
  cut into strips
olive oil, for oiling

1 Preheat the oven to 200°C (400°F/Gas 6). Place the bread in a food processor and whiz to crumbs, then sprinkle in the paprika, a pinch of salt and some black pepper and whiz again. Tip the crumbs onto a baking sheet, spread them out evenly then bake for 3–6 minutes until golden, giving them a gentle stir halfway through.

2 Return the toasted crumbs to the food processor and whiz again until fine. Tip out onto a large plate.

3 Pour the beaten egg onto another large plate and tip the flour onto a third large plate. Toss the chicken pieces in the egg first, then coat them with the flour and finally the breadcrumbs. Oil a baking sheet well with olive oil and sit the coated chicken pieces on it. Bake in the oven for 15–20 minutes or until the chicken is cooked and the coating is golden.

STATISTICS PER SERVING:

Energy 208kcals/880kJ

Carbohydrate 17g

Sugar 0.9g

Fibre 0.5g

Fat 6g
Saturated fat 1g

Salt 0.6g

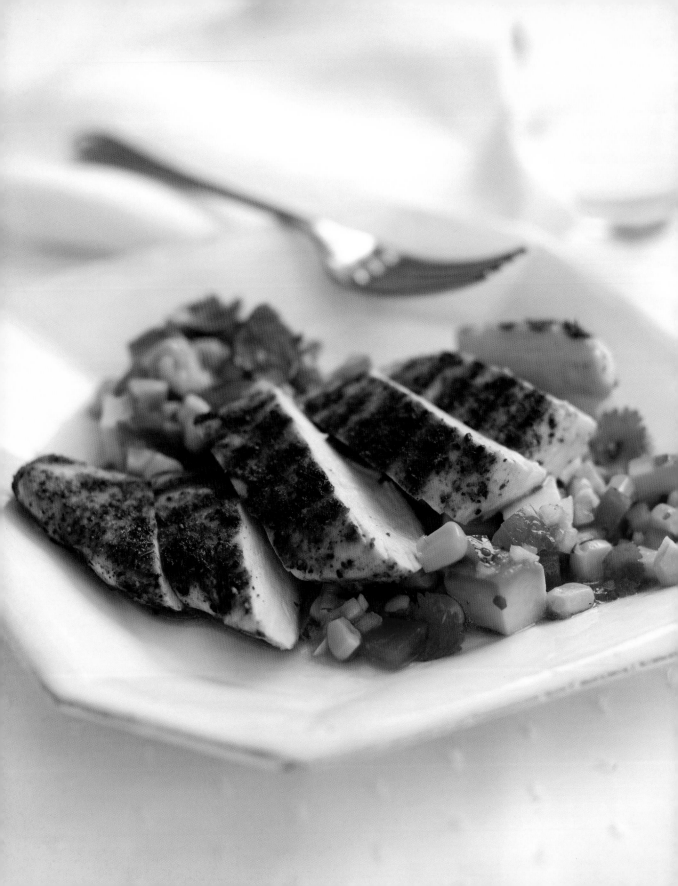

CAJUN CHICKEN WITH SWEETCORN SALSA

GUIDELINES PER SERVING:

● ○ ○ GI

● ● ○ CALORIES

● ● ○ SATURATED FAT

● ○ ○ SALT

SERVES 2   **PREP** 10 MINS   **COOK** 15 MINS

Avocados give the salsa a wonderfully creamy flavour, which helps to balance the fieriness of the chicken.

2 skinless chicken breasts
1 tbsp of Cajun seasoning
1 tbsp olive oil

For the salsa
1 large fresh corn on the cob, stripped
  of husks and threads

½ small red onion, finely chopped
½ red pepper, deseeded and diced
1 red chilli, deseeded and
  finely chopped
1 small hass avocado, diced
1 tbsp olive oil
juice of 1 lime

1 Put the chicken breasts between 2 pieces of cling film and pound with a rolling pin until flattened evenly. Mix the the Cajun seasoning with the oil and brush over the flattened chicken. Leave to marinate for at least 15 minutes.

2 To make the salsa, add the corn to a large pan of boiling water and cook for 5 minutes, then immediately transfer to a bowl of iced water to cool. Drain well, then, using a sharp knife, scrape off all the kernels. Combine with the remaining salsa ingredients, mix well, and set aside.

3 Heat a griddle pan and cook the chicken for 4–5 minutes on one side, pressing the pieces down on the griddle pan, then turn and cook for 4–5 minutes on the other side, or until cooked through.

4 Spoon the salsa onto serving plates and top with the griddled chicken.

STATISTICS PER SERVING:

Energy 442kcals/1,846kJ

Carbohydrate 18g

Sugar 5g

Fibre 3.5g

Fat 23g
Saturated fat 4g

Salt 0.3g

⬤◯◯ GI

⬤◯◯ CALORIES

⬤◯◯ SATURATED FAT

⬤◯◯ SALT

SAFFRON CHICKEN BROCHETTES

SERVES 6 **PREP** 10 MINS **COOK** 10 MINS
PLUS MARINATING

Simple, prepare-ahead food, also suitable for a barbecue.

6 x 175g (6oz) skinless boneless
  chicken breasts, cubed
2 tbsp olive oil
zest and juice of 3 lemons
4 pinches of saffron powder, dissolved
  in 1 tbsp boiling water

salt and freshly ground black pepper
2 red onions, finely sliced
30g (1oz) polyunsaturated margarine
basil leaves, to garnish

1 Put the chicken in a large bowl. Whisk together the oil, lemon zest, the juice from 2 lemons and the saffron in its water. Season to taste with salt and pepper. Add the sliced onions and pour over the chicken. Mix, cover, and chill for 2 hours or overnight.

2 When ready to cook, melt the margarine in a small pan with the remaining lemon juice.

3 Preheat the grill to high. Remove the chicken from the marinade and thread on to skewers. Place under the grill with the onions and grill for 5–6 minutes. Turn, brush with the lemon-margarine mixture, and grill for another 5–6 minutes or until cooked through. Arrange on a heated plate and serve hot, scattered with basil leaves.

COOK'S TIP
If using wooden skewers, soak them in cold water for 30 minutes before using to prevent them burning.

STATISTICS PER SERVING:

Energy 268kcals/1,125kJ

Carbohydrate 2.5g

Sugar 2g

Fibre 0.5g

Fat 10g

Saturated fat 2g

Salt 0.4g

TURKEY KEBABS

MAKES 6 **PREP** 20 MINS **COOK** 10-12 MINS
PLUS MARINATING

GUIDELINES PER SERVING:

GI

CALORIES

SATURATED FAT

SALT

Zingy kebabs served with a refreshing mint yogurt.

60ml (2fl oz) light soy sauce
2 tbsp olive oil
2 garlic cloves, finely chopped
¾ tsp ground ginger
¼ tsp chilli flakes
675g (1½lb) skinless boneless turkey
  breasts, cut into 2.5cm (1in) cubes
1 red pepper, deseeded and cut into
  2.5cm (1in) pieces

1 green pepper, deseeded and cut
  into 2.5cm (1in) pieces
1 large courgette, cut into 2.5cm
  (1in) slices
240ml (8fl oz) plain yogurt
2 tbsp mint, chopped
½ tsp ground cumin

1 Combine the soy sauce, oil, garlic, ginger, and chilli. Add the turkey pieces and toss to coat. Cover, chill, and marinate for at least 1 hour.

2 Thread the turkey, pepper, and courgette onto skewers and brush with any leftover marinade. Grill for 5–6 minutes on each side, or until cooked through.

3 Mix together the yogurt, mint, and cumin in a small bowl. Arrange the kebabs on a serving platter with the mint yogurt on the side.

COOK'S TIP
If using wooden skewers, soak them in cold water for 30 minutes before using to prevent them burning.

STATISTICS PER SERVING:

Energy 207kcals/869kJ

Carbohydrate 7.5g

Sugar 7g

Fibre 1g

Fat 6g
Saturated fat 2g

Salt 2g

● ○ ○ GI

● ● ○ CALORIES

● ○ ○ SATURATED FAT

● ○ ○ SALT

CHICKEN AND ARTICHOKE FILO PIE

SERVES 4   **PREP** 15 MINS   **COOK** 25-30 MINS

Filo pastry is quick and easy to use and a healthier alternative to shortcrust or flaky pastry, as it contains considerably less fat.

3 tbsp vegetable oil
1 large onion, finely chopped
4 skinless chicken breasts, cut into bite-sized chunks
1 clove garlic, crushed
4 sticks celery, chopped
200g (7oz) low-fat soft cheese with garlic and herbs

400g can artichokes, drained and roughly chopped
salt and freshly ground black pepper
6 large sheets of filo pastry
1 tsp sesame seeds

1 Preheat the oven to 190°C (375°F/Gas 5). Heat 2 tablespoons of the oil in a large frying pan and add the onion. Cook, stirring, for 2–3 minutes or until soft. Add the chicken, garlic, and celery and cook for 5 minutes or until the chicken is golden brown all over.

2 Remove from the heat, stir in the soft cheese and artichokes, and season to taste. Transfer the mixture into a shallow ovenproof dish.

3 Lightly brush the sheets of filo pastry with the remaining oil, then scrunch each sheet slightly and place it on top of the chicken mixture. Sprinkle with sesame seeds and bake in the oven for 20–25 minutes or until the pastry is crisp and golden. Serve hot.

STATISTICS PER SERVING:

Energy 327kcals/1,370kJ

Carbohydrate 17g

Sugar 4.5g

Fibre 3g

Fat 11g

Saturated fat 1.5g

Salt 0.4g

CHICKEN PAPRIKASH

SERVES 4   **PREP** 10 MINS   **COOK** 40-45 MINS   **FREEZE** 1 MONTH

Spicy paprika adds both flavour and colour to this hearty stew from Hungary, which gets an extra rush of flavour from cherry tomatoes added at the end.

GUIDELINES PER SERVING:

● ○ ○ GI

● ○ ○ CALORIES

● ○ ○ SATURATED FAT

● ○ ○ SALT

2 tbsp sunflower oil
2 small red onions, sliced
1 garlic clove, finely chopped
1 tbsp sweet paprika
¼ tsp caraway seeds
8 chicken thighs
250ml (9fl oz) hot chicken stock

1 tbsp red wine vinegar
1 tbsp tomato purée
1 tsp sugar
salt and freshly ground black pepper
250g (9oz) cherry tomatoes
1 tbsp chopped flat-leaf parsley, to garnish

1 Heat the oil in a large, flameproof casserole over a medium heat. Add the onion, garlic, paprika, and caraway seeds. Fry, stirring, for about 5 minutes, or until the onion softens. Use a slotted spoon to remove the ingredients from the pan and set aside.

2 Add the chicken thighs, skin-side down, to any oil remaining in the pan and fry for 3 minutes. Turn them over and continue frying for a further 2 minutes. Return the onion mixture to the pan.

3 Mix together the stock, vinegar, tomato purée, sugar, and salt and pepper to taste. Pour over the chicken and bring to the boil, then reduce the heat to low. Cover and leave to simmer for 25 minutes, or until the chicken is tender.

4 Add the cherry tomatoes and shake the casserole vigorously to mix them into the sauce. Cover and simmer for a further 5 minutes. Sprinkle with parsley and serve.

STATISTICS PER SERVING:

Energy 324kcals/1,356kJ

Carbohydrate 9g

Sugar 7g

Fibre 2g

Fat 14g
Saturated fat 2g

Salt 0.9g

DEVILLED TURKEY

SERVES 4   **PREP** 10 MINS   **COOK** 15 MINS

Serve these spicy stir-fried turkey strips as a healthy lunch or supper.

2 tbsp wholegrain mustard
2 tbsp mango chutney
2 tbsp Worcestershire sauce
¼ tsp ground paprika
3 tbsp orange juice
1 red chilli, chopped
2 tbsp olive oil
450g (1lb) turkey breast escalope,
   cut into strips

1 onion, peeled and finely chopped
1 red pepper, cored and cut
   into strips
1 orange pepper, cored and
   cut into strips
1 garlic clove, crushed

1 Mix the mustard, chutney, Worcestershire sauce, paprika, orange juice, and chilli together until well combined.

2 Heat the oil in a frying pan or wok, add the turkey, and cook over a high heat until browned. Remove the turkey from the pan and set aside, covered to keep it warm.

3 Add the onion to the pan and fry for 2–3 minutes, or until beginning to colour. Add the peppers and garlic and fry, stirring constantly, for 3–4 minutes, or until tender.

4 Stir in the mustard mixture and return the turkey to the pan. Cook for 5 minutes or until piping hot and the turkey is cooked through.

STATISTICS PER SERVING:

Energy 234kcals/981kJ

Carbohydrate 13g

Sugar 11g

Fibre 2g

Fat 7.5g

Saturated fat 1g

Salt 0.9g

CHICKEN JALFREZI

GUIDELINES PER SERVING:

● ○ ○ GI

● ○ ○ CALORIES

● ○ ○ SATURATED FAT

● ○ ○ SALT

SERVES 4   **PREP** 20 MINS   **COOK** 25 MINS   **FREEZE** 3 MONTHS

A spicy dish, with chillies and mustard seeds, for those who like their curries hot.

2 tbsp sunflower oil
2 tbsp ground cumin
2 tsp yellow mustard seeds
1 tsp ground turmeric
2 tbsp masala curry paste
2.5cm (1in) piece fresh root ginger, peeled and finely chopped
3 garlic cloves, crushed
1 onion, sliced
1 red pepper, deseeded and sliced

½ green pepper, deseeded and sliced
2 green chillies, deseeded and finely chopped
675g (1½lb) boneless chicken thighs or breasts, skinned and cut into 2.5cm (1in) pieces
225g can chopped tomatoes
3 tbsp chopped coriander

1 Heat the oil in a large pan over a medium heat, add the cumin, mustard seeds, turmeric, and curry paste, and stir-fry for 1–2 minutes.

2 Add the ginger, garlic, and onion and fry, stirring frequently, until the onion starts to soften. Add the red and green peppers and the chillies and fry for 5 minutes.

3 Increase the heat to medium-high, add the chicken, and fry until starting to brown. Add the tomatoes and coriander, reduce the heat, and simmer for 10 minutes, or until the chicken is cooked through, stirring often. Serve hot.

STATISTICS PER SERVING:

Energy	290kcals/1,205kJ
Carbohydrate	9g
Sugar	7g
Fibre	2g
Fat	9g
Saturated fat	1g
Salt	0.6g

● ○ ○   GI

● ● ○   CALORIES

● ○ ○   SATURATED FAT

● ● ○   SALT

QUICK TURKEY CASSOULET

SERVES 6   **PREP** 15 MINS   **COOK** 35 MINS

A hearty, filling supper dish that is high in fibre.

3 tbsp olive oil
1 medium red onion, peeled
  and finely chopped
2 cloves of garlic, peeled and crushed
1 red pepper, deseeded and diced
60g (2oz) smoked back bacon,
  roughly chopped
2 celery stalks, finely chopped
400g can of chopped tomatoes
250ml (8fl oz) chicken stock

2 tsp dark soy sauce
75g (2½oz) wholemeal breadcrumbs
50g (1¾oz) freshly grated Parmesan
  cheese
3 tbsp chopped flat-leaf parsley
2 tsp Dijon mustard
2 x 400g cans of mixed beans,
  rinsed and drained
400g (14oz) cooked turkey breast,
  roughly chopped

1 Heat 2 tablespoons of the oil in a large non-stick saucepan, add the onion, and cook over a low heat for 5 minutes. Add the garlic, red pepper, bacon, and celery and cook for a further 5 minutes, stirring occasionally.

2 Add the tomatoes, stock, and soy sauce. Bring to the boil, then reduce to a fast simmer and cook for 15 minutes or until the sauce begins to thicken.

3 Meanwhile, mix together the breadcrumbs, Parmesan, and parsley.

4 Add the mustard, beans, and turkey to the saucepan and cook for a further 5 minutes until heated through.

5 Transfer the hot mixture into a shallow ovenproof dish. Sprinkle the breadcrumb mixture evenly over the top and drizzle over the remaining olive oil. Place under a medium-hot grill for 5 minutes or until the top is golden brown, then serve immediately.

STATISTICS PER SERVING:

Energy 400kcals/1,600kJ

Carbohydrate 34g

Sugar 6g

Fibre 9g

Fat 13.5g

Saturated fat 4g

Salt 1.6g

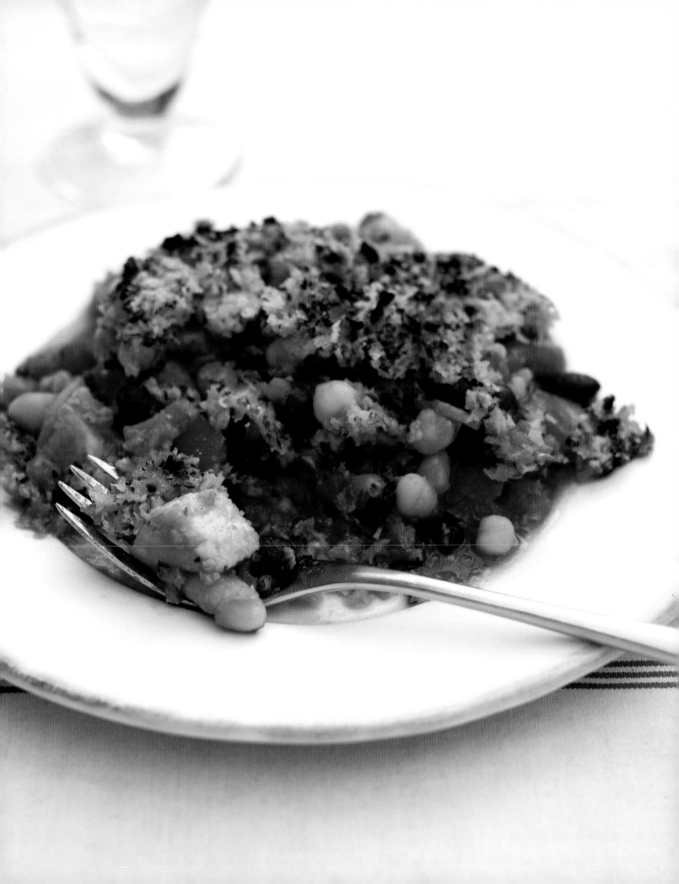

CHICKEN AND APRICOT TAGINE

SERVES 4   **PREP** 15 MINS   **COOK** 35-45 MINS

The dried fruit and warm spices in this dish are the unmistakable flavours of the Middle East.

2 tbsp sunflower oil
1 onion, finely chopped
1 garlic clove, finely chopped
1 tsp ground ginger
1 tsp ground cumin
1 tsp turmeric
pinch of ground cinnamon
pinch of dried chilli flakes
1 tbsp tomato purée

600ml (1 pint) chicken stock
4 tbsp fresh orange juice
150g (5½oz) mixed dried fruit, such
   as apricots and raisins
salt and freshly ground black pepper
675g (1½lb) skinless boneless chicken
   breasts and thighs, cut into
   large chunks
2 tbsp chopped coriander, to garnish

1 Heat the oil in a large flameproof casserole over a medium heat. Add the onion, garlic, ground spices, and chilli flakes and fry, stirring, for 5 minutes, or until the onions have softened. Stir in the tomato purée and stock and bring to the boil, stirring.

2 Add the orange juice, dried fruits, and salt and pepper to taste. Reduce the heat, partially cover the pan, and simmer for 15 minutes, or until the fruits are soft and the juices have reduced slightly.

3 Add the chicken, re-cover the casserole, and continue simmering for 20 minutes, or until the chicken is tender and the juices run clear. Adjust the seasoning, if necessary, then garnish with coriander and serve hot.

STATISTICS PER SERVING:

Energy 380kcals/1,605kJ

Carbohydrate 32g

Sugar 28g

Fibre 1.5g

Fat 9g
Saturated fat 1.5g

Salt 1g

CHICKEN AND CHICKPEA PILAF

SERVES 4   **PREP** 20 MINS   **COOK** 35 MINS

This one-pot rice dish is easy to make and full of flavour.

GUIDELINES PER SERVING:

● ○ ○ GI

● ● ○ CALORIES

● ○ ○ SATURATED FAT

● ● ○ SALT

pinch of saffron threads
2 tsp vegetable oil
6 skinless boneless chicken thighs,
  cut into small pieces
2 tsp ground coriander
1 tsp ground cumin
1 onion, sliced
1 red pepper, deseeded and chopped
2 garlic cloves, peeled and crushed

225g (8oz) long-grain rice
750ml (1¼ pints) hot chicken stock
2 bay leaves
400g can chickpeas, drained
  and rinsed
60g (2oz) sultanas
60g (2oz) flaked almonds
  or pine nuts, toasted
3 tbsp chopped flat-leaf parsley

1 Crumble the saffron threads into a small bowl, add 2 tbsp boiling water, and set aside for at least 10 minutes.

2 Meanwhile, heat half the oil in a large saucepan, add the chicken, coriander, and cumin, and fry over a medium heat for 3 minutes, stirring frequently. Remove from the pan and set aside. Lower the heat, add the rest of the oil, the onion, red pepper, and garlic, and fry for 5 minutes, or until softened.

3 Stir in the rice, return the chicken to the pan and pour in about three-quarters of the stock. Add the bay leaves and saffron with its soaking water and bring to the boil. Simmer for 15 minutes, or until the rice is almost cooked, adding more stock as needed. Stir in the chickpeas and sultanas, and continue cooking until the rice is tender. Transfer to a warm serving platter and serve hot, sprinkled with the toasted nuts and chopped parsley.

STATISTICS PER SERVING:

Energy 621kcals/2,604kJ

Carbohydrate 75g

Sugar 15g

Fibre 2.5g

Fat 13g
Saturated fat 1.5g

Salt 1.1g

● ○ ○ GI

● ● ○ CALORIES

● ○ ○ SATURATED FAT

● ● ○ SALT

CHICKEN BIRYANI

SERVES 4   **PREP** 20 MINS   **COOK** 30 MINS

A subtly spiced, aromatic dish from India.

2 tbsp vegetable oil
30g (1oz) polyunsaturated margarine
1 large onion, thinly sliced
2 garlic cloves, crushed
6 curry leaves
6 cardamom pods
1 cinnamon stick, broken into
   2 or 3 pieces
1 tsp ground turmeric

½ tsp ground cumin
4 skinless boneless chicken breasts,
   cut into 2.5cm (1in) pieces
3 tbsp mild curry paste
300g (10oz) basmati rice
85g (3oz) sultanas
900ml (1½ pints) chicken stock
2 tbsp flaked almonds, toasted

1 Heat the oil and margarine in a large deep saucepan, and gently fry the onion and garlic until softened and starting to turn golden. Add the curry leaves, cardamom pods, and cinnamon stick, and fry for 5 minutes, stirring occasionally.

2 Add the turmeric and cumin, fry for 1 minute, then add the chicken and stir in the curry paste.

3 Add the rice and sultanas, stir well, then pour in enough of the stock to cover the rice. Bring to the boil, lower the heat, and cook gently for 10–12 minutes, or until the rice is cooked, adding more stock if the mixture becomes dry.

4 Transfer to a serving dish, fluff up the rice with a fork, and serve with toasted flaked almonds scattered over the top.

STATISTICS PER SERVING:

Energy 723kcals/3,026kJ

Carbohydrate 80g

Sugar 17g

Fibre 2g

Fat 22g

Saturated fat 3g

Salt 1.9g

ARROZ CON POLLO

SERVES 4   **PREP** 20 MINS   **COOK** 45 MINS

GUIDELINES PER SERVING:

◐○○ GI
◐◐○ CALORIES
◐○○ SATURATED FAT
◐◐○ SALT

This colourful chicken and rice dish from Latin America
is cooked and served in one pot.

2 tbsp olive oil
8 chicken thighs
1 Spanish onion, finely sliced
1 green pepper, deseeded
 and chopped
1 red pepper, deseeded and chopped
2 garlic cloves, finely chopped
1 tsp smoked paprika
1 bay leaf
230g can chopped tomatoes

1 tsp thyme leaves
1 tsp dried oregano
175g (6oz) basmati rice
pinch of saffron threads
750ml (1¼ pints) chicken stock
2 tbsp tomato purée
juice of ½ lemon
salt and freshly ground black pepper
100g (3½oz) frozen peas

1 Preheat the oven to 180°C (350°F/Gas 4). Heat half the oil in a large
flameproof casserole and fry the chicken thighs over high heat, turning
frequently, or until evenly browned. Remove from the casserole, drain,
and set aside.

2 Add the remaining oil, reduce the heat and fry the onion until softened.
Add the chopped peppers and garlic and fry for 5 minutes, or until they
start to soften. Add the paprika, bay leaf, tomatoes, thyme, and oregano,
and stir in the rice. Fry for 1–2 minutes, stirring constantly.

3 Crumble in the saffron, add the stock, tomato purée, and lemon juice,
and season to taste with salt and pepper.

4 Return the chicken thighs to the casserole, pushing them down into the
rice, cover, and cook in the oven for 15 minutes. Add the peas and return
to the oven for a further 10 minutes, or until the rice is tender and has
absorbed the cooking liquid. Serve hot, straight from the casserole.

STATISTICS PER SERVING:

Energy 476kcals/2,000kJ

Carbohydrate 50g

Sugar 10.5g

Fibre 4g

Fat 10g

Saturated fat 2g

Salt 1.2g

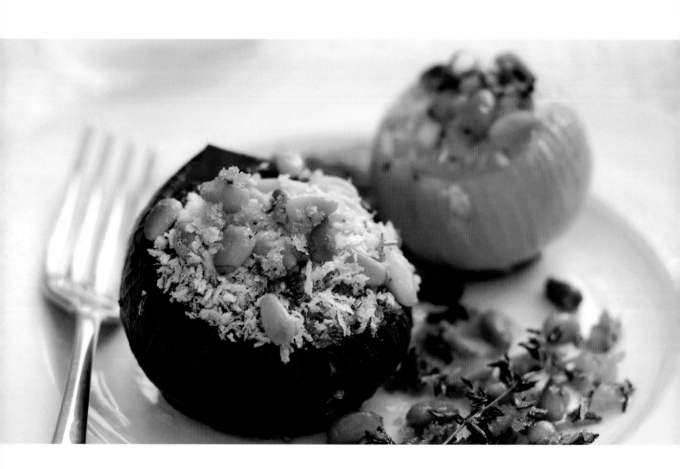

ON THE SIDE

● ○ ○ GI

● ○ ○ CALORIES

● ○ ○ SATURATED FAT

● ○ ○ SALT

CAJUN-SPICED SWEET POTATO WEDGES

SERVES 4   **PREP** 10 MINS   **COOK** 25-30 MINS

A quick, easy and healthier alternative to chips – sweet potatoes are rich in betacarotene, which the body can convert to vitamin A.

3 large sweet potatoes, unpeeled
salt
3 tbsp olive oil
3 tbsp Cajun seasoning mix

1 Preheat the oven to 220°C (425°F/Gas 7). Slice each sweet potato in half lengthways, then cut each half into 3 fat wedges. Cook the sweet potatoes in a pan of salted boiling water for 5 minutes. Drain well.

2 Mix the oil and seasoning together in a small bowl. Using a pastry brush, brush the mixture over the sweet potatoes.

3 Transfer the sweet potatoes to a non-stick roasting tin and bake for 20–25 minutes, or until crisp and nicely browned.

STATISTICS PER SERVING:

Energy 243kcals/1,020kJ

Carbohydrate 34g

Sugar 10g

Fibre 4g

Fat 11g
Saturated fat 3g

Salt 0.7g

COLESLAW WITH POPPY SEEDS

GUIDELINES PER SERVING:

● ○ ○ GI

● ○ ○ CALORIES

● ○ ○ SATURATED FAT

● ○ ○ SALT

SERVES 4   **PREP** 10 MINS

A mayonnaise-free coleslaw that cuts the calorie count of the traditional version but is every bit as delicious.

4 carrots, roughly grated
1 white cabbage, finely shredded
1 red onion, finely sliced
1 orange, segmented and roughly
  chopped
2 apples, halved, cored, and diced
salt and freshly ground black pepper

For the dressing
2–3 tbsp Greek yogurt
1 tbsp poppy seeds
1 tbsp finely chopped flat-leaf parsley

1 Put the carrots, cabbage, onion, orange, and apple in a bowl and stir to combine. Season well with salt and black pepper.

2 Mix the Greek yogurt with the poppy seeds and parsley, then stir into the cabbage mixture.

COOK'S TIP
For ease, you could shred the cabbage and carrots in a food processor fitted with a grater attachment.

STATISTICS PER SERVING:

Energy 117kcals/489kJ

Carbohydrate 23g

Sugar 21g

Fibre 6g

Fat 2g
Saturated fat 1g

Salt 0.2g

BAKED CHICORY WITH GOLDEN BREADCRUMBS

SERVES 4   **PREP** 10 MINS   **COOK** 30 MINS

Baking the leaves allows you to enjoy the wonderful flavour of chicory without the bitterness that you will sometimes find when it is served raw.

6 heads of chicory
25g (scant 1oz) butter
salt and freshly ground black pepper
3 sage leaves, finely chopped

3 slices of wholemeal bread
25g (scant 1oz) Parmesan, finely
  grated

1 Preheat the oven to 180°C (350°F/Gas 4). Halve the chicory lengthways then lay the pieces out in an ovenproof baking dish. Dot all over with the butter and season well with salt and pepper, then sprinkle with the sage.

2 Loosely cover with foil and place in the oven to bake for 20–25 minutes or unit the chicory is soft when poked with a sharp knife.

3 Meanwhile, place the bread in a food processor and whiz to crumbs, then tip out on to a baking tray. Place in the oven for about 5 minutes until golden, then tip the breadcrumbs back into the food processor, add the Parmesan, and whiz until fine and well mixed. Remove the chicory from the oven, cover evenly with the breadcrumbs, then return to the oven for a further 5–10 minutes until golden. Serve as a side dish.

STATISTICS PER SERVING:

Energy 140kcals/587kJ

Carbohydrate 13.5g

Sugar 1g

Fibre 2g

Fat 5g
Saturated fat 4.5g

Salt 0.6g

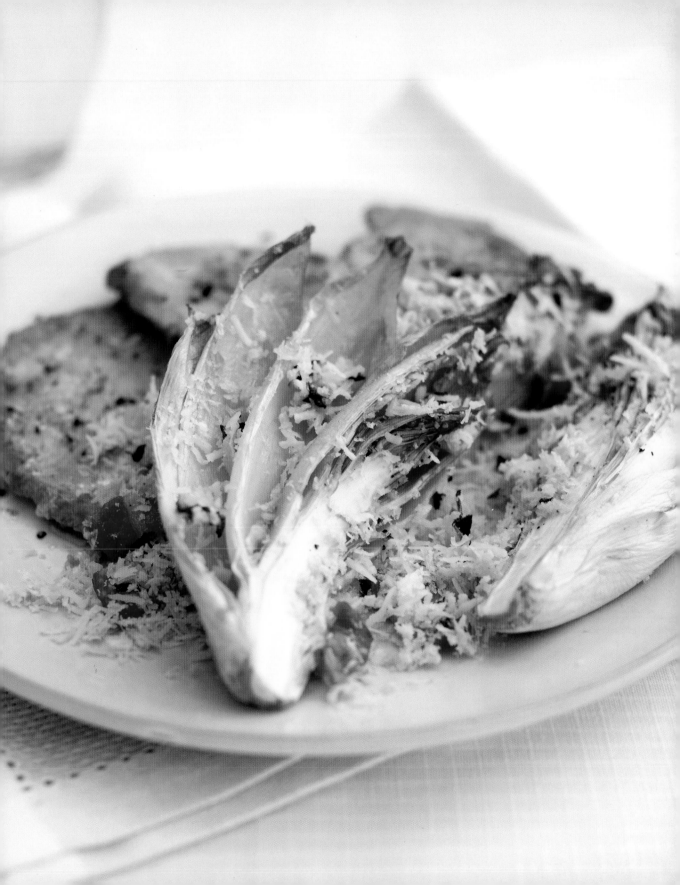

ROAST ARTICHOKES WITH TOMATO AND GARLIC

SERVES 4   **PREP** 5 MINS   **COOK** 1 HOUR

This is a simple accompaniment, but very colourful and tasty, especially if you use ripe, in-season tomatoes.

400g can artichoke hearts,
  drained and halved
8 small plum tomatoes on the vine
12 garlic cloves, unpeeled
2 tbsp olive oil

2 tsp balsamic vinegar
few sprigs of thyme
salt and freshly ground
  black pepper

1 Preheat the oven to 140°C (275°F/Gas 1).

2 Place the artichoke hearts in a roasting tray with the tomatoes, keeping them on the vine, and scatter the garlic cloves in the tray. Drizzle with the oil and balsamic vinegar, add the thyme, and season to taste with salt and pepper.

3 Roast for 1 hour, or until the vegetables are cooked, and serve.

STATISTICS PER SERVING:

Energy 78kcals/324kJ

Carbohydrate 5g

Sugar 2g

Fibre 2g

Fat 5.5g

Saturated fat 0.8g

Salt trace

ROAST SQUASH WITH GINGER

SERVES 4   **PREP** 20 MINS   **COOK** 40 MINS

Spicy vegetables make a punchy side dish.

GUIDELINES PER SERVING:

●●○ GI

●○○ CALORIES

●○○ SATURATED FAT

●○○ SALT

1 butternut squash, peeled
4 tbsp olive oil
½ tsp salt
2 red chillies, deseeded and
  finely chopped

60g (2oz) fresh root ginger, peeled
  and grated or finely sliced
freshly ground black pepper
handful of mint leaves, torn
2 limes, cut into wedges, to serve

1 Preheat the oven to 180°C (350°F/Gas 4). Slice the squash into long thick strips and place in a roasting tin. Mix together 2 tbsp warm water, the olive oil, salt, chillies, ginger, and pepper to taste. Drizzle the sauce over the squash, mixing to coat well.

2 Bake the squash for 40 minutes, or until tender, shaking occasionally during cooking to avoid sticking. If the squash dries out, add a little more olive oil.

3 Transfer the warm squash to a large serving dish, and scatter with the torn mint leaves. Serve with lime wedges to squeeze over.

STATISTICS PER SERVING:

Energy 166kcals/697kJ

Carbohydrate 16g

Sugar 8g

Fibre 3g

Fat 11g
Saturated fat 1.5g

Salt 0.5g

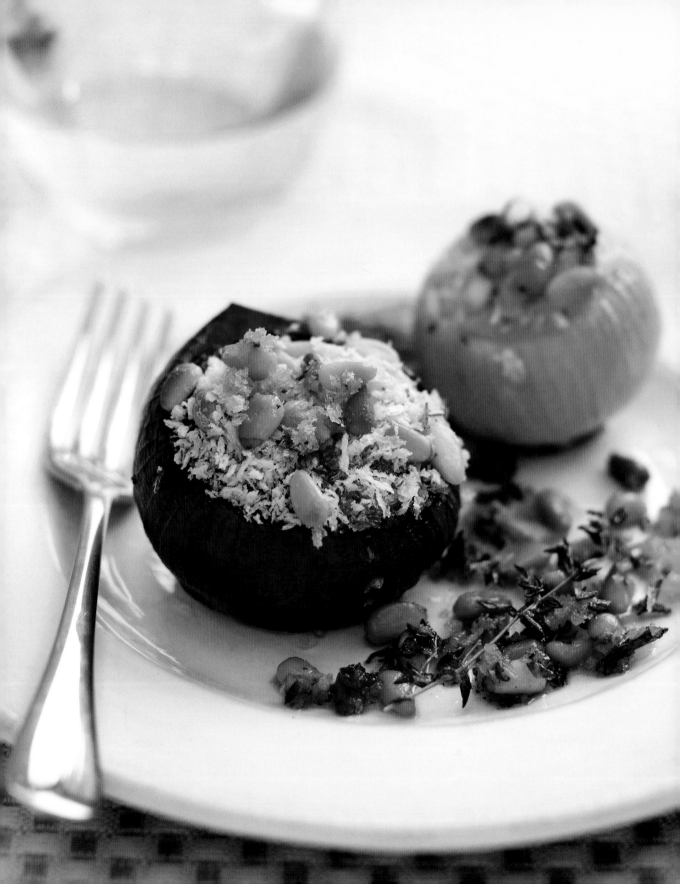

ROASTED ONIONS TOPPED WITH PINE NUTS

GUIDELINES PER SERVING:

● ○ ○ GI

● ● ○ CALORIES

● ○ ○ SATURATED FAT

● ○ ○ SALT

SERVES 4   **PREP** 5 MINS   **COOK** 50 MINS

Onions become meltingly soft when baked.

4 red onions, peeled
4 white or brown onions, peeled
1–2 tbsp olive oil
salt and freshly ground black pepper

few stalks thyme
2 slices bread
few sage leaves
75g (2½oz) pine nuts

1 Preheat the oven to 190°C (375°F/Gas 5). Top and tail the onions and sit them in a roasting tin. Drizzle over the oil and use your hands to coat, then sprinkle with salt and pepper, scatter the thyme over, cover with foil, and put in the oven.

2 Add the bread to a food processor and whiz to breadcrumbs, then add the sage leaves, whiz again, and set aside. When the onions have been in the oven for 40–45 minutes and are starting to soften, remove the foil, sprinkle over the breadcrumbs and pine nuts, and return to the oven for 10 minutes or until the pine nuts are golden. Transfer to plates and serve.

COOK'S TIP
You could toast the pine nuts separately then sprinkle them over at end of cooking to make sure they don't burn.

STATISTICS PER SERVING:

Energy 291kcals/1,210kJ

Carbohydrate 30g

Sugar 14.5g

Fibre 4g

Fat 16.5g
Saturated fat 1g

Salt 0.3g

● ◯ ◯ GI

● ◯ ◯ CALORIES

● ◯ ◯ SATURATED FAT

● ◯ ◯ SALT

RATATOUILLE WITH STAR ANISE

SERVES 6   **PREP** 15-20 MINS   **COOK** 45 MINS

Star anise gives this traditional French dish a delicious oriental twist.

4 tbsp olive oil
2 onions, sliced
4 red peppers, cut into 2cm (¾in) cubes
2 aubergines, cut into 2cm (¾in) cubes
3 courgettes, cut into 2cm (¾in) cubes

450g (1lb) fresh tomatoes, skinned, deseeded, and roughly chopped
2 garlic cloves, crushed
2 tbsp tomato purée
1 star anise
salt and freshly ground black pepper

1 Heat the oil in a large saucepan, add the onions and cook over a medium heat for 5 minutes or until soft.

2 Add the peppers, aubergines, courgettes, tomatoes, garlic, and tomato purée. Fry for 2–3 minutes.

3 Add the star anise, and salt and black pepper to taste, then cover and simmer for 30 minutes or until the vegetables are tender. Remove the lid and cook for 15 minutes more or until the liquid has evaporated. Adjust the seasoning, remove the star anise and serve hot or cold.

STATISTICS PER SERVING:

Energy 223kcals/930kJ

Carbohydrate 23g

Sugar 20g

Fibre 7g

Fat 13g
Saturated fat 2g

Salt 0.2g

HOME-MADE BAKED BEANS

GUIDELINES PER SERVING:

● ○ ○ GI

● ○ ○ CALORIES

● ○ ○ SATURATED FAT

● ○ ○ SALT

SERVES 4   **PREP** 12 MINS   **COOK** 45 MINS

This home-made version is vastly superior to canned baked beans. Grated apple adds a little sweetness.

1 tbsp olive oil
1 onion, finely diced
2 rashers back bacon, chopped
2 garlic cloves, finely chopped
1 apple, grated
½ tbsp Worcestershire sauce

2 tsp Dijon mustard
250ml (8fl oz) passata
2 x 400g cans haricot beans,
   drained and rinsed
salt and freshly ground black pepper

1 Heat the oil in a shallow, heavy pan, add the onion and cook over a low heat until soft. Add the bacon, increase the heat a little and cook until it begins to colour.

2 Stir in the garlic, apple, Worcestershire sauce, and mustard. Pour in the passata and bring to the boil. Reduce to a simmer, add the beans and partially cover the pan. Cook on a gentle heat for 15–20 minutes, topping up with a little hot water as needed. Season to taste.

COOK'S TIP
You could also use dried haricot beans - these need to be soaked overnight and cooked for about 2 hours before they are added to the dish.

STATISTICS PER SERVING:

Energy 243kcals/1,029kJ

Carbohydrate 36g

Sugar 5.5g

Fibre 11g

Fat 6g

Saturated fat 1.5g

Salt 0.6g

● ○ ○ GI

● ○ ○ CALORIES

● ○ ○ SATURATED FAT

● ○ ○ SALT

CHICKPEAS WITH SPINACH

SERVES 4   **PREP** 15 MINS   **COOK** 10 MINS

Chickpeas are widely used in Spain as a basis for a variety of stews such as this one.

3 tbsp olive oil
1 thick slice of crusty wholemeal
  bread, torn into breadcrumbs
750g (1lb 10oz) spinach leaves
240g can chickpeas, rinsed
  and drained

2 garlic cloves, finely chopped
salt and freshly ground
  black pepper
1 tsp paprika
1 tsp ground cumin
1 tbsp sherry vinegar

1 Heat 1 tablespoon of the oil in a frying pan and fry the bread, stirring, until crisp. Remove from the pan, drain on kitchen paper, and reserve.

2 Rinse the spinach and shake off any excess water. Place it in a large saucepan and cook over a low heat, tossing constantly so it does not stick to the pan. When it has wilted, transfer the spinach to a colander and squeeze out as much water as possible by pressing it with a wooden spoon, then place on a chopping board and chop coarsely.

3 Heat the remaining oil in the frying pan, add the spinach and allow it to warm through before stirring in the chickpeas and garlic. Season to taste with salt and pepper. Add the paprika and cumin, then crumble the reserved fried bread into the mixture.

4 Add the vinegar and 2 tablespoons of water and allow to heat through for several minutes. Divide between 4 small serving dishes or ramekins and serve immediately.

STATISTICS PER SERVING:

Energy 202kcals/839kJ

Carbohydrate 15g

Sugar 3g

Fibre 4.5g

Fat 10g
Saturated fat 1.4g

Salt 0.8g

ROSEMARY-SIMMERED WHITE BEANS

GUIDELINES PER SERVING:

●○○ GI

●●○ CALORIES

●○○ SATURATED FAT

●●○ SALT

SERVES 4   **PREP** 5 MINS   **COOK** 2 HOURS
PLUS SOAKING

Fragrant and delicate-tasting beans cooked with woody rosemary and orange zest.

350g (12oz) dried cannellini beans,
  soaked in water overnight
2 garlic cloves, finely chopped
3 rosemary stalks
3 tbsp olive oil

2 tbsp white wine vinegar
pared peel of 1 orange
1.4 litres (2½ pints) vegetable stock
  or chicken stock
salt and freshly ground black pepper

1 Drain the soaked beans, then rinse, drain again, and place in a large heavy-based pan. Add the garlic, rosemary, olive oil, vinegar, orange peel, and stock and season with salt and pepper.

2 Bring to the boil then reduce the heat to a low simmer, cover with a lid and cook gently for 2 hours or until the beans are soft. Top up with more stock if needed. Taste and adjust the seasoning, if required. Remove the rosemary and orange peel. This makes a good side for roast lamb dishes.

COOK'S TIP
Using canned cannellini beans will reduce the cooking time by more than a third but they won't be as tasty, so it is well worth the effort to rehydrate and cook dried beans.

STATISTICS PER SERVING:

Energy 377kcals/1,589kJ

Carbohydrate 41g

Sugar 3g

Fibre 14g

Fat 12g

Saturated fat 2g

Salt 1.8g

SPICY PUY LENTILS

SERVES 4   **PREP** 10 MINS   **COOK** 40-45 MINS

One of the benefits of lentils is that, unlike most pulses, they do not require soaking beforehand.

2 tbsp olive oil
1 large onion, finely chopped
4 celery sticks, chopped
1 red pepper, deseeded and diced
1 clove garlic, finely chopped
1 red chilli, deseeded and finely chopped

225g (8oz) Puy lentils, rinsed and any grit removed
600ml (1 pint) chicken or vegetable stock
salt and freshly ground black pepper
3 tbsp chopped fresh coriander

1 Heat the oil in a large, non-stick saucepan. Put in the onion and cook, stirring, for 2–3 minutes. Add the celery, red pepper, garlic, and chilli. Cook for a further 3–4 minutes.

2 Add the lentils and stock, bring to the boil, reduce the heat and simmer for 40 minutes, or until the lentils are tender, adding a little extra stock or water if necessary. Season to taste with salt and pepper, stir in the chopped coriander and serve.

STATISTICS PER SERVING:

Energy 276kcals/1,164kJ

Carbohydrate 35g

Sugar 6g

Fibre 7g

Fat 8g
Saturated fat 1.5g

Salt 0.7g

SPLIT PEA DHAL

SERVES 4   **PREP** 10 MINS   **COOK** 45 MINS

A delicious comfort food to eat simply – enjoy it with wholemeal chapattis.

GUIDELINES PER SERVING:

⬤◯◯ GI

⬤◯◯ CALORIES

⬤◯◯ SATURATED FAT

⬤◯◯ SALT

2 tbsp vegetable oil
2 large onions, finely chopped
salt and freshly ground black pepper
3 garlic cloves, finely chopped
2.5cm (1in) piece of fresh root ginger, finely chopped

1 tsp turmeric
400g (14oz) yellow split peas, rinsed and drained
2 tbsp garam masala
4 lemon wedges, to serve

1 Heat the oil in a heavy pan, add the onions and cook for 5–6 minutes until just beginning to turn golden. Season with salt and black pepper. Add the garlic and ginger and cook for a further 2 minutes.

2 Stir in the turmeric, then the split peas. making sure they are all coated. Pour in 250ml (9fl oz) hot water and bring to the boil. Reduce to a simmer, partially cover the pan and cook over a low heat for about 20 minutes, adding more water if and when needed.

3 Stir in the garam masala, season, and partially cover the pan. Cook over a low heat for a further 25 minutes, topping up with hot water if needed. Serve with the lemon wedges.

COOK'S TIP
Make this up to a day ahead and refrigerate. Reheat to serve; the taste only gets better.

STATISTICS PER SERVING:

Energy 224kcals/948kJ

Carbohydrate 35g

Sugar 3g

Fibre 4g

Fat 4.5g
Saturated fat 0.6g

Salt 0.3g

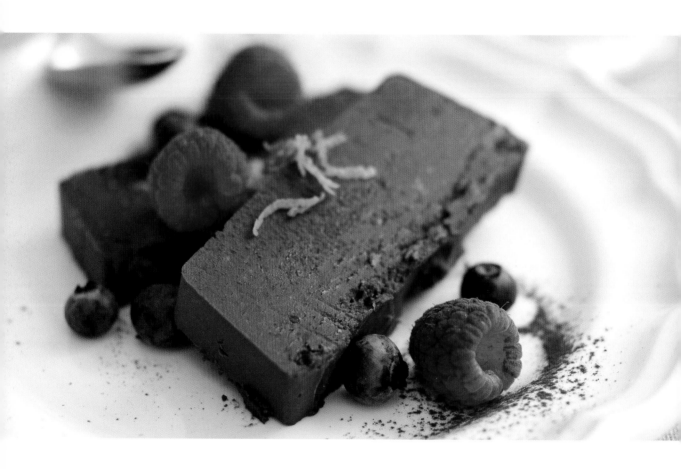

DESSERTS

⬤⬤◯ GI

⬤◯◯ CALORIES

⬤◯◯ SATURATED FAT

⬤◯◯ SALT

SUMMER PUDDING

SERVES 6   **PREP** 15 MINS   **COOK** 3-4 MINS
PLUS FIRMING

When fresh berries aren't in season, you can make this
classic dessert using frozen berries.

900g (2lb) mixed soft fruits,
   e.g. raspberries, strawberries,
   blackberries, pitted cherries,
   or blueberries
50g (1¾oz) fructose (fruit sugar)

8-10 thick slices of day-old
   white bread
15g (½oz) redcurrants, to decorate
15g (½oz) fresh mint,
   to decorate

1 Place the fruit in a saucepan with the fructose and 3 tablespoons of water.
Heat gently and cook for 3–4 minutes or until the juices begin to run from
the fruit. Set aside to cool.

2 Remove the crusts from the bread. Cut a circle from one slice of bread
to fit the bottom of a 1.5 litre (2¾ pint) pudding basin. Arrange the
remaining bread, apart from two slices, around the sides of the basin,
overlapping slightly and leaving no gaps. Place the circle of bread over the
gap at the bottom of the basin.

3 Spoon the fruit mixture, together with enough juice to moisten the bread,
into the basin. Reserve the remaining juice. Seal in the fruit with a final
layer of the remaining bread, trimming to fit as necessary.

4 Cover the pudding with a saucer or small plate and place a heavy
weight on top. Place the pudding in the refrigerator for several hours,
preferably overnight.

5 To serve, remove the weight and the saucer, and invert the pudding onto
a large serving plate. Hold the two together and shake firmly, then carefully
remove the pudding basin. Spoon the reserved juice over the pudding and
decorate with the redcurrants and mint.

STATISTICS PER SERVING:

Energy   149kcals/631kJ

Carbohydrate   30g

Sugar   9g

Fibre   4g

Fat   1g

Saturated fat   0.2g

Salt   0.6g

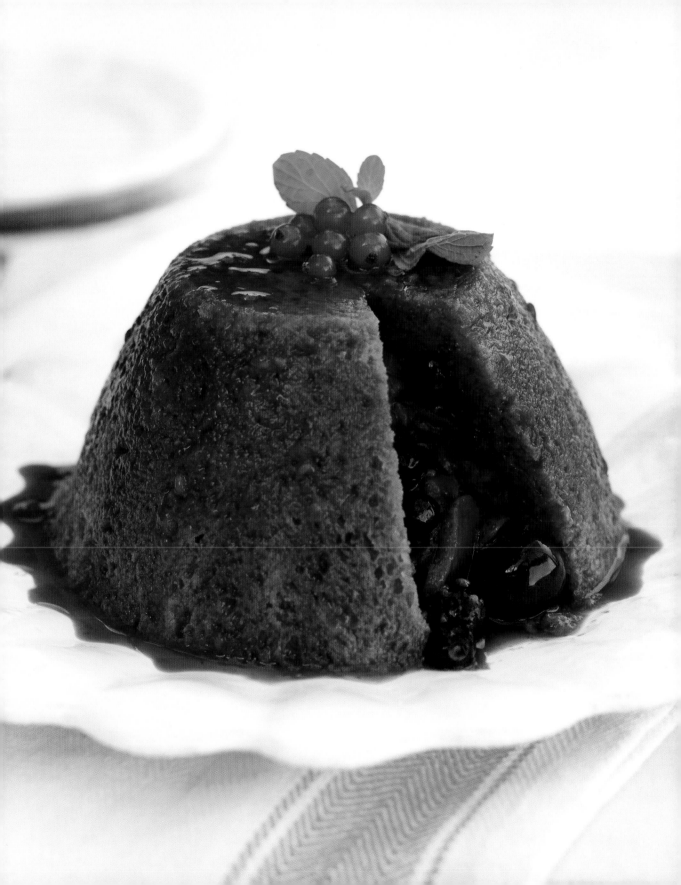

⬤◯◯ GI

⬤◯◯ CALORIES

⬤◯◯ SATURATED FAT

⬤◯◯ SALT

CARPACCIO OF ORANGES WITH PISTACHIO NUTS

SERVES 4 **PREP** 10 MINS
PLUS CHILLING

A deliciously refreshing, Moroccan-inspired dessert that is low in calories but full of flavour.

4 oranges
2 pomegranates
generous pinch ground cinnamon
30g (1oz) shelled pistachio nuts,
  roughly chopped

1 Using a sharp knife, remove the skin and pith from the oranges and slice the flesh into rounds. Sprinkle with the cinnamon and chill for 15 minutes.

2 Remove the seeds from the pomegranates, and discard the white membrane.

3 Place the orange slices on a serving dish, and sprinkle with the pomegranate seeds and pistachio nuts.

STATISTICS PER SERVING:

Energy 125kcals/525kJ

Carbohydrate 18g

Sugar 18g

Fibre 4g

Fat 4g
Saturated fat 0.5g

Salt 0.1g

POACHED PEARS WITH TOASTED ALMONDS

SERVES 4   **PREP** 10 MINS   **COOK** 20 MINS

A classic, elegant dessert that can be made with such ease: treat yourself.

GUIDELINES PER SERVING:

● ○ ○ GI

● ○ ○ CALORIES

● ○ ○ SATURATED FAT

● ○ ○ SALT

juice of 4 oranges
zest of 1 orange
1 cinnamon stick
2 star anise
4 just-ripe pears, halved lengthways
  and cored

50g (1¾oz) blanched almonds
250g (9oz) reduced-fat Greek-style
  yogurt, to serve

1 Put the orange juice and zest in a pan along with 200ml (7fl oz) water, the cinnamon stick, and star anise. Bring to the boil.

2 Reduce to a simmer and add the pears. Cover with a lid and cook for 10–15 minutes, or until the pears are soft and tender. Remove with a slotted spoon and put on a serving plate or plates. Bring the juice to the boil and spoon a little over the pears.

3 Meanwhile, put the almonds in a small frying pan and toast them for a few minutes until golden, stirring occasionally so that they don't burn. Serve the pears topped with the almonds and a spoonful of Greek yogurt.

STATISTICS PER SERVING:

Energy 182kcals/765kJ

Carbohydrate 24g

Sugar 22.5g

Fibre 4.3g

Fat 8g

Saturated fat 1g

Salt trace

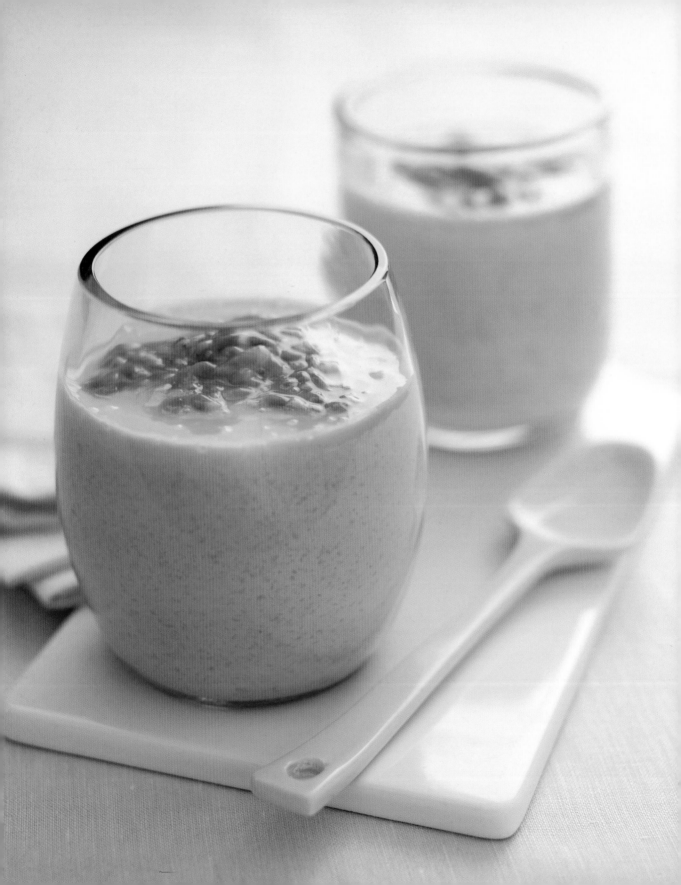

MANGO, ORANGE, AND PASSION FRUIT FOOL

GUIDELINES PER SERVING:

● ● ○ GI
● ● ○ CALORIES
● ● ● SATURATED FAT
● ○ ○ SALT

SERVES 4   **PREP** 10 MINS
PLUS CHILLING

This creamy, golden fruit fool is rich in vitamin C and fibre, and can be whizzed up in minutes.

3 large, ripe mangoes, stoned and
  flesh roughly chopped
zest of 1 large orange
4 tbsp orange juice

400g (14oz) Greek yogurt
sugar-free sweetener, to taste
4 passion fruit, seeds extracted

1 Place the mango, and orange zest and juice in a food processor or blender. Process until smooth. Stir in the Greek yogurt and add sweetener to taste.

2 Divide the mixture among 4 glasses or bowls, and chill for at least 30 minutes.

3 Spoon the seeds from the passion fruit on top of the fool and serve.

STATISTICS PER SERVING:

Energy 229kcals/962kJ

Carbohydrate 28g

Sugar 26g

Fibre 4.5g

Fat 10g
Saturated fat 7g

Salt 0.2g

● ● ○ GI

● ○ ○ CALORIES

● ○ ○ SATURATED FAT

● ○ ○ SALT

SUGAR-FREE PEACH SORBET

SERVES 4   **PREP** 15 MINS
PLUS FREEZING

A refreshing, melt-in-the-mouth dessert. Make the most of juicy peaches when they're in season with this guilt-free summer indulgence.

1.25kg (2¾lb) ripe peaches,
  stoned and chopped
60g (2oz) sucralose sweetener
  (Splenda)
juice of 1 lemon

1 Put the peaches in a food processor or blender and whiz until smooth. Pass through a sieve to make a smooth purée.

2 Tip the purée into a clean food processor or blender along with 180ml (6fl oz) water, the sweetener, and the lemon juice. Whiz again until smooth.

3 Pour the mixture into a freezerproof container with a lid, and put it in the freezer for 1–2 hours until it has almost set. Remove and stir well with a fork to break up the ice crystals, or put back in the food processor and whiz again. Return to the freezer for 4–5 hours until frozen. Serve scoops of sorbet in individual glass dishes.

COOK'S TIP
Choose a shallow container if you can, as the sorbet will freeze more quickly.

STATISTICS PER SERVING:

Energy 83kcals/355kJ

Carbohydrate 19g

Sugar 18g

Fibre 4g

Fat 0g

Saturated fat 0g

Salt trace

CHOCOLATE ESPRESSO POTS

SERVES 4   **PREP** 15 MINS
PLUS CHILLING

These little chocolate pots taste deliciously wicked, but in fact a little chocolate goes a long way and the silky texture comes without any cream being added.

400g can prunes in fruit juice
150g (5½oz) plain chocolate, broken
  into small pieces

2 eggs, separated
25g (scant 1oz) pistachio nuts, finely
  chopped, to serve

1 Strain the prunes, reserving the juice, then press each prune gently between your fingers to eject the stone. Tip the prunes into a food processor or blender with 100ml (3½fl oz) of the juice, and process to a purée.

2 Melt the chocolate in a small heatproof bowl set over a pan of simmering water. Stir in the prune mixture and egg yolks.

3 In a large, clean bowl, whisk the egg whites until they form stiff peaks. Fold the egg whites into the chocolate mixture using a large metal spoon.

4 Spoon the chocolate mixture into 4 espresso cups or individual serving dishes and transfer to the refrigerator to chill for at least 1 hour.

5 Remove from the refrigerator just before serving and scatter with a few chopped pistachio nuts.

GUIDELINES PER SERVING:

● ○ ○   GI
● ● ○   CALORIES
● ● ○   SATURATED FAT
● ○ ○   SALT

STATISTICS PER SERVING:

Energy   315kcals/1,324kJ

Carbohydrate   38g

Sugar   36g

Fibre   2.5g

Fat   16g
Saturated fat   7g

Salt   0.14g

● ● ○ GI

● ● ○ CALORIES

● ● ● SATURATED FAT

● ○ ○ SALT

DARK CHOCOLATE AND YOGURT ICE CREAM

SERVES 6　**PREP** 25 MINS　**COOK** 2 MINS

Rich in taste but lower in calories than ordinary ice cream.

300ml (10fl oz) milk
200g (7oz) dark chocolate (at least 70% cocoa solids), broken into small pieces

calorie-free sweetener
4 egg yolks
250ml (8fl oz) low-fat natural yogurt

1 Put the milk, chocolate, and calorie-free sweetener to taste in a small pan and heat gently, stirring occasionally, until the chocolate has melted. Bring the mixture just to the boil, then remove from the heat.

2 Whisk the egg yolks together, then slowly pour into the chocolate mixture and whisk until the mixture is smooth.

3 Leave to cool for 15 minutes, then whisk in the yoghurt and spoon into a freezer-proof container. Cover with a lid and leave to cool completely, then transfer to the freezer to freeze overnight.

COOK'S TIP
You could use an ice cream maker; the result will be smoother and creamier.

STATISTICS PER SERVING:

Energy 266kcals/1,116kJ

Carbohydrate 30g

Sugar 27g

Fibre 1g

Fat 14g
Saturated fat 7.5g

Salt 0.1g

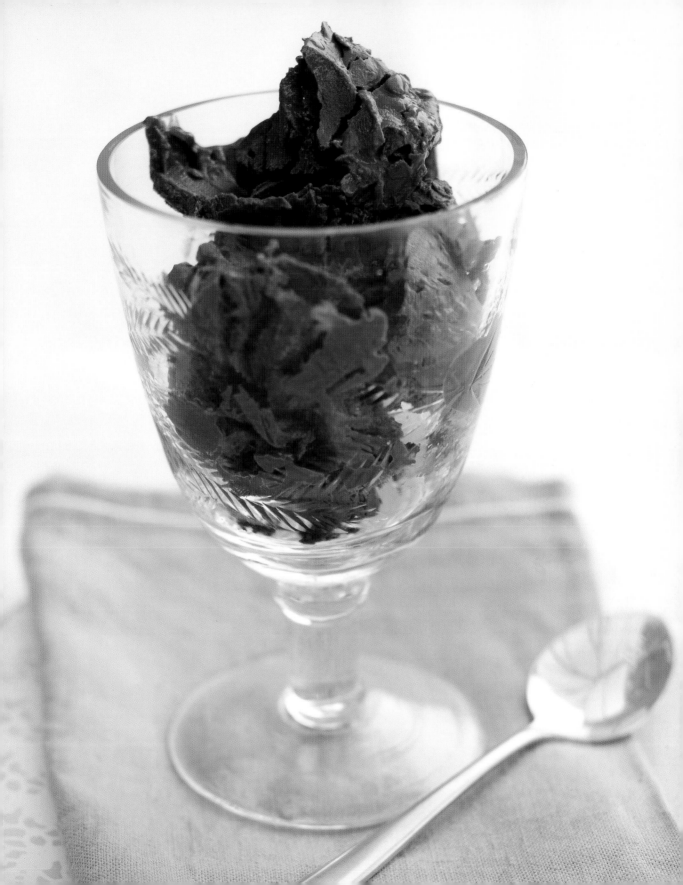

⬤◯◯ GI

⬤◯◯ CALORIES

⬤◯◯ SATURATED FAT

⬤◯◯ SALT

CRANBERRY AND POMEGRANATE JELLY

SERVES 4 **PREP** 10 MINS
PLUS SETTING

These tasty little jellies are perfect for occasions when you fancy something sweet, but healthy.

750ml (1¼ pints) light cranberry juice
1 tbsp powdered gelatine or
  vegetarian equivalent
2 pomegranates, seeds extracted and
  white membranes removed

1 Place 120ml (4fl oz) of the cranberry juice in a small heatproof bowl, sprinkle in the gelatine and leave to soak for 5 minutes. Place the bowl over a pan of simmering water and stir until the gelatine melts and becomes clear. Stir in the remaining juice.

2 Divide the pomegranate seeds between 4 wine glasses, pour in enough of the liquid to just cover the fruit, and then chill for about 30 minutes or until just set.

3 Pour in the remaining liquid and chill for 3 hours, or until set.

COOK'S TIP
If the remaining cranberry juice mixture sets before you add it in the final step, place it over a pan of gently simmering water until it becomes liquid again.

STATISTICS PER SERVING:

Energy 53kcals/221kJ

Carbohydrate 11g

Sugar 11g

Fibre 1g

Fat 0g

Saturated fat 0g

Salt trace

APRICOT CRUMBLE

SERVES 4   **PREP** 10 MINS   **COOK** 20 MINS

By cooking apricots with a little orange, it helps to bring out their flavour and make this a truly moreish crumble.

GUIDELINES PER SERVING:

● ● ○ GI

● ● ● CALORIES

● ● ○ SATURATED FAT

● ○ ○ SALT

700g (1lb 9oz) apricots, stoned
  and cut into quarters
juice and zest of 1 large orange
2-3 tbsp sucralose sweetener
  (Splenda)

60g (2oz) plain white flour
60g (2oz) plain wholemeal flour
60g (2oz) jumbo oats
85g (3oz) polyunsaturated margarine
60g (2oz) fructose

1 Preheat the oven to 180°C (350°F/Gas 4). Place the apricots and the orange juice and zest in a saucepan and cook over a gentle heat until the apricots are soft. Stir in the sweetener and taste to check the sweetness.

2 To make the crumble, mix together both types of flour and the oats. Rub in the margarine until the mixture resembles coarse breadcrumbs. Stir in the fructose.

3 Spoon the apricots into a shallow heatproof dish, sprinkle the crumble topping over them evenly, and bake for 20 minutes or until the topping is golden brown.

STATISTICS PER SERVING:

Energy 399kcals/1,672kJ

Carbohydrate 42g

Sugar 20g

Fibre 6g

Fat 19g
Saturated fat 4g

Salt 0.3g

● ● ○ GI

● ● ○ CALORIES

● ○ ○ SATURATED FAT

● ○ ○ SALT

APPLE AND WALNUT STRUDEL

SERVES 6　　**PREP** 20 MINS　　**COOK** 30 MINS

This strudel is made with filo pastry, and is a good choice if you are looking for a heathier alternative to apple pie.

500g (1lb 2oz) Bramley cooking
　apples, peeled, cored, and thickly
　sliced
zest and juice of 1 lemon
8 large sheets of filo pastry
　(about 200g/7oz)

30g (1oz) polyunsaturated
　margarine, melted
30g (1oz) fresh breadcrumbs
3 tbsp fructose (fruit sugar)
60g (2oz) walnuts, roughly chopped
½ tsp ground cinnamon

1 Preheat the oven to 180°C (350°F/Gas 4). Sprinkle the apples with a little lemon juice to prevent them browning.

2 Lay 4 sheets of filo side by side on a clean tea towel, overlapping the long edges by about 5cm (2in). Brush with a little of the melted margarine. Place the 4 remaining sheets of filo on top and brush again. Cover the filo with a clean, damp tea towel to help prevent it from drying out before you are ready to add the filling.

3 Mix together the apples, breadcrumbs, lemon zest, 2 tablespoons fructose, the walnuts, and cinnamon. Spoon the mixture along one long edge of the pastry. Using the tea towel underneath the pastry to help you, roll up the pastry as you would roll up a Swiss roll.

4 Put the strudel on a non-stick baking sheet, seam-side down, curling it slightly if necessary to fit onto the sheet. Brush with the remaining margarine and sprinkle with the remaining fructose.

5 Place in the oven and bake for 15–20 minutes, or until the pastry is golden brown and the apples are soft. Cover with foil halfway through cooking if necessary.

STATISTICS PER SERVING:

Energy 308kcals/1,288kJ

Carbohydrate 33g

Sugar 17g

Fibre 3.5g

Fat 17g

Saturated fat 2.5g

Salt 0.5g

BANANA, CINNAMON, AND PISTACHIO PARCELS

SERVES 4   **PREP** 15 MINS   **COOK** 15 MINS
PLUS COOLING

A quick and easy dessert guaranteed to satisfy even the sweetest tooth.

4 small, ripe bananas, peeled
  and thickly sliced
30g (1oz) pistachio nuts, chopped,
  plus extra to serve
2 tbsp sucralose sweetener (Splenda)
¼ tsp ground cinnamon

zest of 1 lemon
45g (1½oz) polyunsaturated
  margarine
4 sheets of filo pastry, 40 x 28cm
  (16 x 11in)

1 Place the bananas and pistachio nuts in a bowl and sprinkle with the sweetener and cinnamon. Melt half the margarine in a small pan, add the banana mixture and cook over a low heat for 10 minutes. Remove from the heat, stir in the lemon zest and allow to cool. Chill in the refrigerator.

2 Preheat the oven to 200°C (400°F/Gas 6). Melt the remaining margarine. Lay one sheet of filo pastry on the worksurface, brush lightly with melted margarine, and then fold 3 times, lengthways, to make a long sausage.

3 Spoon a quarter of the banana mixture onto the pastry about 4cm (1½in) from the end. Fold the left corner of the pastry diagonally to the right side of the dough, to cover the filling. Then fold the right corner diagonally to the left, and continue folding alternate corners in the same way until you reach the end of the sheet, forming a little parcel. Repeat with the remaining sheets of filo pastry.

4 Place the parcels on a lightly greased baking sheet, brush with a little more melted butter, and bake for 15 minutes or until golden. Sprinkle with a few chopped pistachio nuts before serving.

STATISTICS PER SERVING:

Energy 252kcals/1,055kJ

Carbohydrate 29g

Sugar 21g

Fibre 1g

Fat 13.5g
Saturated fat 2.5g

Salt 0.3g

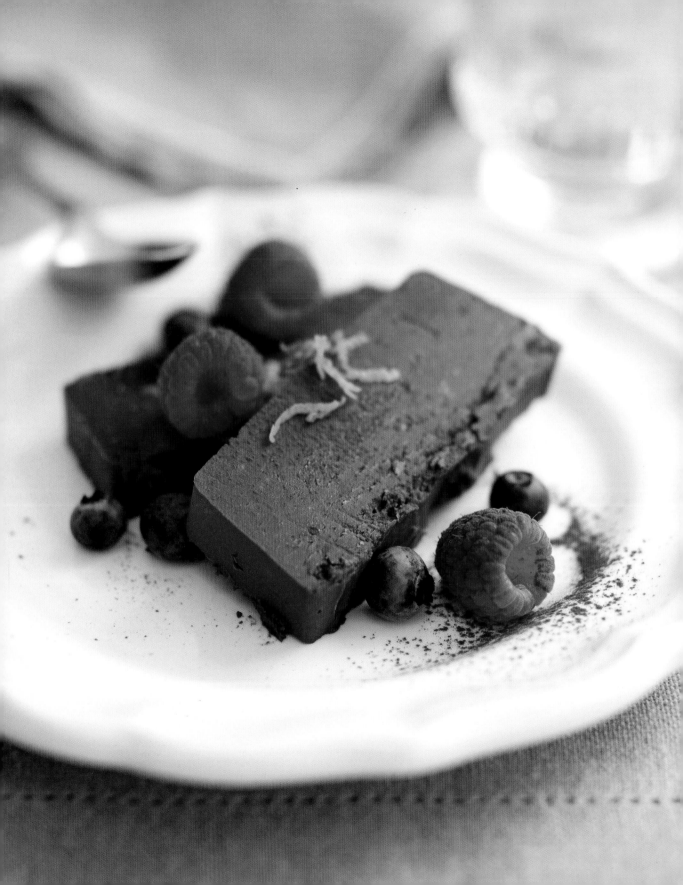

CHOCOLATE AND ORANGE PARFAIT

SERVES 4 **PREP** 15 MINS **COOK** 5 MINS **FREEZE** 1 MONTH

This rich, creamy, chocolatey dessert has a refreshing tang of orange. It looks sophisticated, yet is easy to make and will be a sure-fire winner when entertaining.

GUIDELINES PER SERVING:

● ● ○ GI
● ● ○ CALORIES
● ● ● SATURATED FAT
● ○ ○ SALT

200g (7oz) good-quality
  plain chocolate
2 gelatine leaves, or vegetarian
  equivalent
3 tbsp orange juice or water

3 large oranges
300g (10oz) fat-free fromage frais
150g (5½oz) blueberries, to serve
150g (5½oz) raspberries, to serve

1 Line a 450g (1lb) loaf tin with cling film. Melt the chocolate in bowl set over a pan of boiling water, making sure that the base of the bowl does not touch the water. Allow the melted chocolate to cool slightly.

2 Meanwhile, soak the gelatine leaves in a bowl of cold water for 3–4 minutes, or until softened. Heat the orange juice or water in a small pan until hot, but not boiling. Squeeze excess water out of the gelatine leaves and put them in the pan, then stir to help the gelatine dissolve. Remove from the heat.

3 Remove the zest from the oranges and stir it into the chocolate along with the dissolved gelatine and the fromage frais. Mix well, then spoon into the prepared tin, place in the refrigerator and leave for 2 hours, or until set.

4 Carefully turn out the chocolate mixture onto a plate and remove the cling film. Using a hot knife, cut the parfait into slices and serve with the blueberries and raspberries. (Alternatively, you could use up the oranges and serve them with the parfait instead of the berries. Remove the pith from the oranges and slice the flesh.)

STATISTICS PER SERVING:

Energy 323kcals/1,350kJ

Carbohydrate 39g

Sugar 38g

Fibre 2.5g

Fat 14g
Saturated fat 8.5g

Salt trace

- ●●○ GI
- ●○○ CALORIES
- ●●○ SATURATED FAT
- ●○○ SALT

ROASTED FIGS WITH CITRUS CRÈME FRAÎCHE

SERVES 4   **PREP** 5 MINS   **COOK** 20 MINS

A simple dish with "wow factor" flavour. Figs are a good source of iron.

8 fresh figs, stalks snipped
juice of 2 oranges
2 tsp sucralose sweetener (Splenda)

pinch of ground cinnamon
150g (5½oz) low-fat crème fraîche
juice and zest of ½ lime

1 Preheat the oven to 200°C (400°F/Gas 6). Make a cross at the top of each fig and gently squeeze the fruit apart a little. Place the figs in an ovenproof dish.

2 Pour in the orange juice, and sprinkle with the sweetener and cinnamon. Put in the oven to cook for about 15 minutes until the figs have softened and are beginning to caramelize.

3 Mix the crème fraîche with the lime juice and zest, and spoon it over the figs in the dish. Serve immediately.

COOK'S TIP
For a special occasion, you could drizzle a tiny amount of cassis over the figs before roasting.

STATISTICS PER SERVING:

Energy 111kcals/467kJ

Carbohydrate 13g

Sugar 12g

Fibre 1g

Fat 6g

Saturated fat 4g

Salt trace

LEMON CHEESECAKE

SERVES 8   **PREP** 5 MINS   **COOK** 50 MINS

This low-fat version of a traditional baked cheesecake is just as full of creamy flavour.

GUIDELINES PER SERVING:

⬤◯◯ GI

⬤◯◯ CALORIES

⬤◯◯ SATURATED FAT

⬤◯◯ SALT

100g (3½oz) sucralose sweetener (Splenda)
juice of 2 lemons and zest of 3 lemons
4 eggs, separated
150g (5½oz) low-fat cream cheese

200g (7oz) quark cheese
50g (1¾oz) sultanas
2 tbsp plain flour
butter for greasing

1 Preheat the oven to 170°C (340°F/Gas 3½). In a large bowl, dissolve the sweetener in the lemon juice, then add the egg yolks and whisk until pale and thick. Add the cream cheese and quark and beat until smooth.

2 Empty the lemon juice and zest into the cream cheese mixture, then add the sultanas. Stir to mix. Sprinkle the flour over the mixture and fold it in gently. In a clean bowl, using a clean whisk, whisk the egg whites until stiff, then fold into the cheesecake mixture.

3 Spoon the mixture into a deep, round, 20cm (8in) springform cake tin, greased and lined with greaseproof paper. Bake in the oven for 45–50 minutes or until golden and almost set; it should still wobble slightly in the centre. Leave to cool in the oven with the door open (this should prevent it from cracking too much).

4 Once cooled, run a knife around the edge of tin, release the sides and carefully remove the cheesecake.

STATISTICS PER SERVING:

Energy 121kcals/509kJ

Carbohydrate 9g

Sugar 6g

Fibre 0.3g

Fat 5.5g

Saturated fat 2g

Salt 0.1g

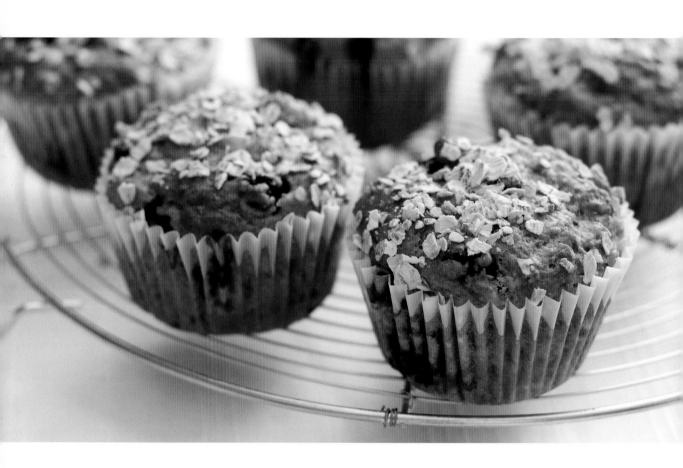

BAKING

● ● ○ GI

● ● ○ CALORIES

● ○ ○ SATURATED FAT

● ○ ○ SALT

BANANA AND THREE-SEED OAT BAKES

MAKES 9   **PREP** 10 MINS   **COOK** 20-30 MINS   **FREEZE** 3 MONTHS

These tasty little bars contain considerably less sugar than most commercial cereal bars, so they'll provide an energy boost without sending your blood sugar levels sky-high.

100g (3½oz) polyunsaturated margarine, plus extra for greasing
3 tbsp maple syrup
150g (5½oz) porridge oats
2 bananas (about 250g/9oz total weight before peeling), roughly diced

100g (3½oz) ready-to-eat dried apricots, roughly chopped
25g (scant 1oz) pumpkin seeds, toasted
25g (scant 1oz) sunflower seeds, toasted
25g (scant 1oz) sesame seeds, toasted

1 Preheat the oven to 180°C (350°F/Gas 4). Lightly grease a 19 x 19cm (7½ x 7½in) baking tin and line the bottom with non-stick baking parchment.

2 Melt the margarine and maple syrup in a heavy saucepan, stirring until dissolved. Remove from the heat and add the oats, bananas, apricots, and seeds. Mix well.

3 Spoon the mixture into the prepared tin, level the surface and bake in the oven for 20–30 minutes, or until golden brown. The mixture will still be very soft in the centre.

4 Leave to cool in the tin for 10 minutes, then cut into 9 squares. When cold, transfer the squares to an airtight container. Don't try to remove the bars from the tin while they are still warm or they will break.

COOK'S TIP
You can divide this into more or fewer than 9 pieces if you wish but bear in mind the effect this will have on the calorie count.

STATISTICS PER BAKE:

Energy 250kcals/1,040kJ

Carbohydrate 15g

Sugar 12g

Fibre 3g

Fat 15g

Saturated fat 3g

Salt 0.2g

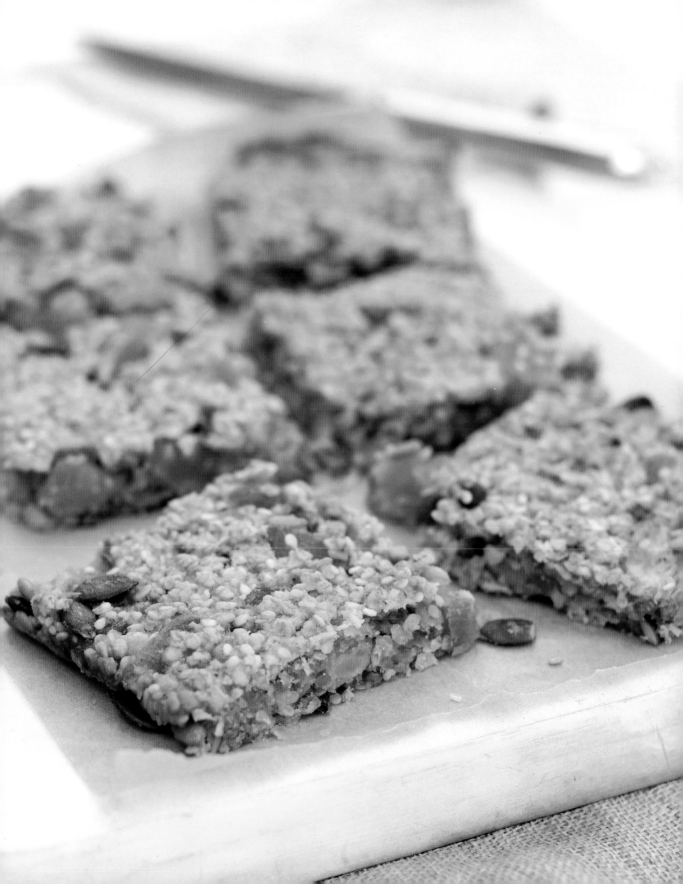

SEVEN-GRAIN BREAD

MAKES 2 LOAVES (20 SLICES)   **PREP** 20 MINS PLUS RISING   **COOK** 35–40 MINS   **FREEZE** 3 MONTHS

Full of healthy wheat, this bread includes millet, rolled oats, polenta, quinoa, brown rice, rye flakes, and wheat.

85g (3oz) bulgur wheat
50g (1¾oz) polenta
50g (1¾oz) millet
50g (1¾oz) quinoa
450g (1lb) strong white flour
250g (9oz) granary flour or
   strong wholemeal flour
75g (2½oz) rolled oats
75g (2½oz) rye flakes

2 x 7g sachets easy-blend dried yeast
2 tsp salt
50g (1¾oz) cooked long-grain
   brown rice
4 tbsp honey, maple syrup
   or treacle, to taste
250ml (8fl oz) milk, warmed
2 tbsp sunflower oil, plus
   extra for brushing

1 Mix the first 4 ingredients in a bowl, stir in 400ml (14fl oz) lukewarm water, cover with a tea towel, and leave to stand for 15 minutes. Mix the next 6 ingredients in a bowl, add the bulgur mixture, and stir in the rice.

2 Heat the honey with the milk until it dissolves and add to the bowl along with the oil. Gradually add up to 200ml (7fl oz) lukewarm water, or until a soft, sticky dough forms. Knead on a lightly floured work surface for 10 minutes or until elastic. Shape into a ball, place in a lightly oiled bowl, then cover the bowl with oiled cling film. Leave to rise in a warm place until doubled in size. Meanwhile, oil and flour 2 x 900g (2lb) loaf tins.

3 Turn the dough out on to a floured surface and knead for 1 minute. (The dough will be sticky again.) Divide into 2 equal-sized balls and, with a floured rolling pin, roll each ball into a rectangle as wide as the tins and twice as long. Fold both ends to the centre and pinch the edges to seal. Place in the tins, cover with tea towels, and leave to rise until the dough reaches the tops of the tins. Preheat the oven to 220°C (425°F/Gas 7).

4 Brush the tops with oil and bake for 10 minutes, then reduce the heat to 190°C (375°F/Gas 5) and bake for a further 25–30 minutes, or until the loaves sound hollow when tapped on the base. Leave to cool on a wire rack.

STATISTICS PER SLICE:

Energy 217kcals/916kJ

Carbohydrate 43g

Sugar 3.5g

Fibre 2.5g

Fat 3.5g

Saturated fat 0.6g

Salt 0.4g

RYE BREAD

MAKES 1 LOAF
(10 SLICES)

PREP 25 MINS
PLUS STANDING
PLUS RISING

COOK 40-45 MINS

FREEZE 3 MONTHS

Breads made with rye flour are very popular in central and eastern Europe.

For the starter
150g (5½oz) rye flour
150g (5½oz) pot live natural yogurt
1 tsp fast-action dried yeast
1 tbsp black treacle
1 tsp caraway seeds, lightly crushed

For the dough
150g (5½oz) rye flour
200g (7oz) strong white flour,
  plus extra for dusting
2 tsp salt
1 egg, beaten
1 tsp caraway seeds, to decorate

1 Mix all of the starter ingredients together with 250ml (8fl oz) tepid water. Cover and leave overnight, until bubbling.

2 The next day, mix the flours together with the salt, then stir into the starter. Mix to make a dough, adding a little extra water if required.

3 Turn out on to a lightly floured surface and knead the dough for 5–10 minutes, or until smooth and springy. Shape into a ball, put into an oiled bowl and cover loosely with oiled cling film. Leave in a warm place for 1 hour, or until doubled in size.

4 Flour a baking tray. Lightly knead the dough again, then form it into a rugby-ball shape. Lift onto the tray, re-cover it loosely with the oiled cling film, and leave to rise again for another 30 minutes. Preheat the oven to 220°C (425°F/Gas 7).

5 Brush the dough with the egg, sprinkle with the caraway seeds, and slash the loaf along its length with a sharp knife. Bake for 20 minutes, then reduce the heat to 200°C (400°F/Gas 6) and bake for another 20–30 minutes, or until dark golden with a hard shiny crust. Cool on a wire rack.

COOK'S TIP
The starter must be made the day before you want to make the loaf.

STATISTICS PER SLICE:

Energy 193kcals/806kJ

Carbohydrate 40g

Sugar 2.3g

Fibre 4.1g

Fat 2.1g
Saturated fat 0.6g

Salt 0.8g

CHAPATTIS

MAKES 8   **PREP** 30 MINS   **COOK** 10 MINS
PLUS RESTING

In India, these flat, unleavened breads would be cooked in a concave pan called a tava. However, a cast-iron frying pan works well.

250g (9oz) chapatti flour or wholemeal plain flour, plus extra for dusting

1 tsp salt
10g (¼oz) ghee or melted butter, for brushing

1 Sift the flour into a bowl and discard any bran left in the sieve. Make a well in the centre of the flour, add 3 tablespoons of cold water and mix in. Work in the salt, then mix in another 4 tablespoons of cold water until a dough starts to form.

2 Gradually add another 4 tablespoons of cold water to make a sticky dough. Keep kneading the dough in the bowl until it becomes firm, elastic, and less sticky.

3 Cover with a tea towel and leave to rest for 15 minutes, or until the dough becomes firmer and is no longer sticky.

4 Dust your hands with flour and pull off egg-sized pieces of dough. Shape these into balls, then roll out into rounds 18cm (7in) in diameter.

5 Heat an ungreased frying pan and cook the chapattis for 30 seconds on each side, or until golden and speckled. As you remove each one from the pan, brush with ghee or melted butter, and set aside in a warm place while you cook the rest.

STATISTICS PER SERVING:

Energy 114kcals/484kJ

Carbohydrate 25g

Sugar 0.5g

Fibre 1g

Fat 1g
Saturated fat 0.7g

Salt 0.3g

LOW-FAT GINGER TEA BREAD

MAKES 1 LOAF
(12 SLICES)

PREP 15 MINS
PLUS SOAKING

COOK 45-60 MINS

FREEZE 3 MONTHS

This low-fat cake is quick and easy to make, and perfect for an afternoon snack that won't pile on the calories.

150g (5½oz) mixed dried fruit
325ml (11fl oz) lemon and ginger tea
  (made with 2 tea bags)
225g (8oz) plain wholemeal flour

2 tsp baking powder
100g (3½oz) fructose
1 egg, beaten

1 Place the dried fruit in a large heatproof bowl, pour the tea over it and leave to stand for at least 2 hours, stirring occasionally.

2 Preheat the oven to 160°C (325°F/Gas 3). Grease and line the bottom of a 900g (2lb) loaf tin with non-stick baking parchment.

3 Place the flour, baking powder, fructose, and egg in a food processor or blender and process for a couple of minutes. Add the dried fruit and tea and whiz again until well mixed.

4 Spoon the mixture into the prepared loaf tin, brush the surface with a little water and bake for 45 minutes–1 hour until the cake looks done and feels springy in the centre. You may need to cover it with foil halfway through cooking if it is browning too quickly.

5 Allow the cake to cool in the tin for 5 minutes, then carefully turn out on to a wire cooling rack.

GUIDELINES PER SLICE:

GI
CALORIES
SATURATED FAT
SALT

STATISTICS PER SLICE:

Energy 106kcals/450kJ

Carbohydrate 23g

Sugar 8g

Fibre 1g

Fat 0.8g
Saturated fat 0.2g

Salt 0.2g

FRUIT AND SEED SODA BREAD

MAKES 1 LOAF   **PREP** 10 MINS   **COOK** 20-25 MINS   **FREEZE** 3 MONTHS
(10 SLICES)

A tasty loaf that helps you get more fruit into your diet.

sunflower oil, for greasing
50g (1¾oz) mixed dried fruit
175g (6oz) wholemeal flour

1 tbsp bicarbonate of soda
60g (2oz) sunflower seeds
150g pot plain yogurt

1 Preheat the oven to 180°C (350°F/Gas 4). Lightly grease a 450g (1lb) loaf tin. Place the dried fruit in a heatproof bowl, pour over 100ml (3½fl oz) boiling water, and set aside for 10 minutes.

2 Mix the flour, bicarbonate of soda, and seeds in a large bowl. Stir in the fruit in its water and the yogurt.

3 Pour the mixture into the prepared tin and bake for 20–25 minutes or until firm. Allow to cool for 10 minutes before slicing.

STATISTICS PER SLICE:

Energy 129kcals/539kJ

Carbohydrate 9g

Sugar 2g

Fibre 2g

Fat 3g

Saturated fat 0.7g

Salt 0.3g

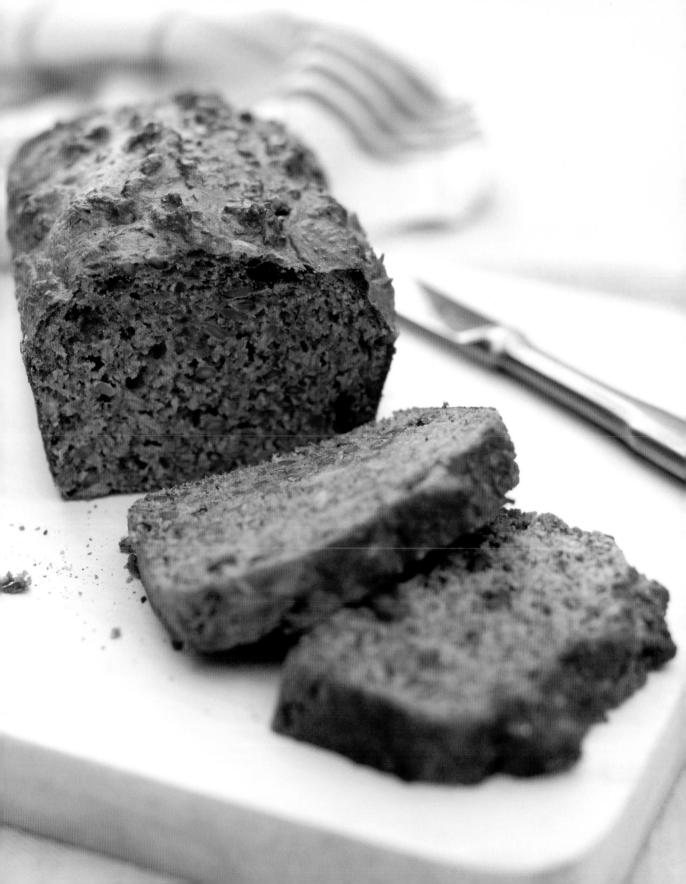

BANANA AND MUESLI BREAD

MAKES 1 LOAF (12 SLICES) **PREP** 15 MINS **COOK** 45–60 MINS **FREEZE** 3 MONTHS

A slice of this bread makes the perfect treat to pop into a packed lunch.

175g (6oz) wholemeal flour
85g (3oz) sugar-free muesli
125g (4½oz) polyunsaturated margarine
85g (3oz) fructose
2 tsp baking power

¼ tsp ground cinnamon
2 large eggs, beaten
4 ripe bananas, about 350g (12oz), mashed
85g (3oz) pecan nuts, roughly chopped

1 Preheat the oven to 160°C (325°F/Gas 3). Grease and line the bottom of a 900g (2lb) loaf tin with non-stick baking parchment.

2 Place the flour, muesli, margarine, fructose, baking powder, cinnamon, and eggs in a large bowl. Beat together until evenly mixed. Stir in the banana and pecan nuts, taking care not to over-mix.

3 Spoon the mixture into the prepared loaf tin and bake for 45 minutes–1 hour, or until the cake looks done and feels springy in the centre. You may need to cover it with foil halfway through cooking if it is browning too quickly. Allow the cake to cool in the tin for 5 minutes, then carefully turn out on to a wire cooling rack.

STATISTICS PER SLICE:

Energy 267kcals/1,118kJ

Carbohydrate 34g

Sugar 17g

Fibre 2.6g

Fat 13g

Saturated fat 3g

Salt 0.5g

BANANA AND PECAN MUFFINS

GUIDELINES PER MUFFIN:

● ● ○ GI

● ● ○ CALORIES

● ○ ○ SATURATED FAT

● ○ ○ SALT

MAKES 6   **PREP** 10 MINS   **COOK** 20-25 MINS   **FREEZE** 3 MONTHS

The banana helps sweeten the muffin mixture, reducing the need for sugar in the recipe.

4 tbsp sunflower oil, plus
  extra for greasing
125g (4½oz) wholemeal flour
3 tbsp caster sugar
2 tsp baking powder
85g (3oz) pecan nuts,
  roughly chopped

generous pinch of ground cinnamon
1 egg, beaten
4 tbsp semi-skimmed milk
2 ripe bananas (about 225g/8oz),
  roughly mashed

1 Preheat the oven to 200°C (400°F/Gas 6). Grease a six-hole muffin tin; alternatively, line the holes with paper muffin cases. Place the flour, sugar, baking powder, pecan nuts, and ground cinnamon in a bowl. Mix them together and make a well in the centre.

2 In a separate bowl, mix together the egg, milk, and oil. Pour the mixture into the dry ingredients and stir until just blended. Stir in the bananas, taking care not to over-mix.

3 Fill the muffin holes or cases two-thirds full, then place the tin in the oven and bake for 20–25 minutes, or until a skewer inserted into the centre comes out clean.

4 Transfer the muffins to a wire rack to cool. Store in an airtight container; the muffins will keep for up to three days.

STATISTICS PER MUFFIN:

Energy 315kcals/1,316kJ

Carbohydrate 32g

Sugar 16g

Fibre 3g

Fat 19g

Saturated fat 2g

Salt 0.4g

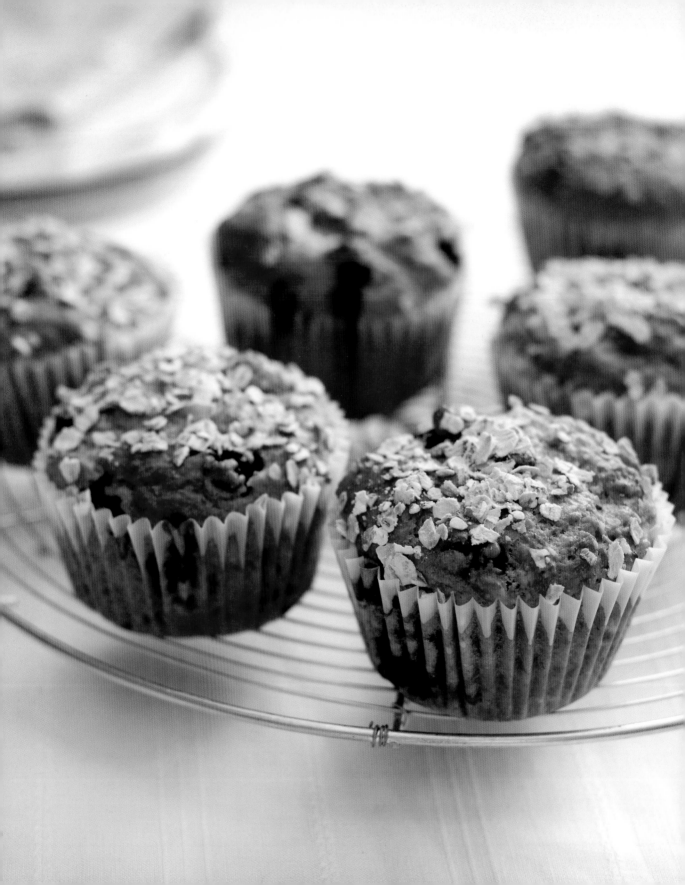

BLUEBERRY AND OAT MUFFINS

GUIDELINES PER MUFFIN:

◑○○ GI

●●○ CALORIES

◑○○ SATURATED FAT

◑○○ SALT

MAKES 6   **PREP** 15 MINS   **COOK** 25–30 MINS   **FREEZE** 3 MONTHS

The combination of wholemeal flour and oats helps to reduce the GI of these muffins.

150g (5½oz) wholemeal flour
45g (1½oz) porridge oats
3 tbsp caster sugar
2 tsp baking powder
1 really ripe banana

150ml (5fl oz) plain yogurt
3 tbsp rapeseed oil
1 egg, beaten
150g (5½oz) fresh blueberries

1 Heat oven to 180°C (350°F/Gas 4). Grease a 6-hole muffin tin well or line with paper muffin cases.

2 Put the flour in a large bowl with 25g (scant 1oz) of the porridge oats, the sugar, and the baking powder. In a separate bowl, mash the banana until nearly smooth, then add the yogurt, oil, and egg and stir together until evenly combined.

3 Make a well in the centre of the flour, pour the banana and yogurt mixture into the well and stir briskly with a wooden spoon. The mixture will look lumpy, but don't be tempted to over-mix. Tip in the blueberries and give it just one more stir.

4 Divide the mix between the muffin cases, sprinkle the tops with the remaining oats, and bake for 25–30 minutes until risen and golden. Transfer to a wire rack to cool.

COOK'S TIP
These muffins can be kept in an airtight container for up to 3 days.

STATISTICS PER MUFFIN:

Energy 260kcals/1,088kJ

Carbohydrate 35g

Sugar 17g

Fibre 3g

Fat 9g

Saturated fat 1g

Salt 0.5g

CARROT AND OLIVE OIL CAKE

SERVES 12　　**PREP** 10 MINS　　**COOK** 1 HOUR 40 MINS　　**FREEZE** 3 MONTHS

This is an incredibly easy cake to make, and it has a wonderfully moist texture.

125g (4½oz) plain flour, sifted
125g (4½oz) wholemeal flour
pinch of cinnamon
1 tsp bicarbonate of soda
250ml (9fl oz) mild olive oil
100g (3½oz) soft brown sugar
4 eggs

2 tbsp runny honey
juice and zest of 1 large orange
400g (14oz) carrots, grated
50g (1¾oz) walnuts, roughly chopped

For the topping
juice of 1 orange

1 Preheat the oven to 160°C (325°F/Gas 3). Put both types of flour in a bowl and add the cinnamon and bicarbonate of soda. Set aside.

2 In another bowl, whisk together the olive oil, sugar, eggs, honey, and orange juice. Pour this mixture into the flour and mix until smooth. Stir in the grated carrots, walnuts, and orange zest.

3 Tip the mixture into a greased 23cm (9in) round, loose-bottomed cake tin. Level the surface and put the tin in the oven to bake for 1 hour 30 minutes, or until it is cooked all the way through. To test whether it is cooked, insert a skewer into the centre: if it comes out clean, the cake is done.

4 Remove the cake from the oven and while it is still hot, pierce all over with a skewer, and then drizzle with the orange juice. Transfer to a wire cooling rack and leave to cool before turning the cake out of the cake tin.

STATISTICS PER SERVING:

Energy 300kcals/1,244kJ

Carbohydrate 28g

Sugar 13g

Fibre 2g

Fat 19g

Saturated fat 3g

Salt 0.4g

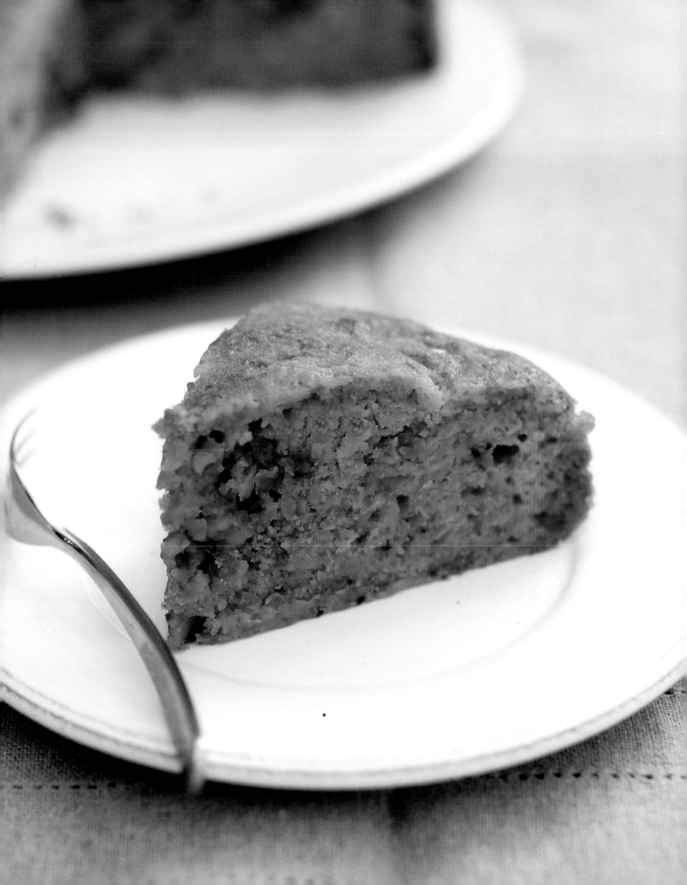

INDEX

ACKNOWLEDGMENTS

ABOUT THE AUTHORS

Fiona Hunter is a food writer and nutritionist of over 25 years' experience. With a degree in Nutrition and a postgraduate diploma in Dietetics, she began her career as a dietician in the NHS before going on to write for magazines including *Good Housekeeping*, *Health and Fitness*, and *BBC Good Food*, as well as making many appearances on television and radio. She is the co-author of several books, including *The Big GL+ Diet Planner*, *101 Fantastic GI Recipes*, and *The Natural Menopause Cookbook*.

Heather Whinney is an experienced food writer and home economist. She has been the food editor of *Family Circle* and *Prima* magazines, freelance food editor of *BBC Good Food* magazine, and has also worked freelance for publications such as *Good Housekeeping* and *Woman and Home*. She is the author of the recipe book *Cook Express*, and is now the contributing food editor for *Prima*. Her food philosophy has always been to write simple recipes for the everyday cook.

Fiona Hunter would like to thank Tim Burkinshaw and her family for their support and encouragement, Heather Whinney for being a wonderful co-author and friend, and the creative team at DK.

Heather Whinney would like to thank Fiona Hunter for her advice and support throughout the book, the photography team, home economists, and all at DK.

Dorling Kindersley would like to thank the following people: art director Luis Peral, food stylist Cara Hobday and assistants Georgie Besterman, Ann Reynolds, Emily Jonzen, and Kelly Bowers; prop stylist Victoria Allen; home economists Richard Harris, Emily Shardlow, and Rachel Wood; out-of-house editors Helena Caldon and Fiona Corbridge.

USEFUL WEBSITES
Diabetes UK
www.diabetes.org.uk

Weight Loss Resources
www.weightlossresources.co.uk

Glycaemic index
www.glycemicindex.com

Satiety index
www.diabetesnet.com/diabetes_food_diet/satiety_index.php

British Heart Foundation
www.bhf.org.uk

The NHS
www.nhs.uk